AF505682

DIABETIC ANGIOPATHY

DIABETIC ANGIOPATHY

Edited by

John E Tooke DM, FRCP

Department of Diabetes and Vascular Medicine
Postgraduate Medical School
University of Exeter, UK

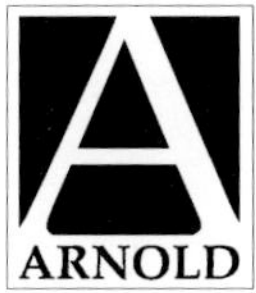

A member of the Hodder Headline Group
LONDON · SYDNEY · AUCKLAND
Co-published in the United States of America by
Oxford University Press Inc., New York

First published in Great Britain in 1999 by
Arnold, a member of the Hodder Headline Group,
338 Euston Road, London NW1 3BH

http://www.arnoldpublishers.com

Co-published in the United States of America by
Oxford University Press Inc.,
198 Madison Avenue, New York, NY10016
Oxford is a registered trademark of Oxford University Press

Whilst the advice and information in this book are believed to be true and
accurate at the date of going to press, neither the authors nor the publisher
can accept any legal responsibility or liability for any errors or omissions
that may be made. In particular (but without limiting the generality of the
preceding disclaimer) every effort has been made to check drug dosages;
however, it is still possible that errors have been missed. Furthermore,
dosage schedules are constantly being revised and new side-effects
recognized. For these reasons the reader is strongly urged to consult the
drug companies' printed instructions before administering any of the drugs
recommended in this book.

British Library Cataloguing in Publication Data
A catalogue record for this book is available from the British Library

Library of Congress Cataloging-in-Publication Data
A catalog record for this book is available from the Library of Congress

ISBN 0 340 74102 3

1 2 3 4 5 6 7 8 9 10

Composition by Photoprint, Torquay, Devon
Printed and bound in Great Britain by The Bath Press, Bath

CONTENTS

List of contributors   xiii

Preface by *Harry Keen*   xv

PART ONE: BACKGROUND   1

1   Introduction   3
    John E. Tooke and William Liddell

    1.1 Historical perspective   3
    1.2 Diabetic angiopathy   4
    1.3 Scope of the text   5

2   Epidemiology of diabetic angiopathy   7
    Rhys Williams and Mark Airey

    2.1 Scope of this chapter   7
    2.2 Making sense of the epidemiological information   7
    2.3 Peripheral vascular disease   8
         2.3.1 Definitions   8
         2.3.2 Practice-based studies   8
         2.3.3 Population-based studies   9
    2.4 Coronary heart disease   9
         2.4.1 Definition   9
         2.4.2 Practice-based studies   10
         2.4.3 Population-based studies   10
    2.5 Cerebrovascular disease   11
         2.5.1 Definition   11
         2.5.2 Practice based studies   11
         2.5.3 Population based studies   12
         2.5.4 World-wide comparisons   12
    2.6 Microvascular disease   12
         2.6.1 Definition   12
         2.6.2 Clinic-based and population-based studies   13
    2.7 Predicting the future   14

PART TWO: THE PATHOGENESIS OF ARTERIAL DISEASE IN DIABETES   19

3   The atherosclerotic process and its exacerbation by diabetes   21
    Hans-Joachim Baumgartl and Eberhard Standl

    3.1 Atherogenesis   21

3.2 The atherosclerotic process in diabetes 22
   3.2.1 Introduction 22
   3.2.2 The AGE hypothesis 23
   3.2.3 Cytokines and growth factors: TGF-β 26
   3.2.4 Inositol depletion 26
   3.2.5 Heparan sulphate proteoglycan depletion 27
   3.2.6 Vascular endothelial growth factor 29
3.3 Future perspectives 30

4 Risk factors for arterial disease in diabetes: hyperglycaemia 37
Amanda I. Adler and H. Andrew W. Neil

4.1 Introduction 37
4.2 Increased risk of cardiovascular disease in diabetes 37
4.3 Role of glycaemia as a cardiovascular risk factor in impaired glucose tolerance and impaired fasting glucose 39
4.4 Evidence for the independent role of glycaemia 40
4.5 Pathophysiologic basis for the role of glycaemia in atherosclerosis 41
4.6 Clinical implications 41
4.7 Conclusions 42

5 Risk factors for arterial disease in diabetes: hypertension 45
James R. Sowers and Murray Epstein

5.1 Summary 45
5.2 Introduction 45
5.3 Hyperinsulinaemia and cardiovascular disease 47
5.4 Platelet abnormalities associated with diabetes and hypertension 48
5.5 Coagulation abnormalities in diabetic hypertensive persons 48
5.6 Other metabolic abnormalities associated with diabetes mellitus and hypertension 49
5.7 Abnormalities of non-esterified fatty acid metabolism in diabetes and hypertension 50
5.8 Endothelial dysfunction in diabetes and hypertension 50
5.9 Kidney disease, diabetes and hypertension: analogy between glomerulosclerosis and atherosclerosis 51
5.10 Treatment of hypertension in patients with diabetes mellitus 53
   5.10.1 Goals of therapy 53
   5.10.2 Non-pharmacological therapy in diabetic hypertensive patients 53
   5.10.3 Pharmacological therapy 55

6 Risk factors for arterial disease in diabetes: dyslipidaemia 65
D. John Betteridge

6.1 Introduction 65
6.2 Atherosclerosis-related disease in diabetes 66
6.3 The physiology of lipid and lipoprotein transport 66
   6.3.1 Exogenous pathway 67
   6.3.2 Endogenous lipoprotein pathway 70

6.3.3 High density lipoprotein and reverse cholesterol transport   71
6.3.4 Lipids, lipoproteins and atherosclerosis   72
6.3.5 Lipoprotein(a)   76
6.4 Lipid and lipoprotein metabolism in diabetes   76
   6.4.1 NIDDM patients   76
6.4.2 IDDM patients   78
6.4.3 Lipid and lipoprotein levels in relation to diabetic macrovascular disease   78
6.5 Management of dyslipidaemia in diabetic patients   79
6.5.1 Screening   79
6.5.2 Treatment targets   81
6.5.3 Treatment   82
6.5.4 Choice of lipid-lowering drugs   84
6.5.5 Choice of lipid-lowering therapy   86
6.5.6 An approach to lipid-lowering therapy in diabetic patients   87

7 Risk factors for arterial disease in diabetes: coagulopathy   93
Peter J. Grant

7.1 Introduction   93
7.2 Mechanisms in thrombosis   93
7.2.1 Coagulation   93
7.2.2 Fibrinolysis   94
7.2.3 Platelets   95
7.3 Diabetes as a hypercoagulable state   95
7.3.1 Introduction   95
7.3.2 Biochemical evidence for a pro-coagulant state in diabetes   96
7.4 Diabetes and atherothrombotic risk   97
7.5 Coagulation   97
7.5.1 Fibrinogen   97
7.5.2 Factor VII   99
7.6 Fibrinolysis   100
7.6.1 Fibrinolysis in NIDDM and IDDM subjects   100
7.6.2 Determinants of fibrinolytic activity in diabetes mellitus   101
7.6.3 Fibrinolysis and vascular disorders   101
7.6.4 Genetics of PAI-1 and diabetes mellitus   101
7.7 Platelets and Von Willebrand factor   102
7.7.1 Platelet function in diabetes mellitus   102
7.7.2 vWF in diabetes mellitus   103
7.8 Conclusions   104

8 Insulin resistance and arterial disease in diabetes: a unifying hypothesis   113
John S. Yudkin

8.1 Introduction   113
8.2 The insulin resistance syndrome: what is it and who belongs?   114
8.2.1 What is insulin resistance?   114
8.2.2 Insulin resistance and the metabolic syndrome   114
8.2.3 The relevance of obesity and physical activity   115

8.2.4 Can insulin resistance explain dyslipidaemia and hypertension?   115
8.2.5 Insulin resistance and CHD   116
8.3 The insulin resistance syndrome club: new applicants for membership   117
8.3.1 Plasminogen activator inhibitor-1   117
8.3.2 Pro-insulin-like molecules   117
8.3.3 Microalbuminuria   119
8.3.4 Fibrinogen   119
8.4 Insulin resistance and its associates: consequences of a common antecedent?   119
8.5 The small baby syndrome   119
8.6 Endothelial dysfunction as a common antecedent of insulin resistance
and the metabolic cluster   121
8.7 Pro-inflammatory cytokines, the acute phase response and insulin resistance   122
8.8 The role of infections and adipose tissue?   125
8.9 A new paradigm for insulin resistance, obesity, endothelial dysfunction
and cardiovascular disease   127
8.10 Conclusions   128

PART THREE: THE PATHOGENESIS OF DIABETIC MICROANGIOPATHY   **135**

9   The role of glycaemia in the pathogenesis of microangiopathy   137
Kenneth M. MacLeod

9.1 Introduction   137
9.2 The glucose hypothesis   137
9.3 Indirect evidence incriminating glucose in the pathogenesis of microangiopathy   138
9.3.1 Studies of individuals with impaired glucose tolerance and those with
newly diagnosed diabetes   138
9.3.2 Patients with maturity onset diabetes of the young   139
9.3.3 Relationship of microvascular complications to duration of disease and
degree of hyperglycaemia   139
9.3.4 Observational studies: diabetic retinopathy in focus   140
9.3.5 Observational studies: diabetic nephropathy in focus   141
9.4 Interventional studies   142
9.4.1 Animal studies   142
9.4.2 Human studies   142
9.4.3 The evidence in insulin-dependent diabetes mellitus   142
9.5 Tight control in type 2 diabetes: the evidence   147
9.6 Glycaemic re-entry   150
9.7 Hypoglycaemia and microangiopathy   152
9.8 More than glucose: the missing links?   153

10   The vascular cellular consequences of hyperglycaemia   161
Joseph R. Williamson and Yasuo Ido

10.1 Functional and structural vascular responses to hyperglycaemia   161
10.1.1 Early vascular dysfunction induced by acute hyperglycaemia
in non-diabetic humans and rats   161

10.1.2 Early vascular dysfunction in diabetic humans and in animals
 with spontaneous or experimentally induced diabetes 162
10.1.3 Vascular structural changes 163
10.2 Pathophysiological significance of increased blood flow and loss of vascular
barrier functional integrity: relationship to vascular structural changes 163
10.3 Metabolic imbalances implicated in mediating vascular changes
induced by hyperglycaemia and the diabetic milieu 164
10.4 Cytosolic free $NADH/NAD^+$ and reductive stress, energy metabolism and
regulation of blood flow 166
 10.4.1 Redox cycling of NAD(H) and ATP synthesis 170
10.5 NADPH: co-factor for aldose reductase, nitric oxide synthase and glutathione
reductase 171
10.6 Metabolic consequences of cytosolic reductive stress 173
 10.6.1 Cytosolic reductive stress, oxidative stress, non-enzymatic glycation,
 and extracellular matrix changes 173
 10.6.2 Cytosolic reductive stress and vascular endothelial growth factor 175
 10.6.3 Cytosolic reductive stress, *de novo* synthesis of diacylglycerol,
 and activation of protein kinase C 176
 10.6.4 Vascular consequences of cytosolic reductive stress in non-vascular
 versus vascular cells 177
 10.6.5 Cytosolic reductive stress, paradoxical responses to ischaemic injury,
 and metabolic suppression 178
10.7 Conclusions 179

11 A pathophysiological framework for the pathogenesis of microangiopathy 187
John E. Tooke

11.1 Introduction 187
11.2 Indirect evidence for microvascular malfunction in diabetes 188
11.3 The haemodynamic hypothesis of diabetic microangiopathy 189
 11.3.1 Direct support for the haemodynamic hypothesis 190
11.4 Reduced microvascular vasodilatory reserve 191
11.5 Alternative pathophysiological concepts 191
 11.5.1 The role of increased microvascular permeability 191
11.6 The pathophysiology of the microcirculation in non-insulin dependent
diabetes 193
11.7 A pathophysiological framework for diabetic microangiopathy 194

12 The endothelium in diabetes 197
Lucilla Poston

12.1 Introduction 197
12.2 Vascular responses to acetylcholine in diabetes 198
12.3 Flow-mediated, endothelium-dependent, dilation in diabetes 200
12.4 Insulin, NO and insulin resistance 202
12.5 Endothelium-dependent constrictors 202
12.6 The diabetic milieu and vascular endothelial function 202
 12.6.1 Hyperglycaemia 203
 12.6.2 Oxidative stress, lipids and endothelial dysfunction 203

13	**Blood rheological changes in diabetes**	**213**
	Alan Jaap and Gordon D.O. Lowe	
	13.1 Introduction	213
	13.2 Rheological changes in diabetes	213
	13.3 White cells and platelets in diabetes	214
	13.3.1 White cells	215
	13.3.2 Platelets	215
	13.4 Rheological, white cell and platelet abnormalities and the pathogenesis of microangiopathy	215
	13.4.1 Early haemodynamic changes	215
	13.4.2 Established microvascular disease	215
	13.5 Conclusions	216
14	**Mechanisms underlying pathophysiological changes in human diabetic microangiopathy**	**219**
	John E. Tooke	
	14.1 Introduction	219
	14.2 The origins of luxury perfusion	219
	14.3 The origins of capillary hypertension	221
	14.4 Limitation in maximal microvascular hyperaemia	222
	14.5 Changes in capillary permeability in diabetes	224
	14.5.1 Determinants of capillary wall permeability	224
	14.5.2 The molecular basis for increased permeability in diabetes	225
	14.6 Conclusions	227

PART FOUR: ORGAN-SPECIFIC VASCULAR CHANGES   **231**

15	**Diabetic retinopathy**	**233**
	Eva M. Kohner and Rakesh Chibber	
	15.1 Introduction	233
	15.2 The evolution of diabetic retinopathy	233
	15.3 Pathogenic mechanisms in diabetic retinopathy	234
	15.3.1 Haemodynamic changes	235
	15.3.2 Direct effect of hyperglycaemia on retinal vascular cells	238
	15.3.3 Capillary occlusion	240
	15.3.4 Vascular proliferation	241
16	**Diabetic nephropathy**	**249**
	Allan Kofoed-Enevoldsen	
	16.1 Introduction	249
	16.2 The nature of diabetic renal disease	249
	16.3 Morphological changes	250
	16.4 Genetic determinants	251
	16.5 Haemodynamic changes	251
	16.5.1 Renin–angiotensin system	252
	16.5.2 Hypertension	253

16.6 Glomerular size and charge selectivity 253
16.7 Derangement of the extracellular matrix 254
  16.7.1 Heparan sulphate proteoglycan (Steno hypothesis) 255
16.8 Cellular and molecular mechanisms 256
  16.8.1 Na^+/H^+ exchanger and sodium-lithium countertransport activity 256
  16.8.2 Polyol pathway and pseudohypoxia 256
  16.8.3 Non-enzymatic glycation 257
  16.8.4 Protein kinase C 257
  16.8.5 TGF-β 258
  16.8.6 Nitric oxide 258
  16.8.7 Growth hormone and IGF-1 259
  16.8.8 Insulin resistance 259
16.9 Diabetic nephropathy in NIDDM versus IDDM 259

17 Organ-specific vascular changes 267
Andrew J.M. Boulton and Rayaz A. Malik

17.1 Introduction 267
17.2 Human structural and functional neurovascular abnormalities 267
17.3 Experimental nerve ischaemia 269
17.4 Evidence from pharmaceutical studies 270
17.5 The role of nitric oxide and endothelin 271
17.6 Conclusions 271

18 The diabetic foot 277
Michael D. Flynn

18.1 Introduction 277
18.2 Pathogenesis: the neuroischaemic and neuropathic foot 277
18.3 The microcirculation of the foot 278
18.4 Regulation of microvascular blood flow 279
18.5 The abnormal circulation in the diabetic foot 280
18.6 Capillary morphological changes in diabetes 281
18.7 Changes in the capillary basement membrane 281
18.8 Is there small vessel disease? 282
18.9 Changes in the capillary endothelium 283
18.10 Functional changes in the microcirculation 284
18.11 Neuropathy and microvascular disease 285
18.12 Capillary flow in the diabetic foot 287
18.13 Do closed capillaries contribute to ischaemia in the skin of the foot? 287
18.14 Clinical implications 288
18.15 Conclusions 289

Index 297

CONTRIBUTORS

Mark Airey
Division of Public Health
Nuffield Institute for Health
71–75 Clarendon Road
Leeds LS2 9PL, UK

Amanda I. Adler
Oxford University
Radcliffe Infirmary
Diabetes Research Laboratories
Nuffield Department of Clinical Medicine
Woodstock Road
Oxford OX2 6HE, UK

Hans-Joachim Baumgartl
Department of Nuclear Medicine
Technical University of Munich
Klinikum Rechts der Isar
Ismaninger Str. 22
D-81675, München, Germany

D. John Betteridge
University College London Medical School
  and Royal Free Hospital School of
  Medicine
Department of Medicine
Sir Jules Thorn Institute
The Middlesex Hospital
Mortimer Street
London W1N 8AA, UK

Andrew J.M. Boulton
Department of Medicine
Manchester Royal Infirmary
Oxford Road
Manchester M13 9WL, UK

Rakesh Chibber
Department of Medicine
St Thomas' Hospital
Lambeth Palace Road
London SE1 7EH, UK

Murray Epstein
Professor of Medicine
Department of Veterans Affairs
Medical Center
1201 Northwest 16th Street
Miami
Florida 33125, USA

Michael D. Flynn
Department of Medicine
Kent and Canterbury Hospital
Ethelbert Road
Canterbury
Kent, CT1 3NG, UK

Peter J. Grant
Unit of Molecular Vascular Medicine
Martin Wing
Leeds General Infirmary
Leeds LS1 3EX, UK

Yasuo Ido
Washington University School of Medicine
Pathology Department, Box 8118
660 South Euclid Avenue
St Louis
MO 63110, USA

Alan Jaap
Diabetic Day Centre
Crosshouse Hospital
Kilmarnock KA2 0BE, UK

Harry Keen
Unit of Metabolic Medicine
Department of Medicine
United Medical and Dental Schools
Guy's Campus
London Bridge
London SE1 9RC, UK

Allan Kofoed-Enevoldsen
Department of Endocrinology
Herlev Hospital
University of Copenhagen
DK-2730 Herlev
Denmark

Eva M. Kohner
Department of Medicine
Department of Endocrinology, Diabetes and
    Metabolic Medicine
St Thomas' Hospital
Lambeth Palace Road
London SE1 7EH, UK

William Liddell
Department of Vascular Medicine
(Diabetes Research)
Postgraduate Medical School
Barrack Road
Exeter, EX2 5AX
Devon, UK

Gordon D.O. Lowe
University Department of Medicine
Royal Infirmary
84 Castle Street
Glasgow G4 0SF, UK

Kenneth M. MacLeod
Department of Diabetes and Vascular
    Medicine
Postgraduate Medical School
Barrack Road
Exeter EX2 5AX
Devon, UK

Rayaz A. Malik
Department of Medicine
Manchester Royal Infirmary
Oxford Road
Manchester M13 9WL, UK

H. Andrew W. Neil
Division of Public Health and Primary
    Health Care
Institute of Health Sciences
University of Oxford
Oxford OX3 7LF, UK

Lucilla Poston
Fetal Health Research Group
Division of Obstetrics and Gynaecology
Guy's, King's and St Thomas' Medical
    School
St Thomas' Hospital
London SE1 7EH, UK

James R. Sowers
Wayne State University School of Medicine
Detroit
MI, USA

Eberhard Standl
Stadt Krankenhaus Schwabing
Kölner Platz 1
Munich D-80804
Germany

John E. Tooke
Department of Diabetes and Vascular
    Medicine
Postgraduate Medical School
Barrack Road
Exeter EX2 5AX
Devon, UK

Rhys Williams
Division of Public Health
Nuffield Institute for Health
71–75 Clarendon Road
Leeds LS2 9PL, UK

Joseph R. Williamson
Pathology Department
Washington University School of Medicine
Washington Medical Center, Box 8118
660 South Euclid Avenue
St Louis
MO 63110, USA

John S. Yudkin
Department of Medicine
University College London
G Block, Archway Wing
Whittington Hospital
Archway Road
London N19 3UA, UK

PREFACE

I willingly accepted the role of the 'veteran diabetologist' when I was invited to write a prologue for this book. The latter half of this century has seen major – in some cases spectacular – advances in knowledge and understanding of diabetic angiopathy at the levels of clinical practice, of pathophysiology and of disordered molecular biology. As we approach the millennium, these advances offer a real prospect of overcoming the problems of the 'complications of diabetes' which have so beset the post-insulin era and clouded the lives of so many people with diabetes.

The clinician is no longer assigned the disagreeable role of being little more than a passive observer as diabetic microvascular disease progressively destroyed visual and renal function and contributed to peripheral and autonomic nerve disease. The importance of sustained hyperglycaemia as a prime mover of these damaging processes had long been suspected on the basis of suggestive clinical correlations between 'control' and 'complications'. A relationship between them approaching, if not including, cause and effect was very strongly supported by the Diabetes Control and Complications Trial (DCCT) which reported early in this decade and effectively settled the 50-year debate on the benefits – and costs – of improved glycaemic control.

However, even the DCCT has not told us how hyperglycaemia does its damage. This is not for want of candidate mechanisms ranging from direct chemical effects of high ambient glucose concentrations on protein/DNA structure and function to more subtle, indirect effects on cell metabolism, rheology and vascular behaviour. We are as yet uncertain whether more than one angiopathic process is involved. Glomerular basement membrane changes, for example, are almost universally present in diabetic humans (and animals), but progression to renal failure, even in those with indifferent metabolic control, appears to affect only a subset of people.

Similarly, retinal capillary microaneurysms are reported in almost 100% of people with insulin-dependent diabetes but the risk of sight-threatening retinal vasoproliferation appears to threaten fewer than half of them. R.D. Lawrence said there is no such thing as diabetic control, only degrees of uncontrol; the degree of uncontrol is clearly one of the determinants of risk, but is unlikely to be the only one or even the main one. However, it appears likely that degrees of glycaemic control are now attainable which greatly delay or even prevent progression of angiopathy to the later stages of tissue damage and organ failure. And even if these later stages are entered, there are physical and pharmacological therapeutic approaches which will conserve vision, renal function and tissue viability. We can surely expect further, increasingly specific 'defences in depth' against these catastrophic outcomes as our knowledge of mechanisms advances.

The situation with macrovascular disease in diabetes is rather different. Here the problem appears to be not so much a direct effect of the diabetic state as a diabetes-induced aggravation of the atherogenic processes operating in the population at large. The jury is still out on whether there is a direct and specific diabetic arteriopathy but what is universally accepted is the role of diabetes as an amplifier of the atherosclerotic process and the impact of the known risk factors for it. As hyperglycaemia is a *mechanism* of microangiopathy, it may only be a *marker* for increased macroangiopathic risk, although there is increasing evidence of a quantitative relationship between the degree of hyperglycaemia and the size of atherosclerotic risk. One model would draw a parallel between tuberculosis and atherosclerosis in diabetes. When tuberculosis is prevalent in the population, the person with diabetes is at much higher risk for the disease than the non-diabetic. The dramatic reduction of tuberculous infection in advanced societies has greatly reduced the risk in people with diabetes, although the susceptibility presumably remains. It can be argued that, in respect of atherosclerosis, improvement in diabetes may reduce the disease. What are the mechanisms of enhanced macrovascular susceptibility in diabetes and are there alternative approaches to its reversal?

All these questions, and many others, are tackled in the chapters which follow. Considerable progress has been made but much remains to be discovered, still lying outside our pool of light. We can, and must, speculate on what lies out there, some of it already half apparent but not really recognizable. Some entirely new factors will doubtless come into view. Not to overstrain the metaphor, the contributors to this book provide an expert and detailed map of our knowledge to date and guidelines to the interesting and important areas of developing thought and experiment for those who travel this road.

Harry Keen
Professor of Metabolic Medicine
Department of Medicine
United Medical and Dental Schools
Guy's Campus
London Bridge
London SE1 9RC, UK

PART ONE

BACKGROUND

INTRODUCTION

John E. Tooke and William Liddell

1.1 HISTORICAL PERSPECTIVE

Although the first description of diabetic retinopathy can be traced back to the mid-1800s [1], authorities in the latter part of that century regarded 'diabetic retinitis' as very rare [2] and readily confused with albuminuric retinitis which was regarded as much more common [3]. This relative rarity no doubt was due in some part to the fact that the outlook for the juvenile form of the condition was such that diabetes of long duration was uncommon. Fox, writing in *Diseases of the Eye* in 1904 recognized that retinopathy was seldom an early occurrence in diabetes but 'usually presents itself near the termination of the affection' [4].

De Schweinitz, writing in the ninth edition of the same title published in 1921, underscored the fact that the occurrence of retinitis was duration-related and, if carefully sought, was seldom absent in long-standing disease. Coexistence with the other vascular complications of gangrene and hemiplegia was also recognized [5].

The association between diabetes and renal disease has a similar history, with several authorities discussing the issue in the mid-1800s, although Dupytren had recognized the link with albuminuria half a century earlier [6]. By the close of the nineteenth century the prognostic importance of albuminuria for the diabetic patient was well recognized [7] and at about the same time the first descriptions of histological changes in the kidney emerged [8], although these concentrated on tubular changes. It was 1936 before Kimmelsteil and Wilson described 'intercapillary lesions' in the glomeruli of the kidney and the concept of glomerulosclerosis emerged [9].

Specific features of diabetic gangrene of the foot were advanced by Marchal de Calvi in 1864 [10], notably moist and warm, (presumably denoting coexistent infection), when compared with ordinary 'senile' gangrene.

The clinical significance of the microvascular complications of diabetes, retinopathy and nephropathy, became much more apparent 10 to 20 years after the introduction of insulin in 1922. Survival carried with it a high price in terms of morbidity, as documented in a series of analyses appearing in the 1940s and 1950s. Root *et al.* coined the term 'triopathy' to emphasize the frequent coexistence of neuropathy, retinitis and nephropathy [11]. In a treatise in 1956, describing the status of 1072 juvenile patients treated at the Joslin Clinic for a period of 20 years or more, White reported that of the 169 that had died, 87.5% had succumbed to 'cardio-renal-vascular' causes, starkly emphasizing the emerging spectre of diabetic vascular disease [12]. Another notable series, that by Lundbaek in 1953 [13], describing the clinical picture in diabetes of 15–25 years' duration in a geographical region of Denmark reported that in young patients (16 to 39 years) isolated retinopathy was common occurring in 66% of patients, whereas 11% had retinopathy, renal disease and heart disease, emphasizing the now well recognized association between nephropathy and heart disease. In middle-aged patients (40 to 59 years) foot disease emerges in combination with the other complications, whereas in the oldest patients (60+ years) isolated retinopathy was very unusual (6%), combined pathology being the norm.

Although the impact of the vascular complications of diabetes in terms of both morbidity and mortality was thus abundantly clear 20–30 years after the development of insulin therapy, the link with the degree of metabolic derangement was far less certain, and has only recently been put beyond reasonable doubt as far as type 1 diabetes is concerned with the publication of the DCCT [14]. The former lack of clarity, despite an abundance of careful clinical observation alluded to above, was arguably due to several factors, notably: (i) the absence of secure means of estimating long-term glycaemic control; (ii) non-uniform susceptibility to the ravages of obviously poor control; and (iii) the fact that the clinical development of clinical complications is a slow process, often taking decades to manifest. Attempts to use a surrogate marker of the microangiopathic process, capillary basement membrane thickening led to considerable controversy, clearly portrayed by Tattersall [15]. Siperstein put forward the intriguing observation that thickened basement membrane occurred in prediabetic individuals [16], observations that were later discounted and attributed to technically induced artefacts.

1.2 DIABETIC ANGIOPATHY

The concept that late complications of diabetes largely represent disease of the blood vessels is thus well established, the term angiopathy being introduced by Lundbaek following his systematic studies [13]. It has been conventional to think in terms of *microangiopathy*, afflicting the vessels between and including the arteriole and venule, and *macroangiopathy* involving the arterial tree. Although such an anatomical distinction may seem to be consistent with the expression of retinopathy and nephropathy on the one hand, and accelerated atherosclerosis on the other, histological changes involving smaller arteries and arterioles in the form of uneven hyalinization are notable findings [17]. Furthermore, recent work suggests that in non-insulin-dependent diabetes the expression of nephropathy may often be associated with sclerosis of interlobular arteries which then questions the conceptual value of subdividing the process according to vessel order [18].

Angiopathy, in theory at least, embraces disease of other elements of the vascular tree, namely the venules, veins and lymphatics. Although the postcapillary segment has commanded far less attention, clinical observation (venous calibre irregularity as a harbinger of sight-threatening retinopathy), physiological [19], and pharmacological [20] studies point to a non-appreciated role for the venous system in the pathogenesis of diabetic complications.

Whereas the generic term angiopathy retains its legitimacy, the prefix diabetic conjures the assumption that the process is the same regardless of the type of diabetes. Epidemiological studies have been plagued by poorly made distinctions between type 1 and type 2, and between insulin-dependent and insulin-treated diabetes. The emergence of the concepts of insulin resistance and the metabolic syndrome have served to emphasize the increased macroangiopathic risk borne by people with type 2 diabetes and its precursors, whereas in the absence of nephropathy the prognosis for type 1 diabetes is relatively benign [21]. Although the majority of type 2 diabetes is likely to represent a polygenic disorder with considerable lifestyle and/or developmental determinants, a minority of cases can be defined genetically. The pattern of microvascular behaviour in subjects with maturity onset diabetes of the young (MODY) is more in accord with that observed in mild type 1 diabetes [22], consistent with the aetiology of this type of diabetes being a β-cell defect rather than due to insulin resistance and relative β-cell failure that is more typically associated with the 'maturity onset' phenotype. As the origins of type 2 diabetes are more closely dissected, so the apparent heterogeneity of angiopathy expression may also be explained.

1.3 SCOPE OF THE TEXT

These considerations aside, this text seeks to draw together current concepts relating to the pathogenesis of diabetic angiopathy. Notwithstanding the comments above, for ease of reference large and small vessel disease are dealt with separately in Parts Two and Three and Part Four deals with the organ-specific manifestations of vascular disease. No attempt has been made to be exhaustive and bias has been shown in emphasizing human observations, with animal work cited when no equivalent human data exist or the implication for our understanding of the process is profound. Reference to treatment is confined to those issues where it may aid the understanding of the underlying disease mechanism.

It is a sobering thought that, 76 years after the introduction of insulin therapy, few specific treatments exist for the prevention of the vascular complications of diabetes. The goal of developing therapies that mitigate the impact of imperfect glycaemic control and the critical features of the metabolic syndrome is an enticing, if elusive, one. Progress towards such a goal will probably depend on resolving the many riddles contained in these pages.

REFERENCES

1 Jaegner, E. *Beitrage zur Retinopatie des Auges,* K.K. Hof und Staadtsdrucherei, Seite 33, Vienna, 1855.
2. Juler, H.E. In *A Handbook of Ophthalmic Science and Practice,* Elder & Co. London, 1884, p. 192.
3. Noyes, H.D. *Textbook of Diseases of the Eye,* William Woods & Co., New York, 1890.
4. Fox, L.W. *Diseases of the Eye,* Sidney Appleton, London, 1904, p. 406.
5. De Schweinitz, G.E. *Diseases of the Eye,* 9th edition, W. B. Saunders, 1921, p. 478.
6. Dupytren and Thenard. Memoire sur le diabète sucre. *Ann. Chim.,* 1806, **59,** 41.
7. Stokvis, B.J. Zur pathologie und therapie des diabetes mellitus. *Verh. Kongr. Int. Med.,* 1886, **5,** 125.
8. Ebstein, W. Ueber drüsenepithelnekrosen beim diabetes mellitus mit besonderer berüchsichtang des diabetischen coma. *D. Arch Klin. Med.,* 1881, **28,** 143.
9. Kimmelstiel, P. and Wilson, C. Intercapillary lesions in the glomeruli of the kidney. *Am. J. Pathol.,* 1935, **11,** 483.
10. Marchal (de Calvi). *Recherches sur les Accidents Diabétiques,* 1864, Paris.
11. Root, H.F., Pote, W.H. and Frehner, H. Triopathy of diabetes : sequence of neuropathy, retinopathy and nephropathy in 155 patients. *Arch. Intern. Med.,* 1954, **94,** 931–41.
12. White, P. Natural course and prognosis of juvenile diabetes. *Diabetes,* 1956, **5,** 445–57.
13. Lundbaek, K. *Long-term Diabetes,* Ejnar Munksgaard, Copenhagen, 1953.
14. The Diabetes Control and Complications Trial Research Group. The effect of intensive treatment of diabetes on the development and progression of long term complications in insulin-dependent diabetes mellitus. *N. Engl. J. Med.,* 1993, **329,** 977–86.
15. Tattersall, R.B. The quest for normoglycaemia: an historical perspective. *Diabet. Med.,* 1994, **11,** 618–35.
16. Siperstein, M.D., Unger, R.H. and Madison, L.L. Studies of muscle capillary basement membranes in normal subjects, diabetic and pre-diabetic patients. *J. Clin Invest.,* 1968, **47,** 1973–99.
17. Goldenberg, S., Alex, M., Joshi, R.A. and Blumenthal, H.T. Nonatheromatous peripheral vascular disease of the lower extremity in diabetes mellitus. *Diabetes,* 1959, **8,** 261–73.
18. Boeri, D., Derchi, L.E., Martinoli, C. *et al.* Intrarenal arteriosclerosis and impairment of kidney function in NIDDM subjects. *Diabetologia,* 1998, **41,** 121–4.
19. Houbens, F.C. *Vascular Compliance and Reactivity in Diabetes Mellitus.* PhD thesis. ISBN 90-901174-3.

20. Bodmer, C.W., Patrick, A.W., How, T.V. and Williams, G. Exaggerated sensitivity to NE-induced vasoconstriction in IDDM patients with micro-albuminuria: Possible aetiology and diagnostic implications. *Diabetes*, 1992, **41**, 209–14.
21. Jensen, T., Borch-Johnsen, K., Kofoed-Enevoldsen, A. and Deckert, T. Coronary heart disease in young type 1 (insulin-dependent) diabetic patients with and without diabetic nephropathy: incidence and risk factors. *Diabetologia*, 1987, **30**, 144–8.
22. Lee, B.C., Shore, A.C., Tooke, J.E. and Hattersley, A.T. Impaired maximum microvascular hyperaemia in subjects with mutations in hepatic nuclear factor -1 alpha gene (MODY 3), in press.

EPIDEMIOLOGY OF DIABETIC ANGIOPATHY

Rhys Williams and Mark Airey

2.1 SCOPE OF THIS CHAPTER

The term 'diabetic angiopathy' as used in this chapter encompasses both the macrovascular and the microvascular manifestations of diabetes. In the former category are peripheral vascular disease (PVD), coronary heart disease (CHD) and cerebrovascular disease (CVD). The latter lead to the diabetic complications of retinopathy, neuropathy and nephropathy. This account deals mainly with the descriptive epidemiology of these conditions. Studies based upon groups of subjects identified through clinical practice (in primary, secondary or tertiary care) are, for most of these entities, contrasted with studies which are population-based.

Following the relevant descriptive studies, some of the factors associated with angiopathy are considered. The description of such associations is usually the first step towards the formulation of aetiological hypotheses. This chapter does not discuss the epidemiology of lipid abnormalities and their relation to diabetic angiopathy – that is covered in Chapter 6. Also, the chapter is not a systematic review. It is reasonably comprehensive but selective in highlighting the information most likely to be of interest in describing the size of the problem on a world-wide scale. The nature of the literature is such that it is not possible to obtain totally comparable studies from every continent. Where relevant, the differences in the approaches that have been taken in disease definition and identification of affected individuals are mentioned.

The concluding section refers to predictions about the likely future epidemiology of diabetes over the next few decades. Such predictions are clearly important in determining the need for health care for the prevention, early detection and treatment of the consequences of diabetic angiopathy. Though they need to be viewed with some scepticism, they are an important aspect of the use of current epidemiological information.

2.2 MAKING SENSE OF THE EPIDEMIOLOGICAL INFORMATION

It is important to distinguish between the clinic-based and population-based studies considered here. The latter are the more useful in judging the size of the problem in the community but then only if the samples chosen have known relationships to the wider populations from which they are drawn. Groups identified through clinical practice are usually more convenient sources of data but their relationship to the population from which they are drawn is frequently unknown. In most cases they suffer, to a greater or lesser extent, from that particular form of selection bias known as referral bias (or 'Berksonian bias'). Not all individuals with a given condition will be represented in those attending for primary, secondary or tertiary care. There is usually selection for the more severely affected or at least those with recognized symptoms or signs.

There is also, usually, a bias introduced by differential retention within a clinic population. This may be due to differential mortality, in which case it is usually the most severe cases that are lost. Alternatively, it may be the result of infrequent or non-attendance, in which case it will usually be the least severe cases that are not available for inclusion.

If findings from clinic-based studies are interpreted with care they can be useful in exploring associations between angiopathy and genetic or environmental factors. Usually the more severe grades of abnormality are represented more frequently in these clinic-based groups than in the general population of people with diabetes from which they are drawn. This fact can be an advantage in any study seeking to identify causal relationships. These studies can also provide a useful indication of workloads in the clinical practices from which they come.

2.3 PERIPHERAL VASCULAR DISEASE

2.3.1 DEFINITIONS

Palumbo and Melton [1] list diminution of peripheral pulses, proneness to infection, ulceration, poor healing, gangrene and amputation as features of PVD. They refer to an international workshop on the assessment of PVD in diabetes [2], the recommendations of which, although sometimes quoted, have not been universally adopted. A standard definition of PVD (and other complications of diabetes) has been considered by a World Health Organization (WHO) Consultation Group. Its proposals for a revision of the diagnostic criteria for diabetes are forthcoming [3]. Publication for consultation of their proposals on the definitions of complications will soon follow.

The sophistication of techniques used for the identification of PVD in people with diabetes varies considerably. Identification may be made by the presence of symptoms (e.g. intermittent claudication), signs (the absence of peripheral pulses, audible bruits), investigations (such as Doppler and ultrasound) or a combination of these.

2.3.2 PRACTICE-BASED STUDIES

A frequently quoted study using Doppler ultrasound for the detection of PVD in people with diabetes is that of Janka *et al.* [4]. Palumbo and Melton [1] list this with four other clinic-based studies. These give a range of prevalence from 5.1% when based on symptoms [5], through to 38.9% when based on Doppler investigation and plethysmography [6]. The estimate of 15.9% from Janka *et al.* [4] falls in between these extremes. The range illustrates the influence on prevalence estimates of different methods used to detect PVD as well as, in all probability, differences in referral and retention bias in the samples included.

A more recent clinic-based study from Madras, India [7], using a combination of symptoms and signs as diagnostic, reported a prevalence of PVD of 15.4%. Given that the subjects included in this study were selected on the basis of having had diagnosed type 2 diabetes of 25 years or more duration, the authors expressed surprise at the low prevalence. Their findings may, however, be the result of lower rates of retention within the clinic population of people with severe PVD. This effect would be expected to be most marked in those who have had diabetes for the longest time.

These clinic-based studies provide little information interpretable beyond the confines of the setting in which they were performed. With their disparate methods of definition and detection, their unknown (but presumably different) degrees of referral and loss to follow-up bias, their wide range of prevalence estimates cannot be used to extrapolate to the size of the problem in the population from which the patients are drawn.

2.3.3 POPULATION-BASED STUDIES

There is also a wide range of prevalence estimates displayed by the population-based studies selected by Palumbo and Melton [1]. For example, within the study by Siitonen *et al.* [8] of people with newly diagnosed type 2 diabetes in Finland, a threefold range of prevalence of PVD is described in the same group of 70 subjects depending on the method by which PVD was defined. When lower/upper extremity blood pressure differences were used it was 7%. When symptoms of claudication were the criterion the prevalence was 9% but when absent foot pulses were used it was 30%.

Estimates of incidence and prevalence of PVD are described in some more recent population-based studies. These studies often use similar, although · rarely identical, methods of detection. An important consideration in drawing comparisons is the means by which diabetic subjects are ascertained.

Two cross-sectional studies, one from the Netherlands [9] and the other from the United Kingdom [10], are examples of the use of similar but not identical methods for the investigation of PVD. They also differed in that the former used oral glucose tolerance tests to identify subjects previously undiagnosed as having diabetes, supplementing those already diagnosed (which made up the group studied by the UK researchers).

Both studies found a greater prevalence of abnormalities in people with diabetes than in those without. In the Dutch population, Duplex scanning, Doppler signal analysis and indirect blood pressure measurements detected vessel obstructions in 31.8% of those with diabetes (known and previously undiagnosed combined) compared with 18.4% in subjects with normal glucose tolerance. The age range of both groups was 50 to 75 years.

The UK workers, using a definition of PVD as an ankle/brachial Doppler pressure ratio of 0.9 or less, found PVD in 23.5% of those with (clinically diagnosed) type 2 diabetes and in 8.7% of those with type 1 diabetes. After adjusting for age, a close correlate of duration of diabetes, the difference between the prevalence in these two groups was not significant: odds ratio (OR) type 2/type 1 = 1.5; 95% confidence interval (CI) 0.8–2.7.

The prevalence of PVD in non-diabetic subjects was 9.6% with a slight excess in males compared to females (11% versus 9%). For type 2 diabetes there was a significant excess prevalence of PVD when compared to those without diabetes in both sexes. For men this was just over twice that in the non-diabetic group (OR 2.47, 95% CI 1.92–10.92) and for women over three times (OR 3.15, 95% CI 1.79–5.56). In people with type 1 diabetes the increased prevalence was significant in men (OR 4.58, 95% CI 1.92–10.92) but not in women (OR 1.78, 95% CI 0.58–5.49) after adjusting for age. The authors commented that there was no difference in whether the PVD was *symptomatic* between diabetic and non-diabetic subjects. This is similar to the conclusions of the Dutch group who qualified their observation of around twice the prevalence of PVD in diabetic subjects compared with non-diabetic subjects by observing that most of the PVD in the former was asymptomatic.

2.4 CORONARY HEART DISEASE

2.4.1 DEFINITION

The influence of definitions is similar to that described above for PVD. As has been observed by Wingard and Barrett-Connor [11], studies of CHD in diabetes have improved in quality in recent years, mainly as a result of the use of standardized definitions of diabetes [12, 13]. They are less enthusiastic about the extent to which standard definitions and methods of detection of CHD have been adopted. These different methods, as they point out, cause practical problems in epidemiological studies. Some, such as angiography, are unsuitable for widespread use in apparently healthy subjects while, at the other extreme, the use of death certificate data suffers from the problems of incomplete and variable recording.

In making comparisons between, in particular, US-based studies and studies based in other countries, the possibility of overdiagnosis of diabetes and CHD needs to be kept in mind. This possibility applies particularly to clinic-based studies and to population-based studies which use self-reported diabetes and/or self-reported CHD as the basis for prevalence estimates. Wingard and Barrett-Connor [11] refer, also, to a form of Berksonian bias which results from the likelihood that people known to have CHD, or who are at risk from CHD, will be more likely to have previously undiagnosed diabetes revealed by case finding. The reverse also may be the case, with more complete identification of CHD in those already known to have diabetes.

2.4.2   PRACTICE-BASED STUDIES

The most informative clinic-based studies are those which have observed, preferably in a prospective fashion, the incidence of well-defined CHD and related events in people with diabetes compared with those of comparable age and sex who do not have diabetes. Such a study has been reported by Jaffe *et al.* [14] who found twice the frequency of congestive heart failure, after myocardial infarction, in 100 patients with diabetes compared with 426 without when followed for two years.

More recent clinic-based studies have highlighted the association between cardiovascular disease, the microvascular complications of diabetes and albuminuria as a risk marker for both. For example, Agardh *et al.* [15] followed up 451 people with type 2 diabetes attending their outpatient clinic in Lund, Sweden. The association they confirmed between CHD, retinopathy and albuminuria

is mentioned below. Their findings in terms of the incidence of CHD among these patients were that 19 developed CHD during the five-year follow-up period. They compared this incidence (of 22.1 events/1000/year) with that predicted from the general population (13.6/1000/year) Their sample was relatively small and, potentially, suffered from the biases described above. However, their ascertainment of incident cases and of death from atherosclerotic vascular disease as a whole in their cohort was probably almost complete.

2.4.3   POPULATION-BASED STUDIES

Estimates of the excess incidence of CHD in people with diabetes are available from a number of population-based studies carried out in the USA. Those which rely on independently verified diabetes and CHD show considerably lower relative risk estimates than do those which use self-reported information on diabetes [11]. In the former category, for example, the Framingham Study [16] and the Honolulu Heart Study [17] report relative risk values of between 1.7 and 2.9, depending on gender and the study concerned. In contrast, the Nurses' Health Study [18], which relied on self-reports of diabetes, found CHD relative risks of 6.7 for type 2 diabetes and 12.2 for type 1.

The US National Health and Nutrition Examination Survey (NHANES) [19] has reported on the prevalence of angina and past myocardial infarction (MI) (both elicited by Rose questionnaire) in people aged 35–74 years with known diabetes, previously undiagnosed diabetes, impaired glucose tolerance, and normal glucose tolerance. As would be expected, the difference in reported past occurrence of myocardial infarction between those with diabetes and those without is greater for women than men. For example, in the 55–74-year age group, 11.3% of women with diabetes (known and previously undiagnosed combined) reported a history of MI compared with 6.3% of those with impaired glucose tolerance and 5.7% of those with normal glucose tolerance. The corresponding figures in men were 10.6%, 7.3% and 7.3%.

The more marked association of MI with diabetes in women than in men is a common finding in population-based studies. The 'Strong Heart Study' [20] of diabetes in three groups of indigenous North Americans found high prevalences of diabetes and significantly increased numbers of people with past histories of MI in those with diabetes compared with those without. Such histories were 3.8-times more common in diabetic women than in non-diabetic women compared with 1.9-times as common in diabetic men compared with non-diabetic men.

In contrast to the above study which was of the prevalence of past history of MI, studies which have prospectively recorded the incidence of MI in people with diabetes have frequently found larger differences between diabetic and non-diabetic risks. For example, Laakso *et al.* [21], reporting on a seven-year follow-up of diabetic and non-diabetic subjects in east and west Finland, showed that women with diabetes had 8–11 times the risk of CHD events (fatal or non-fatal MI) than women without diabetes. Men with diabetes had a three- to fourfold greater risk than their non-diabetic peers.

The issues which need to be considered in comparing the differences between excess risk estimates in different studies include: (1) whether CHD events are self-reported or independently validated; (2) the underlying risk of CHD in the general population; and (3) whether the CHD events are retrospectively or prospectively ascertained. Poorer survival following MI in people with diabetes compared with those without (as suggested, for example, by Jaffe *et al.* [14]) would lead to smaller differences between diabetic and non-diabetic groups in retrospective studies of prevalence compared with prospective studies of incidence. At least part of the difference between the results of Howard [20] and

Laakso *et al.* [21] may be the result of this difference in post-MI survival.

2.5   CEREBROVASCULAR DISEASE

2.5.1   DEFINITION

It is not so much the definition of CVD as its ascertainment which offers the greatest challenge in epidemiological studies. Many CVD events are relatively mild and most occur outside hospital and may remain outside hospital throughout their course. Complete, population-based ascertainment requires comprehensive population-based stroke registers or assiduous follow-up of defined cohorts of individuals. The association of CVD with diabetes is not in dispute, although the excess of CVD in people with diabetes is probably somewhat less than is the case for CHD [22].

2.5.2   PRACTICE BASED STUDIES

As has been pointed out by Kuller [23], the substantial mortality associated with stroke means that prevalence is a misleading indication of its impact on the health of the population. This is particularly true in clinic-based series where the severity of the stroke and the severity of the diabetes are likely to be greater than in the general population. Perhaps for this reason, the literature on stroke and diabetes derived from clinic-based populations is sparse. The Madras study already referred to [7], although it reported the prevalence of PVD and CHD, did not include stroke. In Japan, the country with the world's highest mortality from stroke, the prevalence of past CVD in the Tokyo Metropolitan Geriatric Hospital series [24] was less than that of ischaemic heart disease (18% compared with 23%). This was the case despite the high incidence of stroke in the general population and the strong association between diabetes (in that case type 2 diabetes) and stroke.

Incidence is a better indication of disease burden in this case, but clinic-based incidence studies are of limited use because of the strong likelihood of retention bias. CVD must be a common, but poorly documented, reason for loss to follow-up of patients originally included in hospital clinic-based studies whether because of the resulting immobility or mortality. Autopsy-based series (e.g. that described by Kameyama *et al.* [25]) suggesting associations between poor blood glucose control and the incidence of CVD must be viewed with extreme scepticism. Numbers of cases are small (51 deaths in this case), the likelihood of coming to autopsy is low in most countries, the retrospective investigation of the quality of blood glucose control is problematic and autopsy cases can rarely be related to a defined population.

2.5.3   POPULATION BASED STUDIES

Kuller [23] tabulates mortality from stroke in the diabetic and non-diabetic individuals who participated in the Multiple Risk Factor Intervention Trial (MRFIT) [26]. Though far from a random sample of the US male population, this group did demonstrate a clear 2.8-fold excess risk (95% CI 2.0–3.7) of death from stroke (ICD (International Classification of Diseases) 9th Revision 430–438) in men with diabetes compared to those without. The corresponding figure for CHD was 3.2 (95% CI 2.9–3.5).

In a Finnish study, men and women were followed up for between 15 and 20 years [27]. Men showed a sixfold risk of death from stroke if they had diabetes at baseline. The corresponding figure for women was just over eightfold. In that study, the presence of diabetes was the single most powerful risk factor for stroke mortality. A recently published Swedish study [28] has demonstrated that around 18% of strokes in men in that country and 22% of strokes in women are attributable to diabetes. This represents an annual number of CVD events, attributable to diabetes, of about 50 per 100 000 of the general population aged 35–74 years.

2.5.4   WORLD-WIDE COMPARISONS

Recently published work by Amos *et al.* [29], primarily focused on the prediction of diabetes prevalence in the next millennium (see below), presents a useful summary of studies from every continent describing the prevalence of the major diabetes complications.

Using this material it is possible to compile an overview of the extent to which PVD and CHD and hypertension, the major risk determinant for CVD in diabetes, affect populations in different parts of the world. Using the regions which WHO uses for its own description of the future burden of diabetes [30], Table 2.1 displays selected prevalence estimates for these three conditions. The studies selected are, unless otherwise stated, of type 1 and type 2 diabetes combined, have used similar means of identifying affected subjects and are reasonably recently published. They serve to illustrate the range of estimates being put forward in the current literature.

2.6   MICROVASCULAR DISEASE

2.6.1   DEFINITION

The retinopathy, neuropathy and nephropathy seen in all populations as complications of diabetes have, as their origin, the same pathological changes of the microcirculation [42]. Definitions of retinopathy are widely agreed and extensively used. These may be based on the appearance of the retina or on empirically tested visual function. Definitions of nephropathy vary more widely. They may rely on estimates of urinary albumin excretion rates or, more feasible for population-based studies on a large scale, the detection of

Table 2.1 Prevalence of PVD, CHD and hypertension in five world regions. All diabetes combined unless otherwise stated. (Adapted from Amos *et al.* [29])

| | *Prevalance (%)* | | |
Region	PVD	CHD	Hypertension**
Africa	Zambia: 1.4 [31]	Zambia: 17.2 [31]	Tanzania: 27.0 [40]
Europe	Netherlands: 34.1 [32]	United Kingdom: 43.0 [36]	Netherlands: 54.9 [32]
SE Asia	Korea: 5.9* [33]	Thailand: 10.5* [37]	Thailand: 38.4* [37]
W Pacific	Tonga: 12.0* [34]	Kiribati: 11.9* [38]	Australia: 74.0 [41]
Americas	Jamaica: 13.0 [35]	Cuba: 45.6 [39]	Cuba: 35.9 [39]

* Type 2 diabetes only.
** Systolic BP >160 mmHg and/or diastolic BP >95 mmHg and/or antihypertensive medication.

persistent proteinuria in the absence of urinary tract infection.

2.6.2 CLINIC-BASED AND POPULATION-BASED STUDIES

In selected European countries, for type 1 diabetes, knowledge of the descriptive epidemiology of diabetic microvascular complications has recently been enhanced by the Eurodiab IDDM Complications Study. For example, Sjolie *et al.* [43] have reported on retinopathy and visual loss in 3250 people with type 1 diabetes ascertained through hospital-based diabetes clinics in 31 centres in (mainly western) European countries. Although clinic-based, this large group of subjects was at least selected according to criteria standardized for every centre. Also, given that the study is of people with type 1 diabetes, the majority of whom are likely to be in touch with hospital services, the results may come close to the ideal of truly population-based observations. Bias, if there is any, is most likely towards an overestimation of prevalence. The results suggested that corrected visual acuity was less than or equal to 0.1 in the best eye in 2.3% of subjects, that mild, non-proliferative retinopathy was present in 2.8%, moderate-severe non-proliferative retinopathy in 9.8% and proliferative retinopathy in 10.6%. Univariate analysis showed, unsurprisingly, that age, duration of diabetes and HbA1c were positively associated with visual loss. After adjustment for these factors and albumin excretion rate, blood pressure, serum triglyceride and fibrinogen levels were found to be positively associated with increased risk of retinopathy.

From the USA, observations from the Pittsburgh Epidemiology of Diabetes Complications (EDC) Study [44] and the Wisconsin Study, e.g. [45], have been of considerable interest and importance. The former has been monitoring the incidence and progression of retinopathy (and other diabetic complications) in a cohort of people with childhood onset type 1 diabetes. Their findings suggest that baseline diastolic blood pressure and later HbA$_1$, triglycerides and low-density lipoprotein (LDL) cholesterol and fibrinogen

Table 2.2 Prevalence of microvascular complications in five world regions. All diabetes combined unless otherwise stated. (Adapted from Amos *et al.* [29])

	Prevalance (%)		
Region	*Retinopathy*	*Nephropathy***	*Neuropathy*
Africa	Ethiopia: 37.8 [49]	Egypt: 12.4 [51]	Ethiopia: 9.4 [55]
Europe	Spain: 43.0 [50]	United Kingdom: 5.2 [52]	United Kingdom: 32.1* [56]
SE Asia	Thailand: 32.1* [37]	Thailand: 18.7* [37]	Singapore: 17.2 [57]
W Pacific	Tonga: 32.0* [34]	New Zealand: 11.5* [53]	Tonga: 30.0* [34]
Americas	Jamaica: 34.7 [35]	Mexico: 15.9* [54]	Jamaica: 22.5 [35]

* Type 2 only.
** Persistent proteinuria in absence of urinary tract infection.

concentrations were positively associated with the development of retinopathy. The publication [45] cited from the Wisconsin study had also reported that observation, one which was, of course, endorsed as a result of the intervention carried out in the Diabetes Control and Complications Trial (DCCT) [46].

Information on other complications of diabetes has been made available by Eurodiab (see, for example, [47]). As well as retinopathy, this publication comments on the prevalence of autonomic and sensory neuropathies and nephropathy. Postural hypotension and abnormal heart rate variability were reported in 5.9% (95% CI 5.1–6.7%) and 19.3% (95% CI 17.9–20.7%) respectively. Again, the presence of these complications was found to be positively associated with HbA1c and also with the extent of albuminuria. For some time the association between urinary albumin excretion, not only with nephropathy but also with retinopathy, neuropathy and cardiovascular disease, has been recognized, as has its prognostic value in both clinical and epidemiological terms [48]. These observations strengthen the common pathophysiological origin of not only the microvascular complications of diabetes [42] but also, possibly, including the macrovascular changes.

In a similar manner to the data presented in Table 2.1 for PVD, CHD and hypertension, Table 2.2 presents data for the manifestations of microvascular disease in the same WHO regions.

2.7 PREDICTING THE FUTURE

There is currently considerable interest in the extent to which diabetes prevalence is likely to increase in the next few decades. Zimmet [58] has pointed out that the rise in prevalence seen in developed countries is now affecting developing countries. Quantitative estimates of the likely size of this increase have been produced for Australia [59], The Netherlands [60] and, most recently, for each continent [29].

These and the estimates recently published by WHO [30] agree that the world is likely to see a dramatic rise in diabetes prevalence (Table 2.3). This is partly because of demographic changes, partly as a result of the rising prevalence of obesity and partly

Table 2.3 Estimated and projected prevalence (per thousand total population) of diabetes (type 1 and type 2 combined) in 1995 and 2025, absolute rise in prevalence (per thousand) and relative rise (percentage of 1995 estimates). (Adapted from WHO, 1997 [30])

| | *Prevalance* | | | |
Region	*1995 estimate*	*2025 projection*	*Absolute rise*	*Relative rise**
Africa	2.4	9.8	7.4	308.3%
Europe	32.8	47.5	14.7	44.8%
SE Asia	27.6	79.5	51.9	188.0%
W Pacific	26.4	56.0	29.6	112.1%
Americas	30.7	63.5	32.8	106.8%
E Med	11.2	40.0	28.8	257.1%

* Relative to 1995 prevalence.

because of lifestyle changes including a reduction in physical activity. These epidemiological changes, if they occur as predicted, are certain to increase the burden that the circulatory manifestations of diabetes impose on individuals, families and society as a whole. This gloomy scenario makes it even more important that the mechanisms underlying these effects of diabetes should be more clearly understood and the means by which they can be prevented identified and put into practice.

REFERENCES

1. Palumbo, P.J. and Melton, L.J. Peripheral vascular disease and diabetes. In *Diabetes in America*, 2nd edn, NIH Pub. No. 95-1468, US Government Printing Office, Washington, DC, 1995, 293–338, pp. 401-8.
2. Orchard, T.J. and Strandness, D.E. Assessment of peripheral vascular complications in diabetes. Report and recommendations of an international workshop. *Circulation*, 1993, **88**, 819–28.
3. World Health Organisation Consultation Group. The definition, diagnosis and classification of diabetes mellitus and its complications. Report of a WHO Consultation Group. Part I: the definition, diagnosis and classification of diabetes. *Diabet. Med.* in press.
4. Janka, H.U., Standl, E. and Mehnert, H. Peripheral vascular disease in diabetes mellitus and its relation to cardiovascular risk factors: screening with the Doppler ultrasonic technique. *Diabetes Care*, 1980, **3**, 207–13.
5. Klimt, C.R., Knatterud, G.L., Meinert, C.L. and Prout, T.E. A study of the effects of hypoglycaemic agents on vascular complications in patients with adult-onset diabetes. I: Design, methods and baseline results. *Diabetes*, 1970, **19**, 747–83.
6. Bendick, P.J., Glover, J.L., Keubler, T.W. and Dilley, R.S. Progression of atherosclerosis in diabetics. *Surgery*, 1983, **93**, 834–8.
7. Mohan, V., Vijayaprabha, R. and Rema, M. Vascular complications in long-term south Indian NIDDM of over 25 years' duration. *Diabetes Res. Clin. Pract.*, 1996, **31**, 133–40.
8. Siitonen, O., Uusitupa, M., Pyörälä, K., Voutilainen, E. and Lansinies, E. Peripheral arterial disease and its relationship to cardiovascular risk factors and coronary heart disease in newly diagnosed non-insulin dependent diabetics. *Acta Med. Scand.*, 1986, **220**, 205–12.
9. Mackaay, A.J., Beks, P.J., Dur, A.H. *et al.* The distribution of peripheral vascular disease in a Dutch Caucasian population: comparison of type II diabetic and non-diabetic subjects. *Eur. J. Vasc. Endovasc. Surg.*, 1995, **9**, 170–5.
10. Walters, D.P., Gatling, W., Mullee, M.A. and Hill, R.D. The prevalence, detection and epidemiological correlates of peripheral vascular disease: a comparison of diabetic and non-diabetic subjects in an English community. *Diabet. Med.*, 1992, **9**, 710–15.
11. Wingard, D.L. and Barrett-Connor, E. Heart disease and diabetes. In *Diabetes in America*,

2nd edn, NIH Pub. No. 95-1468, US Government Printing Office, Washington, DC, 1995, 293–338, pp. 429–48.

12. National Diabetes Data Group. Classification and diagnosis of diabetes mellitus and other categories of glucose intolerance. *Diabetes,* 1979, **28,** 1039–57.

13. World Health Organisation. Second report of the WHO experts committee on diabetes mellitus. Technical Report Series No. 646. World Health Organisation, Geneva, 1980.

14. Jaffe, A.S., Spadaro, J.J., Schectman, K., Roberts, R., Gletman, E.M. and Sobel, B.E. Increased congestive heart failure after myocardial infarction of modest extent in patients with diabetes mellitus. *Am. Heart J.,* 1984, **8,** 31–7.

15. Agardh, C.D., Agardh, E. and Torffvit, O. The prognostic value of albuminuria for the development of cardiovascular disease and retinopathy: a prospective 5-year follow-up of 451 patients with type 2 diabetes mellitus. *Diabetes Res. Clin. Pract.,* 1996, **32,** 35–44.

16. Wilson, P.W.F., Cupples, A.D. and Kannel, W.B. Is hyperglycaemia associated with cardiovascular disease? The Framingham Study. *Am. Heart J.,* 1991, **2,** 586–90.

17. Laws, A., Marcus, E.B., Grove, J.S. and Curb, J.D. Lipids and lipoproteins as risk factors for coronary heart disease in men with abnormal glucose tolerance. The Honolulu Heart Program. *J. Intern. Med.,* 1993, **234,** 471–8.

18. Manson, J.E., Colditz, G.A., Stampfer, M.J., Willett, W.C., Krolewski, A.S., Rosmer, B., Arky, R.A., Speizer, F.E. and Hennekens, C.H. A prospective study of maturity-onset diabetes mellitus and risk of coronary heart disease and stroke in women. *Arch. Intern. Med.,* 1991, **151,** 1141–7.

19. Harris, M.I., Hadden, W.C., Knowler, W.C. and Bennett, P.H. Prevalence of diabetes and impaired glucose tolerance and plasma glucose levels in US population aged 20–74 years. *Diabetes,* 1987, **36,** 523–34.

20. Howard, B.V. Risk factors for cardiovascular disease in individuals with diabetes. The Strong Heart Study. *Acta Diabetol.,* 1996, **33,** 180–4.

21. Laakso, M., Ronnemaa, T., Lehto, S., Puukka, P., Kallio, V. and Pyorala. K. Does NIDDM increase risk for coronary heart disease similarly in both low- and high-risk populations? *Diabetologia,* 1995, **38,** 487–93.

22. Tuomilehto, J. and Rastenyté, D. Epidemiology of macrovascular disease and hypertension in diabetes mellitus. In *International Textbook of Diabetes Mellitus,* 2nd edn, (eds K.G.M.M. Alberti, P. Zimmet, R.A. DeFronzo and H. Keen), John Wiley & Sons Ltd, Chichester, 1997, pp. 1560–83.

23. Kuller, L.H. Stroke and diabetes. In *Diabetes in America,* 2nd edn, NIH Pub. No. 95-1468, US Government Printing Office, Washington, DC, 1995, 293–338, pp. 449–56.

24. Ito, H., Harano, Y. and Suzuki, M. Risk factor analyses for macrovascular complications in nonobese NIDDM patients. Multiclinical Study for Diabetic Macroangiopathy (MSDM). *Diabetes,* 1996, **45** (suppl 3), S19–23.

25. Kameyama, M., Fushimi, H. and Udaka, F. Diabetes mellitus and cerebral vascular disease. *Diabetes Res. Clin. Pract.,* 1994, **24** (suppl), S205–8.

26. Stamler, J., Vacarro, O., Neaton, J.D. and Wentworth, D. for the MRFIT Research Group: diabetes, other risk factors, and 12-yr cardiovascular mortality for men screened in the Multiple Risk Factor Intervention Trial. *Diabetes Care,* 1993, **16,** 434–44.

27. Tuomilheto, J., Rastenyté, D., Jousilahti, P., Sarti, C. and Vartiainen, E. Diabetes mellitus as a risk factor for death from stroke. Prospective study of the middle-aged Finnish population. *Stroke,* 1996, **27,** 210–15.

28. Stegmayr, B. and Asplund, K. Diabetes as a risk factor for stroke. A population perspective. *Diabetologia,* 1995, **38,** 1061–8.

29. Amos, A.F., McCarty, D.J. and Zimmet, P. The rising global burden of diabetes and its complications: estimates and projections to the year 2010. *Diabet. Med.,* 1997, **14** (suppl 5), S1–85.

30. World Health Organisation. In *The World Health Report 1997: Conquering Suffering, Enriching Humanity.* World Health Organisation, Geneva, 1997.

31. Rolfe, M. Macrovascular disease in diabetics in Central Africa. *Br. Med. J.* 1998, **296,** 1522–5.

32. Beks, P., Mackaay, A., de Neeling, J., de Vries, H., Bouter, L. and Heine, R. Peripheral arterial disease in relation to glycaemic level in an elderly Caucasian population: the Hoorn study. *Diabetologia,* 1995, **38,** 86–96.

33. Lee, K., Park, J., Kim, S., Lee, M., Kim, G., Park, S. and Park, J. Prevalence and associated features of albuminuria in Koreans with NIDDM. *Diabetes Care,* 1995, **18,** 793–9.

34. Palu, T., Colaiuri, R., Layton, M., Samiu, O., Taufa, S., Eigenmann, C. *et al.* Assessing diabetes complications in Tonga. In *Annual Scientific Meeting of Australian Diabetes Society and Australian Diabetes Educators Association.* Sydney, Australia, 1996, p. 98.

35. Cruickshank, J. and Alleyene, S. Black West Indian and matched white diabetics in Britain compared with diabetics in Jamaica: body mass, blood pressure, and vascular disease. *Diabetes Care,* 1987, **10,** 170–9.

36. Morrish, N., Stevens, L., Fuller, J., Keen, H. and Jarrett, R. Incidence of macrovascular disease in diabetes mellitus: the London cohort of the WHO Multinational Study of Vascular Disease in Diabetics. *Diabetologia,* 1991, **34,** 584–9.

37. Thai Multicenter Research Group on Diabetes mellitus. Vascular complications in non-insulin dependent diabetics in Thailand. *Diabetes Res. Clin. Pract.,* 1994, **25,** 61–9.

38. Tuomilehto, J., Zimmet, P., Nan, L. and Dowse, G. ECG abnormalities in relation to glucose tolerance and other risk factors in men of the developing nation of Kiribati. *Nutr. Metab. Cardiovasc. Dis.,* 1991, **1,** 195–200.

39. Diabetes Drafting Group. The World Health Organization Multinational Study of Vascular Disease in Diabetics. Prevalence of small vessel and large vessel disease in diabetic patients from 14 centres. *Diabetologia,* 1985, **28,** 615–40.

40. Swai, A. and McLarty, D. Diabetes in tropical Africa: a prospective study, 1981–7. *Br. Med. J.,* 1990, **300,** 1103–6.

41. McGill, M., Donnelly, R., Molyneaux, L. and Yue, D. Ethnic differences in the prevalence of hypertension and proteinuria in NIDDM. *Diabetes Res. Clin. Pract.,* 1996, **33,** 173–9.

42. Tooke, J.E. The microcirculation in diabetes. In *International Textbook of Diabetes Mellitus,* 2nd edn, (eds K.G.M.M. Alberti, P. Zimmet, R.A. DeFronzo and H. Keen), John Wiley & Sons Ltd, Chichester, 1997, pp. 1339–48.

43. Sjolie, A.K., Stephenson, J., Aldington, S. *et al.* Retinopathy and vision loss in insulin-dependent diabetes in Europe. The Eurodiab IDDM Complications Study. *Ophthalmology,* 1997, **104,** 252–60.

44. Lloyd, C.E., Klein, R., Maser, R.E., Kuller, L.H., Becker, D.J. and Orchard, T.J. The progression of retinopathy over 2 years: the Pittsburgh Epidemiology of Diabetes Complications (EDC) Study. *J. Diabetes Complications,* 1995, **9,** 140–8.

45. Klein, R., Klein, B.E., Moss, S.E. and Cruickshanks, K.J. Relationship of hyperglycaemia to the long-term incidence and progression of diabetic retinopathy. *Arch. Intern. Med.,* 1994, **154,** 2169–78.

46. The Diabetes Control and Complications Research Group. The effect of intensive treatment of diabetes on the development and progression of long-term complications in insulin-dependent diabetes mellitus. *N. Engl. J. Med.,* 1993, **329,** 977–86.

47. Chaturvedi, N., Stephenson, J.M. and Fuller, J.H. Microvascular and acute complications in IDDM patients: the Eurodiab IDDM Complications Study. *Diabetologia,* 1994, **37,** 278–85.

48. Savage, S., Estacio, R.O., Jeffers, B. and Schrier, R.W. Urinary albumin excretion as a predictor of diabetic retinopathy, neuropathy, and cardiovascular disease in NIDDM. *Diabetes Care,* 1996, **19,** 1243–8.

49. Seyoum, B., Mengistu, Z., Berhanu, P., Abdulkadir, J., Feleke, Y., Worku, Y. and Ayana, G. Prevalence of retinopathy in diabetic patients attending the Tikur Anbessa Hospital (TAH) diabetes clinic (abstract). *Diabetologia,* 1997, **40** (suppl 1), 499.

50. Fernandez-Vigo, J., Macho, J.S., Rey, A.D., Barros, J., Tome, M. and Bueno, J. The prevalence of diabetic retinopathy in Northwest Spain. *Acta Ophthalmol.,* 1993, **71,** 22–6.

51. Al-Kassab, A., Herman, W. and Thompson, T. Albuminuria is an uncommon complication of diabetes in Egypt (abstract). *Diabetes,* 1997, **46** (suppl), 326A.

52. Higgs, E., Kelleher, A., Simpson, H. and Reckless, J. Screening programme for microvascular complications and hypertension in a community diabetic population. *Diabet. Med.,* 1992, **9,** 550–6.

53. Simmons, D., Shaw, L., Scott, D., Kenealy, T. and Scraggs, R. Diabetic nephropathy and microalbuminuria in the community. *Diabetes Care,* 1994, **17,** 1404–10.

54. Paisey, R., Arrendondo, G., Villalobos, A., Lozano, O., Guevara, L. and Kelly, S. Association of differing dietary, metabolic and clinical risk factors with microvascular complications of diabetes: a prevalence study of 503 Mexican Type II diabetic subjects. *Diabetes Care,* 1984, **7,** 428–33.

55. Lester, F. The clinical pattern of diabetes mellitus in Ethiopians. *Diabetes Care*, 1984, **46** (suppl), 326A.
56. Young. M., Boulton, A., Macleod, A., Williams, D.R.R. and Sonksen, P. A multicentre study of the prevalence of diabetic peripheral neuropathy in the United Kingdom hospital population. *Diabetologia*, 1993, **36**, 150–4.
57. Jorgensen, A., Thai, A. A high prevalence of at risk feet for ulceration see at annual review for diabetic complications (Abstract). In *Diabetes Towards the New Millenium*. Third International Diabetes Federation West Pacific Regional Congress, Hong Kong, 1996, p. 77.
58. Zimmet, P. Challenges in diabetes epidemiology – from West to the rest. *Diabetes Care*, 1992, **15**, 232–52.
59. McCarty, D.J., Zimmet, P., Dalton, A., Segal, L. and Welborn, T.A. The rise and rise of diabetes in Australia, 1996: a review of statistics, trends and costs. In *Diabetes – Australia*, International Diabetes Institute, South Caulfield, Victoria, 1996.
60. Ruwaard, D. Forecasting the number of 'diabetic patients in the Netherlands in 2005: an update. In *Diabetes Mellitus: from Epidemiology to Health Policy*. Cip-gegevens Koninklijke Bibliotheek, den Haag, 1996.

PART TWO

THE PATHOGENESIS OF ARTERIAL DISEASE IN DIABETES

Hans-Joachim Baumgartl and Eberhard Standl

3.1 ATHEROGENESIS

Atherosclerosis represents the commonest cause of death in Western countries, typically afflicting the aorta, coronary and cerebral vessels as well as the arteries of the lower extremities. The atherogenic process is complex, involving several key processes and pathological stages. It progresses from the early lesion or fatty streak, to the developing fibrous plaque, leading to the complicated plaque.

It has long been assumed that the infiltration of plasma lipids and lipoproteins into the arterial wall to form the flat or slightly elevated, yellow, lipid-containing intimal lesion or fatty streak was the first stage in atherogenesis. The fatty streaks comprise foam cells (macrophages and smooth muscle cells) that are laden with cholesterol esters, as well as T lymphocytes. Such fatty streaks may be reversible, although the evidence is inconclusive. Lesions which do progress develop a fibrous cap and contain fibrin, elastin and collagen as well as lipid, and the resultant fibrous plaque impinges further on the lumen. Not all atherosclerotic lesions arise from fatty streaks, however. An alternative precursor is more gelatinous and comprises fibrinogen, fibrin and other components of the haemostatic system as well as lipoprotein.

Allied to the concept of infiltration of plasma constituents are the processes of intimal injury and the inflammatory response that follows vessel wall damage and the ingress of various blood components. The concept that atherosclerosis arises in part as a response to endothelial cell injury was suggested by Virchow nearly a century and a half ago and developed by Ross [1]. Several sources of endothelial injury, notably oxidized low density lipoprotein (LDL), homocysteine, various toxins and immunological processes, as well as mechanical injury, have been implicated. In the case of mechanical forces, the haemodynamic localization of arterial lesions at sites of low shear stress and areas of flow separation is of particular clinical significance. The resultant endothelial activation results in the adhesion of monocytes/macrophages and T lymphocytes which migrate through the endothelium, the former becoming lipid-laden foam cells. The activated endothelium may predispose to platelet-rich mural thrombus formation. A variety of growth factors are released from the platelets, white cells and possibly smooth muscle cells which promote proliferation of the smooth muscle cells, creating further plaque thickening. The incorporation of arterial mural thrombi into the developing plaque also stimulates the inflammatory fibroproliferative response.

The fully developed raised plaque is vulnerable to rupture, particularly at the shoulder of the plaque (the so-called unstable plaque). Exposure of plaque contents precipitates further superimposed thrombosis which may be occlusive, resulting in one of the acute syndromes such as myocardial infarction or stroke.

There are clearly many ways in which the metabolic derangement of diabetes and its sequelae may influence the various stages of the atherogenic process. This chapter considers certain key contender mechanisms.

3.2　THE ATHEROSCLEROTIC PROCESS IN DIABETES

3.2.1　INTRODUCTION

Diabetic vascular complications in large vessels arise from an accelerated atherosclerotic process which occurs at a younger age and is more extensive in people with diabetes than in those without. Although the excess of glucose plays an important and specific role in the genesis and exacerbation of the macrovascular disease in diabetes over and above that due to coexisting risk factors such as hypertension and hypercholesterolaemia, it is now commonly known, that the 'prediabetic' metabolic state comprising hyperinsulinaemia, insulin resistance, hypertension and dyslipidaemia is associated with the development of macroangiopathy in individuals who later develop non-insulin-dependent diabetes mellitus (NIDDM) [1, 2]. In both insulin-dependent diabetes mellitus (IDDM) patients and NIDDM patients, however, the duration of the disease as well as the quality of metabolic control are major causes for developing macrovascular disease in conjunction with additional risk factors (e.g. smoking) [2, 3]. In this context, it may be of note that several recent studies have shown the predictive importance of HbA1c values for the development of macrovascular complications, as found in the Munich General Practitioner Project [4, 5] and other studies including the Diabetes Control and Complications Trial [3].

Cardiovascular complications are without doubt the most common cause of death in diabetic patients with no apparent difference

in IDDM and NIDDM [6]. Recent observations show a close interaction between early kidney changes secondary to diabetes and development of complications in large vessels. Microalbuminuria indicates an elevated risk for cardiovascular and other macrovascular morbidity and mortality in NIDDM (Table 3.1) and IDDM patients and, surprisingly, also in non-diabetic persons [7, 8]. As a rule, microalbuminuria precedes the rise of blood pressure and the emergence of hypertension in IDDM patients by 2–3 years [9]. This is in contrast to the situation in NIDDM where, even at clinical diagnosis of NIDDM, as many as three out of four patients already exhibit hypertension and one out of four has micro- or macroalbuminuria and a prevalence rate of co-existing significant macrovascular disease of approximately 50% [10].

In IDDM patients, however, the risk for albuminuria and nephropathy is probably related to a genetic predisposition [11] and data compatible with a genetic predisposition to microalbuminuria have also been accumulated in patients with NIDDM. It is not completely understood what the precise impact of glucose, insulin, insulin resistance and microalbuminuria might be within the framework of early atherogenesis and atherosclerosis, although a specific contribution of diabetes to the accelerated development of macrovascular disease is widely recognized. The atherosclerotic process in diabetic patients does not appear to be principally different from that of non-diabetic subjects, but it starts earlier, progresses in a faster manner and is localized more peripherally [12].

Glucose may affect large vessels via at least three pathways (Figure 3.1):

- The glycation process
- The activation of protein kinase C
- The sorbitol pathway

The following sections deal with these chemical processes and associated cellular and molecular events.

Table 3.1 Predictors of vascular death during the 5 years of follow-up in a representative sample of 290 non-insulin-dependent diabetes mellitus patients

Predictor	Deceased (n=30)	Alive (n=219)	Significance* (P value)
Haemoglobin A_{1c}	9.2	7.6	<0.01
Fasting blood glucose (mg/dl)	190.0	136.0	0.03
Urinary albumin (mg/dl)	34.1	9.7	<0.01
Serum $ß_2$ microglobulin (mg/l)	2.14	1.74	<0.01
Knowledge (no. of correct answers)	8/21	11/21	<0.01
Carotid stenosis (%)	21.4	5.6	0.01
Peripheral vascular disease	72.4	37.8	0.01

The median values are given. *Multiple regression or logistic regression analysis: duration of diabetes, blood pressure, lipids and smoking were not significant.

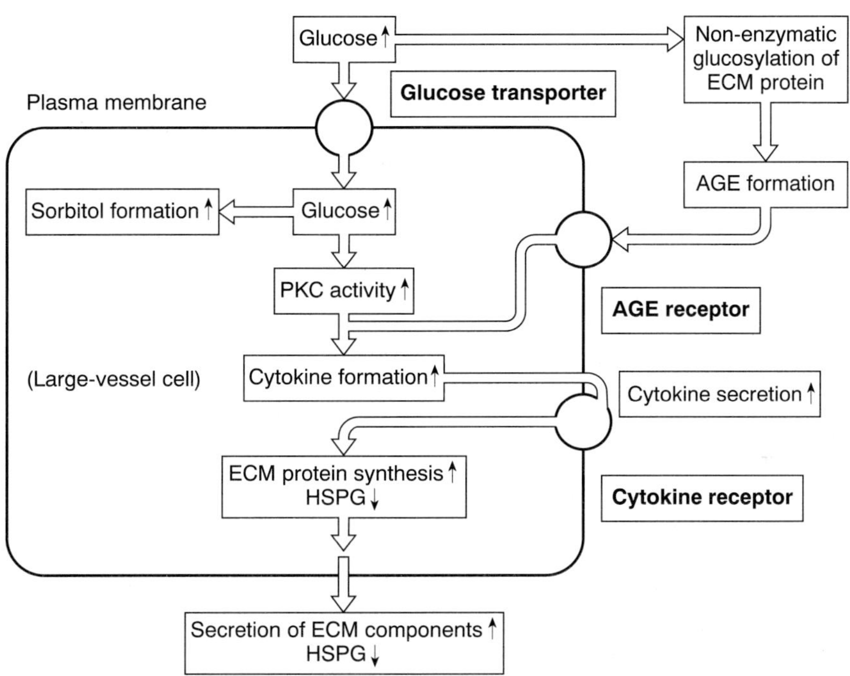

Figure 3.1 Glucose pathways in diabetic macroangiopathy. AGE, Advanced glycosylation endproducts; ECM, extracellular matrix; HSPG, heparan sulphate glycoprotein; PKC, protein kinase C.

3.2.2 THE AGE HYPOTHESIS

In the glycation pathway, reducing sugars such as glucose react non-enzymatically with the amino groups of macromolecules to initiate a chemical modification process known as advanced glycosylation [13]. This process proceeds from reversible Schiff base products to a heterogeneous group of irreversibly-bound, cross-linking moieties which are called advanced glycosylation endproducts or AGEs. AGEs are present on a variety of vascular wall, lipoprotein and lipid constituents. AGEs form in large amounts in the tissues and serum components of patients with diabetes. With a sensitive AGE-specific immunoassay serum, AGE-levels have been found to correlate clearly with renal function [14]. Serum and tissue proteins in non-diabetic individuals also become altered by AGEs, however, and there is evidence to suggest that several of the pathological complications of normal aging, such as atherosclerosis, also result from advanced glycosylation [13, 15–18].

An AGE-specific cell-surface receptor complex (AGE-R or RAGE) is specific for the recognition and uptake of AGE-modified proteins [19]. It has been identified on many cell types such as for circulating monocytes, endothelial cells and renal mesangial cells and other cellular systems [20, 21, 22]. AGEs are chemotactic for monocytes, and the uptake of AGE-modified proteins by specific receptors starts a cytokine-mediated process that promotes tissue repair and protein turnover [23]. Vascular permeability increases, the anticoagulant factor thrombomodulin begins to be down-regulated and the synthesis of the procoagulant tissue factor is elevated [13, 21]. Exposure of cultured mouse mesangial cells to AGE–bovine serum albumin results in a AGE receptor-mediated upregulation of mRNA formation of matrix proteins, such as fibronectin, type IV collagen and laminin [19, 24].

An important mediator of the arterial tone and regional blood flow is nitric oxide (NO), a radical species produced by endothelium after stimulation with acetylcholine and other humoral factors [25, 26]. NO crosses the subendothelial space and nitrosylates smooth muscle cell guanylate cyclase, thus increasing its activity and producing vascular smooth muscle relaxation and vasodilatation. Several years ago Bucala *et al.* [27] proposed that the accumulation of electrophilic, protein-bound AGE moieties might act to chemically quench endothelial cell-derived NO activity (Figure 3.2).

Observations were made that defective endothelium-dependent relaxation occurs commonly in the coronary and systemic circulation in situations where high levels of AGEs occur such as in diabetes [28, 29]. Bucala *et al.* and Vlassara *et al.* demonstrated the specific, chemical inactivation of NO by AGEs in different experiments *in vitro* and *in vivo* [27, 30]. It could be shown that the addition of increasing amounts of either lysine-derived or protein-derived AGEs to a solution of authentic NO produced an apparent first-order inactivation curve for NO. Invasive blood pressure monitoring confirmed that rats with experimentally induced diabetes exhibited defective NO-dependent vasodilatory responses. As the impairment in vascular responsiveness occurred in response to both endothelial cell-derived NO (induced by acetylcholine) and to NO pro-drugs (e.g. nitroglycerin), the vasodilatory defect in the resistance vessels of diabetic animals appears to be primarily a post-endothelial cell phenomenon. The defective vascular relaxation developed over a period of two months and indicated that the vasodilatatory impairment in diabetes requires a structural or physiological modification that develops over weeks to months, consistent with the subendothelial accumulation of AGEs.

In more recent studies by Vlassara *et al.* [19], the diabetes-related syndrome of vascular dysfunction has been induced in normal, non-diabetic animals by the direct, intravascular administration of AGE-modified proteins. AGE administration produced a greater than six-fold increase in vascular wall AGE content without the complex metabolic derangements following a chronic hyperglycaemic process. The increase was associated with many of the vascular changes that occur both in experimentally induced and in human diabetes, such as an increase in vascular permeability and mononuclear cell migratory activity. AGE-treated animals also developed a specific impairment in NO-mediated vaso-

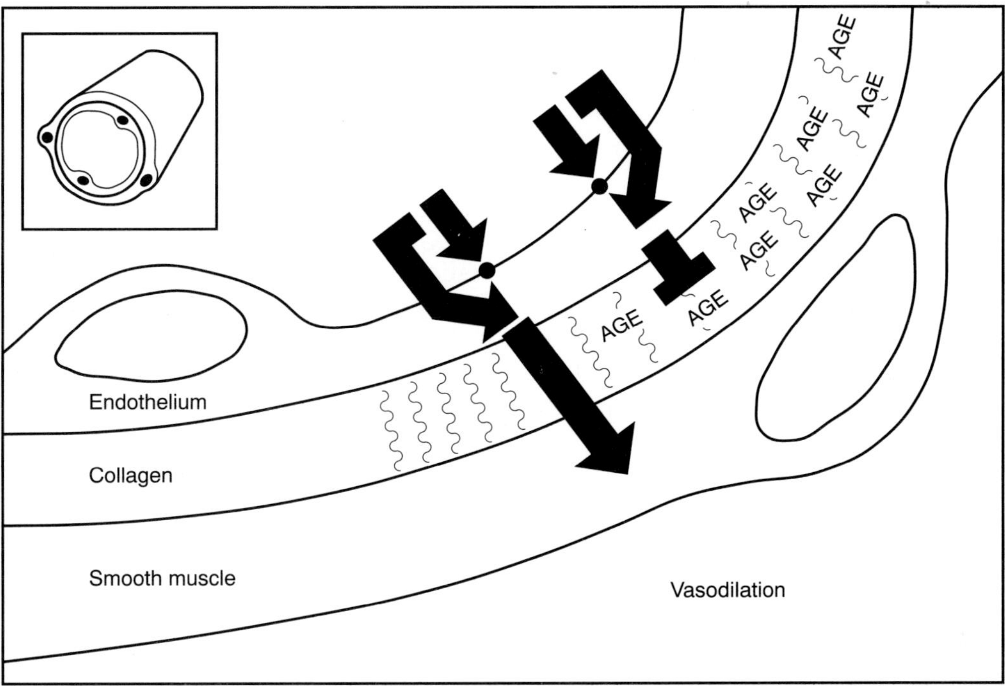

Figure 3.2 Hypothesis of inactivation of nitric oxide by advanced glycosylation endproducts. (Redrawn from reference 13, with permission).

dilatation, consistent with the inactivation of NO by AGEs at the subendothelial level.

The NO effect of the AGEs may also represent a possible mechanism in the evolution of hypertension in diabetes. The rate at which blood pressure increases with age is enhanced in patients with diabetes, and the prevalence of arterial hypertension is more than twofold higher in the diabetic than in the non-diabetic population [31]. This enhances the risk for the rapid development of macrovascular and microvascular diabetic complications. Endothelial-derived NO appears to be necessary for the maintenance of normal vascular tone and blood pressure [32]. Subendothelial AGE-accumulation may increase the loss of NO responsiveness in diabetic individuals (Figure 3.2). Endothelial derived NO is known to affect anti-proliferation of different cell types. Experimental damage of endothelium is associated with proliferation of underlying smooth muscle cells. Subendothelial AGEs might also act to functionally eliminate the anti-proliferative effects of NO. Cell culture studies have confirmed that NO displays potent cytostatic effects in different mesenchymal cell types [33]. AGE-modified matrix proteins were observed to specifically block the anti-proliferative effect of NO on vascular smooth muscle cells and kidney mesangial cells [33]. In this case, AGEs are important modulators of NO-mediated cytostasis *in vivo*, and suggest a new pathway for the development of the proliferative vascular lesions in diabetes mellitus.

In view of additional risk factors in vascular disease, tobacco smoke was described as a source of advanced glycosylation [34]. Immunostaining of human carotid arteries from smokers with vascular disease revealed extensive accumulation of AGEs. Serum AGEs in healthy rats exposed to cigarette

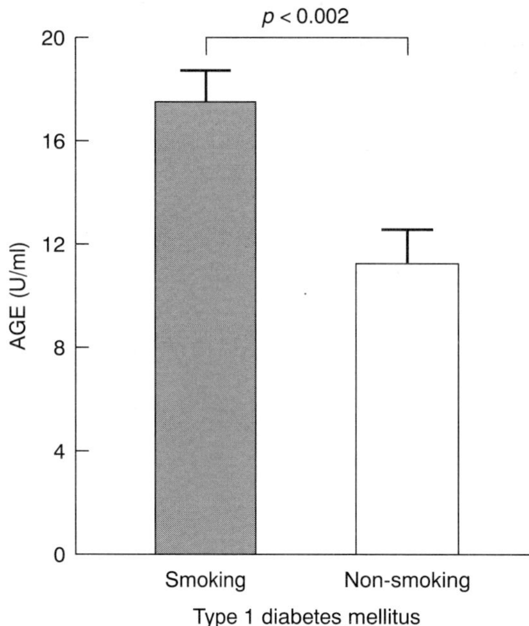

Figure 3.3 Serum level of advanced glycosylation endproducts in insulin-dependent diabetes mellitus patients, comparing smoking (20 patients) with non-smoking (25 patients).

smoke increased nearly 75% above non-smoking control levels. AGEs from cigarette smoke were found to react and attach to human serum proteins *in vitro*, increasing serum AGE level over control serum. Our group found significantly elevated serum AGE levels in smoking versus non-smoking IDDM patients [35] (Figure 3.3). This additional source of AGE accumulation may modify vascular tissues resulting in dysfunction and contributing to the accelerated vascular disease of smoking diabetic patients.

3.2.3   CYTOKINES AND GROWTH FACTORS: TGF-β

Of course, the pathobiochemistry of macrovascular disease in diabetes is much more complex than the hypothesis above would suggest. There is an impressively long and growing list (Table 3.2) of cytokines and growth factors that may be delivered from macrophages and other blood cells entering the vessel wall or that may be released from vessel wall cells of large arteries on activation.

In the context of diabetic macroangiopathy one of the most outstanding factors seems to be TGF-β. TGF-β regulates repair and regeneration following tissue injury, and controls the synthesis and degradation of extracellular matrix and the expression of integrins. Evidence has been accumulated that TGF-β also plays an important role in the pathogenesis of diabetic nephropathy in the experimental animal as well as in human diabetes [36]. High glucose levels are able to induce the transcription and secretion of TGF-β in mesangial cells and elevate cellular transcripts of TGF-β in vascular smooth muscle cells [36, 37]. Whether TGF-β gene expression also occurs in vascular cells of large arteries exposed to hyperglycaemia is at present under investigation. Recently, it could be demonstrated that the early characteristic features of diabetic renal involvment, which include hypertrophy and increased matrix mRNAs, are largely mediated by increased endogenous TGF-β activity in the kidney and that they can be significantly attenuated by treatment with neutralizing anti-TGF-β antibodies [38]. Another interesting feature of TGF-β is the fact that it exclusively binds HSPG (heparan sulphate proteoglycan) at the vessel lining, suggesting that TGF-β-derived effects are increased in the case of a decrease in the number of ligands and an increase in TGF-β formation in the case of hyperglycaemia.

3.2.4   INOSITOL DEPLETION

Another possibility involves the direct action of high glucose levels on endothelial and myomedial cells (Fig. 3.1). In endothelial cells of large arteries, it is of interest that acutely elevated glucose concentrations of 10 mmol or more competitively inhibit the uptake of myoinositol in culture *in vivo*, thus suggesting

Table 3.2 Growth factors and cytokines which may be released from infiltrating leucocytes or an activation of arterial wall cells in connection with the arteriosclerotic process

Growth factor or cytokine sources	Abbreviation	Cellular sources
Epidermal growth factor	EGF	P
Basic fibroblast growth factor	bFGF	EC, M, SMC
Granulocyte–macrophage colony-stimulating factor	G-MCSF	EC, M, SMC, T
Insulin growth factor 1	IGF-1	EC, M, P, SMC
Interferon-γ	IFN-γ	T
Interleukin-1	IL-1	EC, M, SMC, T
Interleukin-2	IL-2	T
Monocyte colony-stimulating factor	MCSF	EC, M, SMC
Monocyte chemotactic protein	MCP-1	EC, M, SMC
Platelet-derived growth factor	PDGF	EC, M, P, SMC
Platelet-derived endothelial growth factor	PDEGF	P
Transforming growth factor-α	TGF-α	M
Transforming growth factor-β	TGF-β	EC, M, P, SMC, T
Tumour necrosis factor-α	TNF-α	EC, M, SMC, T
Tumour necrosis factor-β (lymphotoxin)	TNF-β	T
Vascular endothelial cell growth factor	VEGF/VPF	M, SMC

EC, Endothelial cells; M, macrophages; P, platelets; SMC, smooth muscle cells; T, T lymphocytes.

a mechanism for an intracellular depletion of inositol. Both glucose and myoinositol have been shown by Olgemöller *et al.* to compete for the same carrier [39]. Preincubation experiments with elevated glucose concentrations have indicated that the carrier mechanism can be upregulated to a higher transport rate and that in the long-term hyperglycaemic situation even more inositol will be taken up and at least normal amounts of phosphoinositol will be formed along with an increasing uptake of glucose. It may be stated in this context that neither the previously discussed osmotic effects of elevated intracellular sorbitol concentrations nor a decreased uptake of myoinositol secondary to high intercellular sorbitol appear to play a significant role in precipitating damage to large vessel intima cells.

3.2.5   HEPARAN SULPHATE PROTEOGLYCAN DEPLETION

Induced activation of protein kinase C seems to be a key event in how hyperglycaemia exerts its effects on endothelial, myomedial and mesangial cells [40] (Fig. 3.1). In cultured endothelial cells of porcine aorta, acute stimulation of protein kinase C leads to an increase synthesis of heparan sulphate proteoglycan (HSPG), whereas chronic stimulation results in a 50% drop in HSPG synthesis [41, 42]. A decreased formation of HSPG by endothelial cells of large arteries exposed to permanent hyperglycaemia also seems to be relevant for the *in-vivo* situation of human diabetes, as a significant reduction of HSPG has been described in coronary arteries of NIDDM patients and a decreased ratio of heparan sulphate/dermatan sulphate in the intima layer of aortas from diabetic patients was most pronounced in (diabetic) plaques [43, 44].

Functions of HSPG have also been studied particularly in relation to microvascular disease, and microalbuminuria as a sign of diabetic microangiopathy is thought to be a consequence of a specific loss of HSPG within the extracellular matrix network of the glomerular basement membrane [45, 46] (Fig. 3.4). HSPG is the main anionic component of the glomerular basement membrane and a

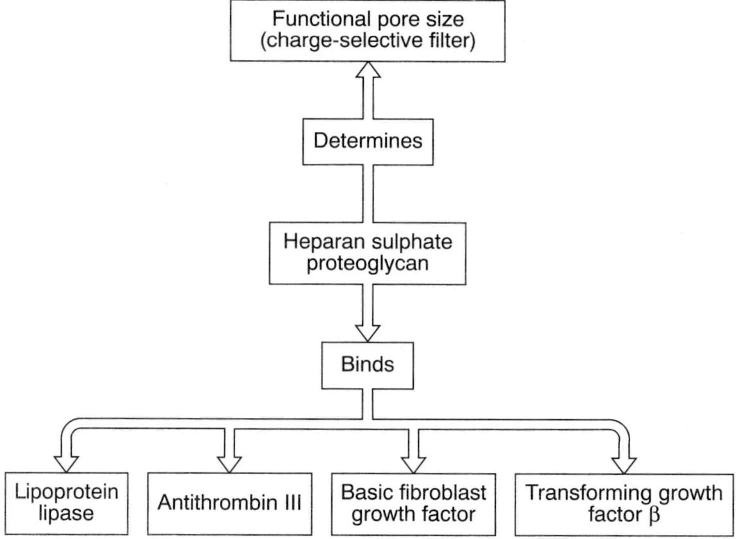

Figure 3.4 The role of heparan sulphate proteoglycan in diabetes.

decrease is followed by an increased leakage of albumin. It has long been known that increased leakage of albumin across the vessel wall is a much more generalized phenomenon in diabetes and that the so-called trans-capillary escape rate of albumin is doubled at the stage of microalbuminuric incipient nephropathy [47]. It has been shown that administration of heparin or other glycosaminoglycans is preventive in diabetic rats in terms of maintaining a normal glomerular basement thickness and anionic charge density in parallel with the prevention of albuminuria [48–50]. Even a significant reduction of albuminuria has been observed in diabetic patients with micro- and macroalbuminuria after treatment with glycosaminoglycans [51–53].

Nevertheless, other important functions of HSPGs have become apparent as specific binding ligands for anti-thrombin III, lipoprotein lipase, TGF-ß and basic fibroblast growth factor (bFGF) [36, 44]. In large vessels, anti-atherogenic properties have been attributed to HSPG, and a negative correlation has been demonstrated between heparan sulphate and the cholesterol content of human large vessel walls [47, 48]. HSPG contributes to the structural integrity of the interendothelial clefts of large vessel walls, across which lipoproteins and other macromolecules are transported. Finally, HSPG has been reported to maintain myomedial cells in the resting state and prevents their activation and migration [54, 55].

In contrast to the decrease of HSPG, other components of the basement membrane of large vessels show an increase. This pertains quite remarkably to collagen IV, collagen VI, fibronectin and laminin [56, 57]. This increase of extracellularly deposited collagens and related proteins further exacerbates the imbalance between low HSPG and collagen (Table 3.3). They comprise both a delayed catabolism of collagens and gene activation, and an increase of specific mRNA formation for the collagen synthesizing pathways. It is clear that not only collagen IV, but also collagen VI and fibronectin are involved [58]. Fibronectin expression is mediated by glucose and probably triggered by protein kinase C since the concomitant induction of protein kinase C isoforms was observed [59]. These findings also apply to endothelial cells of large arteries and to the myocardial extracellular matrix of

Table 3.3 Mechanisms for heparan sulphate proteoglycan (HSPG)-related anionic charge reduction in the extracellular matrix of diabetic patients

---

Decreasing density of HSPG
- Decreased synthesis of HSPG
- Increased gene expression and secretion of collagen IV, collagen VI and fibronectin
- Decreased turnover of glycated collagen I
- Decreased binding of HSPG to glycated collagen IV

Decreased sulphation of heparan sulphate

---

rats [60]. Whatever consequences might emerge from the excessive extracellular matrix deposition are still unknown. It might be speculated that platelet activation might occur more easily and a tissue stiffening would take place, as might be clinically represented by mediasclerosis of arteries and a decreased end-diastolic relaxation of the myocardium.

3.2.6 VASCULAR ENDOTHELIAL GROWTH FACTOR

The vascular permeability factor (VPF) was originally described as a protein secreted from tumours causing substantial vascular leakage [61, 62]. This protein was later called vascular endothelial growth factor (VEGF) because growth-promoting effects on endothelium in culture were observed [63]. Elevated concentrations of VEGF were found in the ocular fluid of diabetic patients with proliferative diabetic retinopathy [64]. VEGF is present in the ocular membranes of those patients, and hypoxia stimulates the secretion of VEGF in retinal pigment epithelial cells [65, 66]. Beside diabetic retinopathy, an involvement was observed in wound healing as shown by the overexpression of its receptor on the endothelium of regenerating vessels, and a variety of other diseases such as rheumatoid arthritis [67, 68]. It was hypothesized that VEGF may also initiate neovascularization in the heart, targeting the growth of blood vessels into ischaemic myocardial regions. Indeed, expression of VEGF in cultured myocardial cells was upregulated by hypoxia *in vitro* and significantly augmented in the ischaemic territory of the myocardium [69]. The role of VEGF in the genesis of diabetic macrovascular disease is currently unclear although it could contribute to the distal prediction of peripheral arterial disease. In distal arteries the vessel wall thickness: lumen radius ratio rises and the media becomes more dependent upon vaso vasorum for oxygen supply. Hypoxic smooth muscle releases VEGF which may promote an increased vascular permeability thereby accelerating the local atherosclerotic process.

Early dysfunctions in platelet regulation, endothelial proteins, coagulation factors and a decreased fibrinolysis play an important role for an increased cardiovascular mortality in diabetic patients [70]. The Munich General Practitioner Project demonstrated dysregulation of the von Willebrand factor protein as a high risk factor for the vascular mortality of NIDDM-patients [71]. Interestingly, the secretion of von Willebrand factor is enhanced by VEGF, and the migration of monocytes and activity of fibrogenesis is also stimulated. In addition, VEGF has been shown to increase monocyte migration through endothelium in culture, possibly due to increased expression of endothelial cell surface P-selectin [72]. Roberts and Palade presented the first evidence of VEGF directly and promptly inducing fenestrae of endothelium [62]. Fenestrated endothelium occurs also in the capillaries of kidney glomeruli [49, 62]. In this context it is of interest that VEGF strongly binds heparin and heparan sulphate, and that heparin enhances the binding of VEGF to its receptor [62, 74]. Since microalbuminuria is a independent risk factor for cardiovascular disease in diabetic patients, and the administration of heparin or other gycosaminoglycans prevents the onset of albuminuria in animals, future studies are necessary to eludicate the possible role of VEGF in this context to the genesis of diabetic angiopathy.

3.3 FUTURE PERSPECTIVES

In terms of the hypotheses presented above, it will be of major interest to define clearly whether there is a genetic predisposition for microalbuminuria or for low HSPG. The Steno group has contributed enormously to the field and is looking into the genetics of *N*-deacetylase, the key enzyme in the sulphation of HSPG [75].

Another area of present and future investigations is the problem of how leucocytes and macrophages receive the first signal to enter the vessel wall. A whole family of specific proteins has been disclosed, which enables some kind of dialogue between the corpuscular blood constituents on the one side, and the vessel wall, especially the endothelial cells, on the other [76, 77]. So-called selectins are expressed by endothelial cells, and integrins by leucocytes. Of particular note might be E-selectin which seems to be exclusively produced by endothelial cells. Circumstantial evidence suggests a key role for E-selectin in early atherogenesis and the term 'atheroselectin' has been suggested [76]. A doubling of circulating levels of E-selectin has been described in diabetes with the limitation, however, that it is as yet clearly to be shown what circulating levels of selectins actually mean in terms of macrophage adhesion [76]. Recent results suggest that the concentration of soluble adhesion molecules and especially of E-selectin may also be related to metabolic control since plasma E-selectin was positively correlated with glycated haemoglobin level [78].

The possibility of an abnormal cellular calcium metabolism in diabetes has recently attracted much interest [79]. Intracellular calcium levels are increased in most tissues in diabetes and may potentially contribute to the pathogenesis of diabetes and its vascular complications. Alterations of the membrane-associated ATPase have been shown in connection with protein kinase C activity and endothelin-1 release. Endothelin concentrations circulating in blood have been found to be significantly elevated in diabetes and it has been suggested that insulin plays a role in this respect. Notable in this context is a recent study that has demonstrated a close relationship between intracellular free-calcium concentrations in erythrocytes with increasing physiological insulin concentrations, using an *in-vitro* system and nuclear magnetic resonance techniques [80]. A variety of insulin effects on cellular calcium metabolism have also been described for smooth muscle cells and diabetes [79]. This brings up the final and still unresolved issue of how detrimental insulin and its precursors may actually be in terms of vessel wall damage of large arteries [81]. It was initially thought that insulin increases renal tubular resorption of sodium *in vivo* [82]. Although this is true for the acute experiment with insulin being administered intravenously, it could not be substantiated in long-term studies in animals or in humans [83, 84]. In addition, activation of the sympathetic nervous system and increased plasma noradrenaline levels have been repeatedly found on intravenous delivery of supraphysiological amounts of insulin [83]. However, this may simply represent a baroreceptor reflex response to vasodilatation and a slight decrease in arterial pressure occurring at the same time [85]. The mechanisms mediating vasodilatation during insulin infusion have yet to be defined [86]. Well proven are the effects of insulin on the activation of lipoprotein lipase bound to the basement membrane of blood vessels. The insulin effects represent a continuing challenge for further research on their importance in macrovascular disease in diabetes (Table 3.4).

More scientists today are inclined to ascribe to insulin resistance a role in diabetic macroangiopathy. This, again, may be seen in the context of increased cellular free-calcium in diabetes, in particular in skeletal muscles but also in smooth muscle cells of large arteries [79]. Intracellular calcium has an optimal

Table 3.4 Hypothetical insulin effects on the components of large blood vessels

---

- Increased free intracellular calcium
- Increased endothelin-1 release
- Increased macrophage lipid accumulation
- Increased lipoprotein lipase activity
- Increased smooth muscle cell proliferation and migration
- Increased smooth muscle cell synthesis of lipids and extracellular matrix
- Increased local Insulin growth factor 1 release
- Increased plasminogen activator factor

---

range for mediating insulin action, and higher or lower levels are associated with impaired insulin action [87]. Chelation of intracellular calcium prevents insulin-stimulated glucose transport, whereas sustained elevations of intracellular calcium decrease insulin-stimulated glucose uptake in both human and rat adipocytes [88, 89]. Part of this effect may be due to inhibition of insulin-receptor dephosphorylation by high intracellular calcium levels and/or activation of protein kinase C. In arteries, calcium is involved in most processes associated with atherogenesis such as LDL permeation, platelet aggregation, smooth muscle cell proliferation and extracellular matrix turnover. It has, therefore, been proposed that the abnormality underlying the association of insulin resistance, diabetes mellitus and macroangiopathy is a primary abnormality of divalent cation flux [90]. Alternatively, evidence is accumulating which suggests a link between hypertrophic structural changes of the vessel wall and insulin resistance. In patients with NIDDM, a decreased insulin-induced vasodilatation has been observed that correlated with a reduced glucose uptake [91]. Interestingly, insulin-mediated glucose uptake, as well as the insulin-mediated rise in skeletal-muscle blood flow, have recently been found to be inversely related to basal blood pressure in normotensive subjects with a wide range of blood pressures [92]. As a whole, this area seems to

respresent another very important field for intriguing and rewarding further research effort.

REFERENCES

1. Ross, R. The pathogenesis of atherosclerosis – an update. *N. Engl. J. Med.*, 1986, **314**, 488.
2. Despres, J.P., Lamarche, B., Mauriege, P. *et al.* Hyperinsulinaemia as an independent risk factor for ischemic heart disease. *N. Engl. J. Med.*, 1996, **334**, 952–7.
3. The Diabetes Control and Complication Trial Research Group. The effect of intensive treatment of diabetes on the development and progression of long-term complications in insulin-dependent diabetes mellitus. *N. Engl. J. Med.*, 1993, **329** 977–86.
4. Janka, H.U., Balletshofer, B., Becker, A. *et al.* Das metabolische Syndrom als potenter kardiovaskulärer Risikofaktor für vorzeitigen Tod bei Typ-II-Diabetikern. Die Schwabinger Studie II. Untersuchungen nach 9 Jahren. *Diab. Stoffw.* 1992, **1**, 2–7.
5. Stiegler, H., Standl, E., Schulz, K. *et al.* Häulhkeit, Risikoprofil und Letalitätsrate einer Stichprobe von Type-II Diabetikern mit Albuminurie in der ärztlichen Praxis. Eine prospektive 5-Jahres-Verlaufsuntersuchung. *Diab. Stoffw.* 1993, **2**, 62–7.
6. Standl, E. Cellular and molecular mechanisms in the macroangiopathy of diabetics. In *Diabetes Mellitus and Cardiovascular Disease*, (eds C.J. Schwartz and G.V.R. Born), Current Science, San Antonio, 1995, pp. 124–31.
7. Morrish, N.J., Steven,s L.K., Head, J. *et al.* A prospective study of mortality among middle-aged diabetic patients (the London cohort of the WHO multinational study of vascular disease in diabetics). II: Asscociated risk factors. *Diabetologia*, 1990, **33**, 542–8.
8. Standl, E., Stiegler, H., Janka, H.U. and Mehnert, H. Risk profile of macrovascular disease in diabetes mellitus. *Diabetes Metab.*, 1988, **14**, 505–11.
9. Mathiesen, E.R., Ronne, B., Jensen, T. Relationship between blood pressure and urinary albumin excretion in the development of microalbuminuria. *Diabetes*, 1990, **39** , 245–9.
10. Standl, E. and Stiegler, H. Microalbuminuria in a random cohort of recently diagnosed type 2

(non-insulin-dependent) diabetic patients living in the Greater Munich Area. *Diabetologia*, 1993, **36**, 1017–20.

11. Marre, M., Bernadet, P., Gallois, Y. *et al.* Relationship between angiotensin I converting enzyme gene polymorphism, plasma levels, and diabetic retinal and renal complications. *Diabetes*, 1995, **43**, 384–8.

12. Donahue, R.P. and Orchard, T.J. Diabetes melitus and macrovascular complications: an epidemiological perspective. *Diabetes Care*, 1992, **15**, 1141–55.

13. Bucala, R., Vlassara, H. and Cerami, A. Advanced glycosylation endproducts: role in diabetic and non-diabetic vascular disease. *Drug Dev. Res.*, 1994, **32**, 77–89.

14. Makita, Z., Radoff, S. and Rayfield, E.J. Advanced glycosylation endproducts in patients with diabetic nephropathy. *N. Engl. J. Med.*, 1991, **325**, 836–42.

15. Brownlee, M., Cerami, A. and Vlassara, H. Advanced glycosylation endproducts in tissue and the biochemical basis of diabetic complications. *N. Engl. J. Med.*, 1992, **318**, 1315–21.

16. Baumgartl, H.J. and Standl, E. Advanced glycosylation endproducts: role in diabetic complications. *Diab. Stoffw.*, 1996, **5**, 177–82.

17. Makita, Z., Radoff, S., Rayfield, E.J., Yang, Z., Skolnik, E., Delaney, V., Friedmann, E.A., Cerami, A. and Vlassara, H. Advanced glycosylation endproducts in patients with diabetic nephropathy. *N. Engl. J. Med.*, 1991, **325**, 836–42.

18. Bucala, R., Makita, Z., Koschinsky, T., Cerami, A. and Vlassara, H. Lipid advanced glycosylation: pathway for lipid oxidation *in vivo*. *Proc. Natl Acad. Sci U.S.A.*, 1993, **90**, 6434–8.

19. Vlassara, H. and Bucala, R. Recent progress in advanced glycation and diabetic vascular disease: role of advanced glycation end product receptors. *Diabetes*, 1996 **45**, (suppl 3), 65–6.

20. Vlassara, H., Brownlee, M. and Cerami, A. High-affinity receptor-mediated uptake and degradation of glucose-modified proteins: a potential mechanism for the removal of sensecent macromolecules. *Proc. Natl Acad. Sci U.S.A.*, 1985, **82**, 5588–92.

21. Esposito, C., Gerlach, H., Brett, J., Stern, D. and Vlassara, H. Endothelial receptor-mediated binding of glucose-modified albumin is associated with increased monolayer permeability and modulation of cell surface coagulant properties. *J. Exp. Med.*, 1989, **170**, 1387–407.

22. Skolnik, E.Y., Yang, Z., Makita, Z., Radoff, S., Kirstein, M. and Vlassara, H. Human and rat mesangial cell receptors for glucose-modified proteins: potential role in kidney tissue remodelling and diabetic nephropathy. *J. Exp. Med.*, 1991, **174**, 931–8.

23. Vlassara, H., Brownlee, M., Manogue, K., Dinarello, C. and Cerami, A. Cachetin/TNF and IL1 induced by glucose-modified proteins: Role in normal tissue remodeling. *Science*, 1988, **240**, 1546–8.

24. Doi, T., Vlassara, H., Kirstein, M. *et al.* Receptor-specific increased mesangial cell extracellular matrix production is mediated by PDGF. *Proc. Natl Acad. Sci U.S.A.*, 1992, **89**, 2873–7.

25. Ignarro, L.J., Buga, J.M., Wood, K.S., Byrns, R.E. and Chaudhuri, G. Endothelium-derived relaxing factor produced and released from artery and vein is nitric oxide. *Proc. Natl Acad. Sci U.S.A.*, 1987, **84**, 9265–9.

26. Palmer, R.M.J., Ferrige, A.G. and Moncada, S. Nitric oxide release accounts for the biological activity of endothelium-derived relaxing factor. *Nature*, 1987, **327**, 524–6.

27. Bucala, R., Tracey, K. and Cerami, A. Advanced glycation products quench nitric oxide and mediate defective endothelium-dependent vasodilatation in experimental diabetes. *J. Clin. Invest.*, 1991, **87**, 432–8.

28. de Tejada, I.S., Goldstein, I., Azadzoi, K., Krane, R.J. and Cohen, R.J.R. Impaired neurogenic and endothelium-mediated relaxation of penile smooth muscle in diabetic men with impotence. *N. Engl. J. Med.*, 1989, **320**, 1025–30.

29. Oyama, Y., Kawasaki, H., Hattori, Y. and Kanno, M. Attenuation of endothelium-dependent relaxation in aorta from diabetic rats. *Eur. J. Pharmacol.*, 1986, **131**, 75–8.

30. Vlassara, H., Fuh, H., Makita, Z., Krungkrai, S., Cerami, A. and Bucala, R. Exogenous advanced glycosylation endproducts induce complex vascular dysfunction in normal animals: a model for diabetic and aging complications. *Proc. Natl Acad. Sci U.S.A.*, 1992, **89**, 12043–7.

31. Sowers, J.R., Levy, J. and Zemel, M.B. Hypertension and diabetes. *Med. Clin. North Am.*, 1988, **72**, 1399–1414.

32. Vallance, P., Collier, J. and Moncada, S. Effects of endothelium derived nitric oxide on peripheral arteriolar tone in man. *Lancet*, 1989, **ii**, 997–1000.

33. Hogan, M., Cerami, A. and Bucala, R. Advanced glycosylation endproducts block the antiproliferative effect of nitric oxide. *J. Clin. Invest.*, 1992, **90**, 1110–15.

34. Founds, H.W., Giordano, D., Mitsuhashi, T. *et al.* Tobacco smoke is a source of advanced glycation endproducts (AGEs): possible role in the accelerated vascular disease of smokers. *Biomed. (Wash.)*, 1996, **5**, 96 (abstract).

35. Baumgartl, H.J., Hofmann, H. and Standl, E. Erhöhung der Serum AGEs bei Rauchern unter den Typ-I-Diabetikern. *Diab. Stoffw.*, 1996, **5**, B7 (abstract).

36. Yamamoto, T., Nakamura, T., Noble, N.A. *et al.* Expressions of transforming growth factor beta is elevated in human and experimental diabetic nephropathy. *Proc. Natl Acad. Sci U.S.A.*, 1993, **90**, 1814–18.

37. Nakamura, T., Fukui, M., Ebihara, I. *et al.* mRNA expression of growth factors in glomeruli from diabetic rats. *Diabetes*, 1993, **42**, 450–6.

38. Sharma, K., Jin, Y., Guo, J. and Ziyadeh, F.N. Neutralization of TGF-beta by anti-TGF-beta antibody attenuates kidney hypertrophy and the enhanced extracellular matrix gene expression in STH-induced diabetic mice. *Diabetes*, 1996, **45**, 522–30.

39. Olgemöller, B., Schleicher, E., Schwaabe, S. and Gerbitz, K.D. Upregulation of myoinositol transport compensates for competitive inhibition by glucose. *Diabetes*, 1993, **42**, 1119–25

40. Ayo, S.H., Radnik, R., Garoni, J.A. *et al.* High glucose increases diacylglycerol mass and activates protein C in mesangial cells. *Am J. Physiol.*, 1991, **261**, F571–7.

41. Olgemöller, B., Schwaabe, S., Gerbitz, K.D. *et al.* Elevated glucose decreases the content of a basement membrane associated proteoglycan in proliferating mesangial cells. *Diabetologia*, 1992, **35**, 183–6.

42. Olgemöller, B. Gerbitz, K.D. and Schleicher, E.D. Veränderungen der Basalmembran als biochemisches Korrelat diabetischer Spätkomplikationen. *Diab. Stoffw.*, 1993, **2**, 261–5.

43. Dybdahl, L. and Ledet, T. Diabetic macroangiopathy. Quantitative histopathological studies of the extramural coronary arteries from type 2 (non-insulin-dependent) diabetic patients. *Diabetologia*, 1987, **30**, 882–6

44. Wasty, F., Alavi, M.Z. and Moore, S. Distribution of glycosaminoglycan in the intima of human aortas: changes in atherosklerosis and diabetes mellitus. *Diabetologia*, 1993, **36**, 316–22

45. Deckert, T., Kofoed-Enevoldsen, A., Norgaard, K. *et al.* Microalbuminuria: implication for micro- and macrovascular disease. *Diabetes Care*, 1992, **15**, 1181–91

46. Deckert, T., Feldt-Rasmussen, B., Borch-Johnsen, K. *et al.* Albuminuria reflects widespread vascular damage: the Steno hypothesis. *Diabetologia*, 1989, **32**, 219–26

47. Norgaard, K., Jensen, T. and Feldt-Rasmussen, B. Transcapillary escape rate of albumin in hypertensive patients with type 1 (insulin-dependent) diabetes mellitus. *Diabetologia*, 1993, **36**, 57–61.

48. Dedov, I., Shestakova, M., Vorontzov, A. and Palazzini, E. An open, controlled study of sulodexide therapie for the treatment of diabetic nephropathy. *Nephrol. Dial. Transplant.*, 1997, **121**, 2285–3000.

49. Gambaro, G., Cavazzana, A.O., Luzi, P. *et al.* Glycosaminoglycans prevent morphological renal alterations and albuminuria in diabetic rats. *Kidney Int.*, 1992, **42**, 285–91.

50. Gambaro, G., Venturini, A.P., Noonan, D.M. *et al.* Treatment with a glycosaminoglycan formulation ameliorates experimental diabetic nephropathy. *Kidney Int.*, 1994, **46**, 797–806.

51. Solini, A., Carraro, A., Barzon, I. *et al.* Therapy with glycosaminoglycans lowers albumin excretion rate in non-insulin dependent diabetic patients with macroalbuminuria. *Diab. Nutr. Metab.*, 1994, **7**, 304–7.

52. Myrup, B., Hansen, P.M., Jensen, T. *et al.* Effect of low-dose heparin on urinary albumin excretion in insulin–dependent diabetes mellitus. *Lancet*, 1995, **345**, 421–2.

53. Velussi, M., Cernigoi, A.M., Dapas, F. and De Monte, A. Glycosaminoglycans oral therapy reduces microalbuminuria, blood fibrinogen levels and limb arteriopathy clinical signs in patients with non-insulin dependent diabetes mellitus. *Diab. Nutr. Metab* ,1996, **9**, 53–8.

54. Deckert, T., Jensen, T. and Feldt-Rasmussen, B. Albuminuria, a risk marker of atherosclerosis in insulin dependent diabetes melitus. *Cardiovasc. Risk Factors*, 1991, **1**, 347–60.

55. Hollmann, J., Schmidt, A. and von Basewitsch, D.B. Relationship of sulfated glycosaminoglycan and cholesterol content in normal and arteriosclerotic human aorta. *Arteriosclerosis*, 1989, **9**, 154–8.

56. Danne, T., Spiro, M.J. and Spiro, R.G. Effect of high glucose on type IV collagen production by cultured glomerular epithelial, endothelial and mesangial cells. *Diabetes,* 1993, **42,** 170–7.

57. Wakisaka, M., Spiro, M.J. and Spiro, R.G. Synthesis of type VI collagen by cultured glomerular cells and comparison of its regulation by glucose and other factors with that of type IV collagen. *Diabetes,* 1994, **43,** 95–103.

58. Andresen, J.L., Rasmussen, L.M. and Ledet, T. Diabetic macroangiopathy and atherosclerosis. *Diabetes,* 1996, **45,** Suppl. 3, 91–4.

59. Mueller, H.K., Fritsche, U., Haslinger, A. and Landgraf, R. Glucose-induced fibronectin expression in endothelial cells is mediated by protein kinase C. *Exp. Clin. Endocrinol. Diabetes,* 1997, **105,** 32–8.

60. Spiro, M.J. and Crowley, T.J. Increased rat myocardial type IV collagen in diabetes mellitus and hypertension. *Diabetologia,* 1993, **36,** 93–8.

61. Senger, D.R., Galli, S.J., Dvorak, A.M *et al.* Tumor cells secrete a vascular permeability factor that promotes accumulation of ascites fluid. *Science,* 1983, **219,** 983–5.

62. Roberts, W.G. and Palade, G.E. Increased microvascular permeability and endothelial fenestration induced by vascular endothelial growth factor. *J. Cell Sci.,* 1995, **108,** 2369–79.

63. Leung, D.W., Cachienes, G., Kuang, W.J. *et al.* Vascular endothelial growth factor is a secreted angiogenetic mitogen. *Science,* 1989, **246,** 1306–9.

64. Aiello, L.P., Avery, R.L., Arrig, P.G. *et al.* Vascular endothelial growth factor in ocular fluid of patients with diabetic retinopathy and other retinal disorders. *N. Engl. J. Med.,* 1994, **331,** 1480–7.

65. Malecaze, F., Clamens, S. and Mathis, A. Expression of angiogenetic growth factors in diabetic neovascular membranes. *Invest. Ophthalmol. Vis. Sci.,* 1993, **34,** 1039 (abstract).

66. Shima, D., Adamis, A.P., Yea, K.T. *et al.* Hypoxic regulation of vascular permeability factor (vascular endothelial growth factor) mRNA and protein secretion by human retinal pigment epithelial cells. *Invest. Ophthalmol. Vis. Sci.,* 1993, **34,** 900 (abstract).

67. Koch, A.E., Harlow, L.A., Haines, G.K. *et al.* Vascular endothelial growth factor. A cytokine modulating endothelial function in rheumatoid arthritis. *J. Immunol.,* 1994, **152,** 4149–56.

68. Peters, K.G., De Vries, C. and Williams, L.T. Vascular endothelial growth factor receptor expression during embryogenesis and tissue repair suggests a role in endothelial differentiation and blood vessel growth. *Proc. Natl Acad. Sci U.S.A.,* 1993, **90,** 8915–19.

69. Banai, S., Shweiki, D., Pinson, A. *et al.* Upregulation of vascular endothelial growth factor expression induced by myocardial ischaemia: implications for coronary angiogenesis. *Cardiovasc. Res.,* 1994, **28,** 1176–9.

70. Ingerslev, J. Research methodologies in measurement of platelet functions, endothelial proteins, coagulation factors and fibrinolysis. In *Research Methodologies in Human Diabetes,* Part 2, (eds C.E. Mogensen and E. Standl), De Gruyter, Berlin, New York, 1995, pp. 125–146.

71. Standl, E., Balletshofer, B., Dahl, B. *et al.* Predictors of 10-year macrovascular and overall mortality in patients with NIDDM. The Munich General Practitioner Project. *Diabetologia,* 1996, **39,** 1540–5.

72. Clauss, M., Gerlach, M., Gerlach, H. *et al.* Vascular permeability factor: a tumor derived polypeptide that induces endothelial cell and monocyte procoagulant activity, and promotes monocytes migration. *J. Exp. Med.,* 1990, **172,** 1535–45.

73. Bearer, E.L. and Orci, L. Endothelial fenestral diaphragms: a quick-freeze, deep-etch study. *J. Cell Biol.,* 1985, **100,** 418–28.

74. Gitay-Goren, H., Soker, S., Vlodavsky, I. *et al.* The binding of vascular endothelial growth factor to its receptors is dependent on cell surface-associated heparin-like molecules. *J. Biol. Chem.,* 1992, **267,** 6093–8.

75. Kofoed-Enevoldsen, A., Noonan, D. and Deckert, T. Diabetes mellitus induced inhibition of glucosaminyl *N*-deacetylase: effect of short-term blood glucose control in diabetic rats. *Diabetologia,* 1993, **36,** 310–5.

76. Gearing, A.J.H. and Newman, W. Circulating adhesion molecules in disease. *Immunol. Today,* 1993, **14,** 506–12.

77. Rösen, P., Schwippert, B. and Tschöpe, D. Adhesive proteins in platelet-endothelial interactions. *European J. Clin. Invest.,* 1994, **24,** Suppl. 1, 21–4.

78. Cominacini, L. *et al.* Elevated levels of soluble E-selectin in patients with IDDM and NIDDM: relation to metabolic control. *Diabetologia,* 1995, **38,** 1122–4.

79. Levy, J., Gavin, III J.R. and Sowers, J.R. Diabetes mellitus: a disease of abnormal cellular

calcium metabolism? *Am J. Med.*, 1994, **96,** 260–73.

80. Barbagallo, M., Gupta, R.K. and Resnick, L.M. Cellular ionic effects of insulin in normal human erythrocytes: a nuclear magnetic resonance study. *Diabetologia,* 1993, **36,** 146–9.

81. Stout, R.W. Insulin and atheroma. A 20-yr perspective. *Diabetes Care,* 1990, **13,** 613–25.

82. DeFronzo, R.A., Cooke, C.R., Andres, R. *et al.* The effects of insulin on renal handling of sodium, potassium, calcium, and phosphate in man. *J. Clin. Invest.,* 1975, **55,** 845–55.

83. Gans, R.O.B., van der Toorn, L., Bilo, H.J.G. *et al.* Renal and cardiovascular effects of exogenous insulin in healthy volunteers. *Clin. Sci.,* 1991, **80,** 219–25.

84. Vargas, F., Sabio, J.M., Castillo, M.A. *et al.* Chronic insulin treatment in rats – evidence against a role for insulin as a pressor agent. *Clin. Sci.,* 1993, **84,** 281–6.

85. Anderson, E.A. and Mark, A.L. The vasodilator action of insulin – implications for the insulin hypothesis of hypertension. *Hypertension,* 1993, **21,** 136–41.

86. McVeigh, G.E., Brennan, G.M., Johnston, G.D. *et al.* Impaired endothelium-dependent and independent vasodilation in patients with type 2 (non-insulin-dependent) diabetes mellitus. *Diabetologia,* 1992, **35,** 771–6.

87. Draznin, B., Sussman, K., Kao, M. *et al.* The existence of an optimal range of cytosolic free calcium for insulin-stimulated glucose transport in rat adipocytes. *J. Biol. Chem.,* 1987, **262,** 14385–8.

88. Pershadsingh, H.A., Shade, D.L., Delfert, D.M. *et al.* Chelation of intracellular calcium blocks insulin action in the adipocyte. *Proc. Natl Acad. Sci U.S.A.,* 1987, **84,** 1025–9.

89. Draznin, B., Lewis, D. and Houlder, N. Mechanisms of insulin resistance induced by sustained levels of cytosolic free calcium in rat adipocytes. *Endocrinology,* 1989, **125,** 2341–9. .

90. Resnick, L.M., Gupta, R.K., Gruenspann, H. *et al.* Hypertension and peripheral insulin resistance. Possible role of mediating intracellular free magnesium. *Am. J. Hypertens.,* 1990, **3,** 373–9.

91. Laakso, M., Edelmann, S.V., Brechtel, G. *et al.* Impaired insulin-mediated skeletal muscle blood flow in patients with NIDDM. *Diabetes,* 1992, **41,** 1076–83. .

92. Baron, A.D., Brechtelhook, G., Johnson, A. *et al.* Skeletal muscle blood flow – a possible link between insulin resistance and blood pressure. *Hypertension,* 1993, **21,** 129–35.

RISK FACTORS FOR ARTERIAL DISEASE IN DIABETES: HYPERGLYCAEMIA

Amanda I. Adler and H. Andrew W. Neil

4.1 INTRODUCTION

Cardiovascular disease defined as coronary artery disease, cerebrovascular disease, and peripheral vascular disease is the principal cause of morbidity and mortality in diabetes, a condition characterized by hyperglycaemia due to absolute or relative insulin deficiency. Nevertheless, the role of hyperglycaemia in the pathogenesis of long-term vascular complications, the so-called 'glucose hypothesis' remains controversial. There is, however, accumulating epidemiological evidence which, together with a number of biologically plausible mechanisms, support the contention that hyperglycaemia may be a cardiovascular risk factor. If hyperglycaemia is an independent cardiovascular risk factor, then lowering blood glucose should result in fewer cardiovascular events in patients with diabetes. Conclusive proof of this hypothesis depends on evidence from long-term clinical trials that near-normoglycaemia reduces cardiovascular events; the impending results of the United Kingdom Prospective Diabetes Study (UKPDS) may provide this [1].

Many large prospective studies in different populations have documented that diabetes increases the risk of coronary artery disease (CAD); the relative increase is greater for women than it is for men [2–7]. The Framingham Study of over 5000 adult residents of the Massachusetts city of the same name, followed subjects from 1948 forward and found that adults with diabetes were two to three times more likely to develop CAD than adults without diabetes [2]. Diabetes has also been shown to increase the risk for stroke [3, 4] and peripheral vascular disease [8, 9]. The ensuing discussion will be limited to prospective population-based or occupation-based studies because cross-sectional studies that include individuals with diagnosed cardiovascular disease skew estimates and cannot be used to determine the incidence of cardiovascular disease. The relative risks (RR) presented in this chapter provide an estimate of how much more likely one group with particular characteristics – or an individual within the group – is to develop the cardiovascular complications of diabetes when compared to those without those characteristics.

4.2 INCREASED RISK OF CARDIOVASCULAR DISEASE IN DIABETES

Both hypertension and dyslipidaemia frequently accompany diabetes [10, 11]. One potential explanation for the increased cardiovascular risk associated with diabetes is that subjects with diabetes are more likely to have co-existing cardiovascular risk factors than those without diabetes. Fortunately, an estimate of the independent effect of diabetes can be extricated using analytical techniques including multivariate modelling which simultaneously addresses both cardiovascular risk factors and diabetes. Several epidemiological studies have measured cardiovascular risk factors, and controlled for them in analyses. Not suprisingly, these studies differ in the criteria for the diagnosis of diabetes and cardiovascular disease. Different studies measure different risk factors, and studies which measure the same risk factors may categorize them differently. One should therefore interpret comparisons between studies with caution.

Among these studies is the Multiple Risk Factor Intervention Trial (MRFIT) which showed that men in the USA with diabetes were slightly more than three times (RR = 3.2) as likely to die from CAD than were men without diabetes adjusting for age, race, cholesterol, blood pressure and smoking. The study size ($n = 5163$ with diabetes and $n = 342\,815$ without diabetes) and length (11–13 years) permitted the investigators to provide a fairly precise range of the probable values of the increase in risk (95% confidence interval, CI, 2.9–3.5) [6]. The strength of the observed diabetes–CAD association could overestimate the true effect, because participants with diabetes in MRFIT were limited to those taking medication and might not be representative of individuals with diabetes not receiving treatment.

The Atherosclerosis Risk in Communities (ARIC) study, also in the USA, controlled for differences between individuals with and without diabetes with regard to: sex, age, race, smoking, drinking, education, fitness, waist to hip ratio, fibrinogen, total and high density lipoprotein (HDL) cholesterol, triglycerides, systolic blood pressure, and antihypertensive medicine use. This study found that diabetes remained associated with incident coronary heart disease (definite, probable or silent myocardial infarction or death due to the same) with a RR for men of 1.8 (1.2–2.6), suggesting an 80% increase in the risk of new coronary events due to diabetes *per se* [12].

Unlike the ARIC study which classified an individual as having diabetes on the basis of a fasting plasma glucose concentration ($\geq$7.8 mmol/l), medical history and medications, the large ($n = 12\,220$) Chicago Heart Association Detection in Industry Study included only men and defined diabetes by self-report. It found a RR of 2.5 (2.1–3.0) for cardiovascular disease for white men and 1.6 (0.6–4.3, non-significant) for black men when taking into account similar variables assessed in ARIC (but excluding fitness and drinking) [5]. In a separate study, diabetes doubled the risk of death from ischaemic heart disease after adjusting for cardiovascular risk factors (RR 1.9, 95% confidence interval CI 1.3–2.8) among elderly men in southern California [13]. These data suggest that diabetes increases the risk of CAD in men approximately twofold.

In women, the occupationally-based Nurses' Health Study cohort was based on analysis of 116 177 women in the USA and controlled for cardiovascular risk factors. It showed that diabetes independently increased the risk of non-fatal myocardial infarction and fatal CAD by 3.1 (2.3–4.2) [4]. This magnitude of risk was very similar to that observed in a separate study in elderly women in southern California (RR = 3.3, CI 2.0–5.6) when controlling for cardiovascular risk factors. In ARIC, controlling for the same risk factors as for men in addition to hormone replacement therapy, the risk in women for incident coronary heart disease was doubled (RR 2.0, CI 1.2–3.4). This suggests that the risk could be as high as 3.5 times that of women without diabetes [12]. In general, then, diabetes increases the risk of CAD in women approximately threefold.

There is also evidence that diabetes increases the risk of stroke and peripheral vascular disease independently of other cardiovascular risk factors. The Framingham Study showed a doubling of risk for stroke associated with diabetes. This was observed for both men and women and took into account differences in age, systolic blood pressure, smoking, cholesterol and left ventricular hypertrophy [2]. Among women, diabetes increased the risk of ischaemic stroke by 3.0 (1.6–5.7), controlling for multiple cardiac risk factors including lipids and hypertension, which was very similar to the increased risk of coronary disease [4]. Diabetes doubles the risk of peripheral vascular disease independent of age, systolic blood pressure, body mass, serum lipids and smoking, among other factors [8].

4.3 ROLE OF GLYCAEMIA AS A CARDIOVASCULAR RISK FACTOR IN IMPAIRED GLUCOSE TOLERANCE AND IMPAIRED FASTING GLUCOSE

Since diabetes, independent of cardiovascular risk factors, unequivocally increases the risk for cardiovascular disease, glycaemia may be deleterious, itself increasing the risk of cardiovascular disease. Supporting this possibility is the observation that an increased risk of cardiovascular disease has been observed in individuals whose plasma glucose levels exceed normal levels while not yet in the range consistent with diabetes. This is consistent with blood glucose being harmful across a broader range. In British male civil servants (Whitehall Study) the risk for death from CAD was 1.6 times higher in men with impaired glucose tolerance – defined as blood glucose between 5.4–11.0 mmol/l two hours following 50 g of oral glucose. This risk persisted even after controlling for age, smoking, blood pressure, body mass index and cholesterol in multivariate analysis [14].

An interesting possibility is that a threshold of blood glucose exists above which one is at markedly increased risk for CAD, although defining this hypothetical threshold is difficult. However, in the Whitehall Study a sharp increase in risk was noted above a blood glucose of 5.4 mmol/l two hours after a 50 g oral glucose tolerance test. Framingham investigators noted that the lowest CAD rates were observed at random blood sugar levels under 4.9 mmol/l and that the risk had doubled by the time the blood sugars were in the range 7.2–11.1 mmol/l [15]. Based on a

20-year follow-up of the combined cohorts of working men from the Paris Prospective Study (6629 men) and the Helsinki Policemen Study (631 men), non-diabetic men in the upper 2.5% of values for fasting glucose in the respective studies were at significantly increased risk (RR = 1.9, CI 1.2–3.1) for death from CAD, taking into account possible differences in cardiovascular risk factors [16]. No associations were observed for fasting blood glucose values below the 97.5th percentile – defined as 6.9 mmol/l in the Parisian cohort and 6.0 mmol/l in the Finnish cohort. It is notable that, according to diagnostic criteria, a fasting blood glucose value of 6.00 mmol/l is not even within the range of impaired fasting glucose, but rather is considered normal [17].

Not all studies find an association between glucose intolerance and CAD. Investigators in Chicago found no increased risk in individuals with impaired glucose tolerance. In working men in Chicago with plasma glucose values between 8.9 and 11 mmol/l one hour after a 50 g oral glucose tolerance test, the study showed that they were not more likely to die of cardiovascular disease than men with blood glucose values <8.9 mmol/l [5]. Yet, as the fasting or two-hour post-load measurements are more conventional, it is difficult to compare the studies. The ARIC study found no increased risk for incident coronary disease in men or women with fasting glucose levels between 6.4 and 7.8 mmol/ l when compared with men or women with fasting blood glucose less than 5.1 mmol/l – the lowest category fasting blood glucose. However, a comparison of fasting glucose levels between 6.4 and 7.8 mmol/l with fasting values less than 6.4 mmol/l was not performed [12].

The increased risk in glucose-intolerant, but not yet diabetic, individuals was also observed for fatal stroke in the Whitehall study. A significant rise in incidence was seen above the same blood glucose level, >5.3

mmol/l, as was observed for coronary disease mortality [14]. The increased risk associated with blood glucose values between 5.4 and 11.0 mmol/l doubled the risk even when controlling for other risk factors. Death caused by cerebrovascular disease was twice as likely to occur for individuals with two-hour blood glucose values above the 97.5th percentile compared with less than the 80th percentile in the combined Whitehall, Paris and Helsinki cohorts [16].

4.4   EVIDENCE FOR THE INDEPENDENT ROLE OF GLYCAEMIA

Ideally, rigorous studies should be done to disentangle the complex associations between glucose, the factors to which it is putatively associated, and the risk for cardiovascular disease. However, there are potential analytical difficulties relating to potentially causal relationships between hyperglycaemia, and, for example, plasminogen activator inhibitor, PAI-1, or to any other variable which is thought to directly or indirectly result from hyperglycaemia. When two variables in a causal path are both present in a regression model, the interpretation can be problematic [18].

Notwithstanding, many studies have directly addressed the role of relative hyperglycaemia to newly detected cardiovascular disease in individuals with diabetes. These include the Wisconsin Epidemiologic Study of Diabetic Retinopathy in which, for each 1% increase in glycohaemoglobin, the risk of death from ischaemic heart disease rose 10% (RR = 1.10, CI 1.04–1.17) and the risk of death from stroke rose 17% (RR = 1.17 CI 1.05–1.30) [19]. These analyses took into account possible differences in age, sex, hypertension and former cardiovascular disease. In Japanese men in Hawaii, serum glucose one hour following 50 g of oral glucose, not simply the presence of diabetes, was significantly associated with a risk of death from cardiovascular disease and CAD when controlled for

established cardiovascular risk factors [20]. Glycohaemoglobin values predicted death from macrovascular disease in multivariate analyses among general practice patients in Munich [21]. The United Kingdom Prospective Diabetes Study showed that HbA1c values ≥7.5% increased the risk of CAD by 1.4–1.7 times for CAD, any myocardial infarction or fatal myocardial infarction when compared with individuals with HbA1c values <6.2 % [22]. This increase in risk was independent of other risk factors for CAD. From the same cohort, HbA1c similarly categorized and compared was associated with a 2.2 increase in newly diagnosed peripheral vascular disease (CI 1.3–3.7) when also controlling for cardiovascular risk factors [23]. However, no independent association between hyperglycaemia and stroke was noted in this cohort [24]. In a Finnish prospective study, in patients with type 2 diabetes, elevated fasting plasma glucose significantly increased the risk of mortality due to ischaemic heart disease independently of, among other factors, age, sex and plasma lipids [25].

Discussion of hyperglycaemia cannot omit mention of the debate regarding a separate role for hyperinsulinaemia, either endogenous or exogenous, in the development of cardiovascular disease. Insulin may interact with hyperglycaemia, as is suggested by hyperinsulinaemia being a risk factor only when accompanied by hyperglycaemia [26]. McKeigue and Davey have suggested that associations between insulin levels and cardiovascular disease are confounded by the many physiological and clinical factors associated with elevated insulin: central obesity, raised triglycerides, lowered HDL, raised total cholesterol [27]. They, and others [28] have concerns about the causal role of hyperinsulinaemia because some studies fail to show an association between insulinaemia and cerebrovascular disease even in univariate analyses. Others note that prospective studies addressing the question of hyperinsulinaemia and heart disease are 'inconsistent and unconvincing' [29].

4.5 PATHOPHYSIOLOGIC BASIS FOR THE ROLE OF GLYCAEMIA IN ATHEROSCLEROSIS

There is ample biological evidence that supports the role of hyperglycaemia in atherosclerosis. Hyperglycaemia is related to many of the metabolic abnormalities in diabetes which constitute cardiovascular risk factors. The lipid and lipoprotein abnormalities are well-recognized and, in untreated type 1 and type 2 diabetes, decreased activity of lipoprotein lipase due to absolute or relative insulin deficiency produces a defect in triglyceride catabolism and exacerbates the hyper-triglyceridaemic effect of increased hepatic lipogenesis. This accounts for the hypertriglyceridaemia of poorly controlled or untreated diabetes [30].

In well-controlled diabetes, however, relatively normal serum lipid and lipoprotein concentrations may mask abnormalities in lipoprotein composition which include higher concentrations of atherogenic small dense low density lipoprotein (LDL) and intermediate density lipoprotein (IDL) [30]. It has been suggested that the larger IDL particles may more readily be trapped in the arterial intima and share with LDL the potential for promoting atherosclerosis [31]. Increased non-enzymatic glycation of LDL has also been demonstrated in diabetes. Some of the early glycosylation products undergo a slow, complex series of chemical rearrangements to form irreversible advanced glycosylation end-products (AGE) [32]. The rate of this accumulation is proportional to the time-integrated blood glucose levels over long periods of time. AGE can bind LDL, and the LDL trapped in arterial wall collagen may accelerate the atherosclerotic process. Hyperglycaemia may also increase the susceptibility of LDL to oxidation as non-enzymatically glycated proteins are a source of free radicals [32]. These may result in oxidative stress, so depleting serum antioxidant levels and increasing the susceptibility of LDL to oxidation. This would be consistent with the inverse relationship between ascorbic acid levels and glycaemic control reported in diabetes [33]. Both oxidized LDL and glycated LDL can induce transformation of macrophages into foam cells, which constitute a major source of secretory products that can promote progression of atherosclerotic process [34].

Hyperglycaemia also induces changes in the coagulation system, affecting all stages of coagulation including : thrombus formation and its inhibition, fibrinolysis, platelet and endothelial function [35]. Reported changes in fibrinolysis appear apparently conflicting, but most studies point to reduced fibrinolytic activity in type 2 diabetes due to increased PAI-1 levels and either normal or increased levels in patients with type 1 diabetes. It is clear that diabetes is associated with increased fibrinogen levels, although the results of studies examining the relation between fibrinogen and microvascular complications are contradictory [36]. Both non-enzymatic glycation and increased oxidative stress have been suggested as mechanisms that may induce these changes in the coagulation system [35]. By contrast, hyperglycaemia does not increase blood pressure, although hypertension is more common in diabetes than in the absence of diabetes [37] and has been reported to be present in 39% of individuals recently diagnosed with type 2 diabetes [38]. The 'insulin hypothesis' proposes that the compensatory hyperinsulinaemia which occurs with insulin resistance raises blood pressure by increasing sodium retention and stimulating sympathetic activity [39].

4.6 CLINICAL IMPLICATIONS

It follows that if hyperglycaemia is an independent risk factor for cardiovascular disease, then therapies aimed at lowering blood glucose should also lower the risk of cardiovascular disease. Intensive treatment of type 1 diabetes aiming at near normal levels of blood glucose is recognized to substantially reduce the risk of renal, neuropathic and retinal complications [40] and may also lower the risk of cardiovascular disease, although this remains unproven. The application of similar standards to type 2 diabetes remains contentious. It has been argued that, even if glycaemia were clearly a risk factor for cardiovascular disease, hypertension and dyslipidaemia should merit priority for treatment as they are modifiable risk factors for which treatment has proved effective in diabetes [41]. The evidence that blood glucose is associated with an increased risk of cardiovascular disease in the range which is higher than normal, but not high enough to be diagnostic of diabetes, brings greater importance to the impaired fasting glucose and impaired glucose tolerance as diagnostic categories. Lastly, it is not yet clear whether the patients with glucose intolerance at high risk for cardiovascular disease include only those who ultimately develop diabetes [42].

4.7   CONCLUSIONS

In summary, there are biologically plausible mechanisms for supposing that hyperglycaemia may be a cardiovascular risk factor, but this does not exclude the possibility that hyperinsulinaemia is also atherogenic. Accumulating epidemiological evidence based on multivariate analyses suggests that hyperglycaemia is an independent risk factor for cardiovascular disease. The evidence that glucose may be a risk factor for cardiovascular disease at levels below those diagnostic of diabetes, and possibly even in the upper range of normal, is compelling. It raises the possible importance of identifying glucose-intolerant individuals. The possibility of a threshold value for blood glucose is intriguing. However, since most epidemiological studies excluded measurement of many potentially important risk factors, caution is necessary before concluding that hyperglycaemia *per se* is an independent cardiovascular risk factor. Conclusive evidence depends on evidence from long-term clinical trials demonstrating that near-normoglycaemia reduces cardiovascular events.

RERERENCES

1. UKPDS Group. UK Prospective Diabetes Study VIII: study design, progress and performance. *Diabetologia*, 1991, **34**, 877–90.
2. Kannel, W. and McGee, D. Diabetes and cardiovascular disease. The Framingham study. *J. Am. Med. Assoc.*, 1979, **241**, 2035–8.
3. Kannel, W. and McGee, D. Diabetes and glucose tolerance as risk factors for cardiovascular disease: the Framingham study. *Diabetes Care*, 1979, **2**, 120–6.
4. Manson, J. E., Colditz, G. A. *et al.* A prospective study of maturity-onset diabetes mellitus and risk of coronary heart disease and stroke in women. *Arch. Intern. Med.* 1991, **151**, 1141–7.
5. Lowe, L. P., Liu, K. *et al.* Diabetes, asymptomatic hyperglycemia, and 22-year mortality in black and white men: The Chicago Heart Association Detection Project in Industry. *Diabetes Care*, 1997, **20**, 163–9.
6. Stamler, J., Vaccaro, O. *et al.* Diabetes, other risk factors, and 12 year cardiovascular mortality for men screened in the Multiple Risk Factor Intervention Trial. *Diabetes Care*, 1993, **16**, 434–44.
7. Koskinen, P., Manttari, M. *et al.* Coronary heart disease incidence in NIDDM patients in the Helsinki Heart Study. *Diabetes Care*, 1992, **15**, 820–5.
8. Brand, F., Abbott, R. *et al.* Diabetes, intermittent claudication, and risk of cardiovascular events. The Framingham Study. *Diabetes*, 1989, **38**, 504–9.
9. Osmundson, P., O'Fallon, W. *et al.* Course of peripheral occlusive arterial disease in diabetes. Vascular laboratory assessment. *Diabetes Care*, 1990, **13**, 143–52.
10. Reaven, G., Lithell, H. *et al.* Hypertension and associated metabolic abnormalities – the role of insulin resistance and the sympathoadrenal system. *N. Engl. J. Med.*, 1996, **334**, 374–81.

11. Reaven, G. Banting lecture 1988. Role of insulin resistance in human disease. *Diabetes*, 1988, **37**, 1595–607.

12. Folsom, A. R., Szklo, M. *et al.* A prospective study of coronary heart disease in relation to fasting insulin, glucose, and diabetes: the Atherosclerosis Risk in Communities (ARIC) Study. *Diabetes Care*, 1997, **20**, 935–42.

13. Barrett-Connor, E. L., Cohn, B. A. *et al.* Why is diabetes mellitus a stronger risk factor for fatal ischemic heart disease in women than in men? *J. Am Med. Assoc.*, 1991, **265**, 627–31.

14. Fuller, J., Shipley, M. *et al.* Mortality from coronary heart disease and stroke in relation to degree of glycaemia: the Whitehall study. *Br. Med. J.*, 1983, **287**, 867–70.

15. Wilson, P., Cupples, L. *et al.* Is hyperglycemia associated with cardiovascular disease? The Framingham Study. *Am. J. Med.*, 1991, **121**, 586–90.

16. Balkau, B., Shipley, M. *et al.* High blood glucose concentration is a risk factor for mortality in middle-aged nondiabetic men. *Diabetes Care*, 1998, **21**, 360–7.

17. Expert Committee on the Diagnosis and Classification of Diabetes Mellitus. Report of the expert committee on the diagnosis and classification of diabetes mellitus. *Diabetes Care*, 1998, **21**, S5–19.

18. Hennekens, C. and Buring, J. *Epidemiology in Medicine*, Little, Brown, and Company, 1987.

19. Moss, S., Klein, R. *et al.* The association of glycemia and cause-specific mortality in a diabetic population. *Arch. Intern. Med.*, 1994, **154**, 2473–9.

20. Yano, K., Kagan, A. *et al.* Glucose intolerance and nine-year mortality in Japanese men in Hawaii. *Am. J. Med.*, 1982, **72**, 71–80.

21. Standl, E., Balletshofer, B. *et al.* Predictors of 10-year macrovascular and overall mortality in patients wtih NIDDM: the Munich General Practitioner Project. *Diabetologia*, 1996, **39**, 1540–5.

22. Turner, R., Milln, H. *et al.* Risk factors for coronary artery disease in non-insulin dependent diabetes mellitus: United Kingdom Prospective Diabetes Study (UKPDS: 23). *Br. Med. J.*, 1998, **316**, 823–8.

23. Adler, A. and Stevens, R. Degree of hyperglycaemia increases the risk of peripheral vascular disease in patients with type 2 diabetes in a large prospective study. Proceedings European Epidemiology Study Group, 1998.

24. United Kingdom Prospective Diabetes Study Group. Risk factors for stroke in type 2 diabetes. Abstract. IDF, Helsinki, 1997.

25. Lehto, S., Ronnemaa, T. *et al.* Dyslipidemia and hyperglycemia predict coronary heart disease events in middle-aged patients with NIDDM. *Diabetes*, 1997, **48**, 1354–9.

26. Welborn, T. and Wearne, K. Coronary heart disease incidence and cardiovascular mortality in Busselton with reference to glucose and insulin concentrations. *Diabetes Care*, 1979, **2**, 154–60.

27. McKeigue, P. and Davey, G. Associations between insulin levels and cardiovascular disease are confounded by comorbidity. *Diabetes Care*, 1995, **18**, 1294–8.

28. Jarrett, R. Why is insulin not a risk factor for coronary heart disease? *Diabetologia*, 1994, **37**, 945–7.

29. Wingard, D., Barrett-Connor, E. *et al.* Is insulin really a heart disease risk factor? *Diabetes Care*, 1995, **18**, 1299–304.

30. Durrington, P. Secondary hyperlipidaemia. In *Hyperlipidaemia Diagnosis and Management*. Butterworth-Heinemann, Oxford, 1995, pp. 293–314.

31. Nordestgaard, B. The vascular endothelial barrier-selective retention of lipoproteins. *Curr. Opin. Lipidol.*, 1996, **7**, 269–73.

32. Ceriello, A., Quatraro, A. *et al.* New insights on non-enzymatic glycosylation may lead to therapeutic approaches for the prevention of diabetic complications. *Diabet. Med.*, 1992, **9**, 297–9.

33. Sinclair, A., Taylor, P. *et al.* Low plasma ascorbate levels in patients with type 2 diabetes mellitus consuming adequate dietary vitamin C. *Diabet. Med.*, 1994, **11**, 893–8.

34. Bowie, A., Owens, D. *et al.* Glycosylated low density lipoprotein is more sensitive to oxidation: implications for the diabetic patient? *Atherosclerosis*, 1993, **102**, 63–7.

35. Ceriello, A. Coagulation activation in diabetes mellitus: the role of hyperglycaemia and therapeutic prospects. *Diabetologia*, 1993, **36**, 1119–25.

36. Gough, S. and Grant, P. The fibrinolytic system in diabetes mellitus. *Diabet. Med.*, 1991, **121**, 1274–82.

37. Cowie, C. and Harris, M. Physical and metabolic characteristics of persons with diabetes. In *Diabetes in America*. (eds M. I. Harris, C. C.

Cowie, M. P. Stern *et al.*) U.S. Government Printing Office, Washington, DC, 1995.

38. Hypertension in Diabetes Study Group. Hypertension in Diabetes Study (HDS): I. Prevalence of hypertension in newly presenting type 2 diabetic patients and the association with risk factors for cardiovascular and diabetic complications. *J. Hypertens.*, 1993, **11**, 309–17.

39. Ferrannini, E. and Natali, A. Essential hypertension, metabolic disorders and insulin resistance. *Am. Heart J.*, 1991, **121**, 1274–82.

40. Diabetes Control and Complications Trial Research Group. The effect of intensive treatment of diabetes on the development and progression of long-term complications in insulin-dependent diabetes mellitus. *N. Engl. J. Med.*, 1993, **329**, 977–86.

41. Barrett-Connor, E. Does hyperglycemia really cause coronary heart disease? *Diabetes Care*, 1997, **20**, 1620–3.

42. Haffner, S. Impaired glucose tolerance – is it relevant for cardiovascular disease? *Diabetologia*, 1997, **40**, 138–40.

RISK FACTORS FOR ARTERIAL DISEASE IN DIABETES: HYPERTENSION

5

James R. Sowers and Murray Epstein

5.1 SUMMARY

Hypertension is often accompanied by a panoply of metabolic defects. There is an association between central obesity, insulin resistance, hyperinsulinaemia and hypertension. Recent interest has focused on the fact that untreated hypertensives have compensatory hyperinsulinaemia, are resistant to insulin-mediated glucose uptake and frequently have co-existing lipid abnormalities. Data from prospective studies suggest that fasting hyperinsulinaemia may be an independent predictor of coronary artery disease. Additionally, there is evidence that hyperinsulinaemia and diabetes eliminate the normal gender differences in the prevalence of coronary artery disease. Clinical and epidemiological evidence have linked elevated blood pressure to disturbances in lipoprotein metabolism, fibrinolytic activity, plasminogen activity inhibitor levels and dyslipidaemia. The salutary effects of aggressive treatment of hypertension on cardiovascular disease and microvascular disease in diabetic persons are well established. There are data suggesting that certain antihypertensive agents may have special beneficial effects on lessening diabetic renal disease. Further, as diabetes is a disease characterized haemodynamically by attenuated nitric oxide action, recent studies indicating angiotensin-converting enzyme (ACE) inhibitors may improve this abnormality are particularly relevant. Diabetic hypertensive persons often have a very abnormal lipid profile, and there is increasing evidence that aggressive treatment is important. This review presents the current understanding of various metabolic disturbances associating the co-morbid conditions of hypertension and diabetes, the pathophysiologic mechanisms involved and the significance of therapeutic approaches to lessen the risk of macrovascular and microvascular disease.

5.2 INTRODUCTION

Diabetes mellitus and hypertension are interrelated diseases, which increase in prevalence with obesity and aging in industrialized societies, and which predispose to both micro- and macrovascular disease [1–11]. Lifestyle and genetic factors contribute to the pathogenesis of both diabetes and hypertension. Hypertension is about twice as frequent in persons with diabetes as those without [1]. Data from death certificates indicated that hypertension was implicated in 4.4% of deaths coded to diabetes, and diabetes was involved in 10% of deaths coded to hypertension-related disease [1, 2]. An estimated 35% to 75% of diabetes-related cardiovascular and microvascular (including renal) complications may be attributed to hypertension [1, 2]. Macrovascular disease is the major cause of mortality in type 2 diabetes and hypertension in association with dyslipidaemia, hyperglycaemia and perhaps hyperinsulinaemia is a very strong risk factor for coronary artery disease (CAD) and stroke mortality in this population [1–21].

A common underlying factor that powerfully contributes to the increasing prevalence of diabetes and hypertension in industrialized societies is obesity, particularly visceral or android obesity [1, 2, 21–28]. Visceral fat, localized around omental and mesenteric tissues, is relatively resistant to the antilipolytic actions of insulin [22–24]. The enhanced lipolytic activity of this fat mass results in increased entry of free fatty acids (FA) into the portal circulation. The resultant increased FA may, in turn, contribute to skeletal muscle insulin resistance [29] by substrate competition between glucose and free FA into the glucose–FA cycle. FA inhibit hepatic clearance of circulating insulin and stimulate hepatic gluconeogenesis [22–24]. In addition, increased delivery of FA to the liver stimulates hepatic synthesis and the release of the triglyceride-rich very low-density lipoproteins (VLDL). Because of peripheral insulin resistance, there is reduced activity of endothelial bound lipoprotein lipase (LPL) in skeletal muscle and adipocytes, and it is this LPL that is responsible for the metabolism of triglyceride-rich particles like VLDL and chylomicrons. Thus, triglyceride levels rise because of increased hepatic production of triglycerides coupled with reduced peripheral metabolism of VLDL. Because of inefficient triglyceride metabolism, HDL levels are also deceased.

In a population-based random sample of 2475 adult Israelis, 52.9% of persons with hypertension had glucose intolerance by National Data Group criteria [21]. Interestingly, glucose intolerance was more severe in hypertensive persons taking antihypertensive medication. Further, the majority of hypertensive persons were obese (59%), and 83.4% of hypertensive persons were either obese or glucose intolerant. It can be ascertained that 23.4% of the persons with hypertension and glucose intolerance were lean (body mass index <25 kg/m^2) and 76.5% were obese. Accordingly, the ratio of obese to lean persons within the hypertensive group with glucose intolerance was 3 to 1. Thus, although carbohydrate intolerance is more common in obese hypertensive persons, glucose intolerance is relatively common even in lean persons with hypertension. Other studies have corroborated this finding, observing reduced tissue insulin sensitivity in lean persons with hypertension [5, 30]. One of these studies demonstrated [30] a strong inverse correlation between systolic blood pressure and total body glucose uptake. This insulin insensitivity was confined solely to attenuated non-oxidative glucose disposal, sparing the liver.

Persons with hypertension have other metabolic abnormalities besides carbohydrate intolerance, *per se*. Persons with hypertension, matched by age and body mass index (BMI) with normotensive persons have lower levels of high-density lipoproteins (HDL), higher levels of triglyceride and low-density lipoprotein (LDL), as well as increased postprandial insulin levels [2, 5]. Other metabolic abnormalities in hypertensive persons include elevated VLDL and abnormal small dense, more atherogenic LDL particles [2, 5] (Table 5.1). Genetics studies, including parent-child, large scale family, twin and candidate gene studies have yielded evidence for a genetic basis for the relationship between hypertension and the accompanying metabolic abnormalities [31,32]. For example, there are higher heritability estimates in twins than in pedigrees for blood pressure, LDL, VLDL, and BMI [31]. Almost 70% of adults with hypertension before age 55 years have siblings or parents with hypertension, and 12% of all hypertensive patients have familial dyslipidaemic hypertension [32]. Accordingly, both hypertensive and dyslipidaemic states probably have a genetic basis, and both conditions have been linked to insulin resistance.

Table 5.1 Metabolic abnormalities seen in diabetes mellitus associated with hypertension

---

Elevated plasma levels of VLDL, LDL and LpA
Decreased plasma HDL cholesterol
Increased lipoprotein oxidation
Increased lipoprotein glycation
Increased small dense LDL cholesterol products
Decreased lipoprotein lipase activity
Increased fibrinogen and plasminogen activation inhibitor (PAI-1)
Decreased plasminogen activator PA and fibrinolytic activity
Increased insulin and proinsulin levels

5.3   HYPERINSULINAEMIA AND CARDIOVASCULAR DISEASE

Large prospective studies have demonstrated that hyperinsulinaemia is a predictor of CAD [12–20, 33, 34], with a few prospective reports not demonstrating such a relationship. The greatest association of hyperinsulinaemia with CAD has been found in Finland, in a population with a very high frequency of CAD [12]. Results of a prospective investigation of 2103 men from Quebec [15] clearly showed that high fasting insulin concentrations are an independent predictor of CAD. This important study utilized an insulin assay without cross-reactivity with pro-insulin; thus avoiding that confounding influence. Recent studies have shown a relationship between carotid wall atherosclerotic lesions, angina, and insulin levels/resistance [16–20]. A recent report suggested that insulin levels predicted blood pressure elevations in children [35]. A positive correlation between serum insulin and both systolic and diastolic blood pressures was described after standardizing for age and weight, suggesting that insulin appeared to regulate actual blood pressure within the normal range and also to predict future blood pressure, independent of age and weight. Collectively, although these observations fall short of establishing a causal link, they suggest that cardiovascular interactions of high levels of insulin may aggravate hypertension and increase the risk of cardiovascular mortality in both men and women [36].

Hyperinsulinaemia associated with hypertension may promote atherosclerosis by a number of mechanisms. For example, insulin stimulates the synthesis of plasminogen activator inhibitor (PAI-1) in hepatocytes, and there is a strong relationship between plasma insulin levels and PAI-1 as well as fibrinogen [4]. Thus, hyperinsulinaemia may interfere with the fibrinolytic process. Insulin increases mitogenic signalling pathways and increases thymidine incorporation into DNA in vascular endothelial and smooth muscle cells [21, 37, 38]. Many of the effects of insulin on vascular growth and remodelling are probably mediated through an insulin-like growth factor (IGF-1) receptor in endothelial/vascular smooth muscle cells (VSMC) [36–38] or indirectly by stimulating IGF-1 synthesis by VSMC [36]. Insulin and IGF-1 are structurally related, share receptors and have similar post-receptor actions. Unlike insulin, which must traverse the endothelium before acting on VSMCs *in vivo*, IGF-1 is synthesized by VSMCs and is more likely to act in an autocrine and paracrine process. In addition to stimulating vascular cell mitogenesis and growth, IGF-1 enhances proteoglycan synthesis by microvascular and macrovascular endothelial cells [36]. Both IGF-1 and insulin function as progression factors or co-factors and promote proliferative properties of several cytokines including tumour necrosis factor [36]. VSMC production of IGF-1 is stimulated by sustained or cyclic stretch as may occur as a function of exerted pulse pressure [36, 38]. The cyclic-stretch-induced IGF-1 production is accompanied by growth and this growth effect of IGF-1 can be attenuated using IGF-1 antibodies [36, 38]. There is also increasing evidence that enhanced IGF-1 expression/ synthesis may play an important role in mesangial hyperplasia and in the development of left ventricular hypertrophy, all of which are characteristic manifestations of diabetes and hypertension [36, 38]. Thus, it is likely that many of the growth and atherosclerotic effects that have been attributed to insulin are mediated through an IGF-1 receptor either directly by IGF-1 or indirectly by high concentrations of insulin.

5.4   PLATELET ABNORMALITIES ASSOCIATED WITH DIABETES AND HYPERTENSION

Platelet aggregation and platelet adhesion are characteristically accentuated in both diabetes mellitus and hypertension [2] (Table 5.2). The aetiology of increased platelet reactivity associated with both diseases is complex, but data suggest several possible underlying mechanisms. For example, exaggerated elevations in platelet intracellular calcium $[Ca^{2+}]_i$, phosphoinositide turnover, intracellular Ca^{2+} mobilization and protein phosphorylation occur in type 2 diabetic and hypertensive persons [2, 39–41]. Enhanced platelet $[Ca^{2+}]_i$ responses to low density lipoprotein (LDL) cholesterol exists in type 2 diabetic persons with and without hypertension [40]. These enhanced responses of platelet $[Ca^{2+}]_i$ to agonists such as LDL cholesterol [40] and thromboxane [39] appear to occur only in those persons who manifest exaggerated platelet aggregation. Platelets from persons with diabetes have reduced membrane fluidity, thought to be due to an increased molar ratio of cholesterol to phospholipid in membranes [42]. Another process that may contribute to enhanced platelet aggregation is the increased non-enzymatic glycosylation of platelet membrane proteins [43] in persons with diabetes and hypertension. Finally, the dyslipidaemia that accompanies diabetes and hypertension contributes directly and indirectly to enhanced platelet aggregation [44].

Table 5.2 Abnormalities of platelet function in diabetes mellitus and hypertension

Increased platelet adhesiveness
Increased platelet aggregation
Decreased platelet survival
Increased platelet generation of vasoconstrictor prostanoids
Reduced platelet generation of prostacyclin and other vasodilator prostanoids
Altered platelet divalent cation homeostasis (i.e. decreased $[Mg^{2+}]_i$ and increased $[Ca^{2+}]_i$)
Increased non-enzymatic glycosylation of platelet proteins
Decreased platelet polyphosphoinositide content
Decreased platelet production of nitric oxide

5.5   COAGULATION ABNORMALITIES IN DIABETIC HYPERTENSIVE PERSONS

In persons with diabetes and hypertension, the balance between coagulative and fibrinolytic activity is affected in a number of ways [2, 45] (Table 5.3). A procoagulant state in diabetes appears to be mediated, in part, by higher than normal levels of a number of coagulation factors. For example, an increase in several components of coagulation, including the endothelial-derived von Willebrand's factor, occurs in diabetes mellitus, particularly in association with micro- and macrovascular damage, and poor diabetic control [45, 46]. Overall, these reports suggest that high concentrations of factor VIII components are related to hyperglycaemia, accelerate the rate of thrombin formation, and contribute to occlusive vascular disease in diabetic patients. Levels of fibrinogen, factor VII, and thrombin–antithrombin complexes have also been reported to be elevated in diabetic patients [45–47]. Levels of these factors, particularly fibrinogen, are important for increasing the survival of the provisional clot matrix upon transformation of fibrinogen to fibrin at the site of injured endothelium [45, 47]. Indeed, increased levels of thrombin–antithrombin complexes have been observed in diabetic patients in association with enhanced thrombin generation [47].

Table 5.3 Coagulation and fibrinolytic abnormalities seen in patients with hypertension and diabetes mellitus

---

Elevated plasma levels of factor VII and VIII
Increased fibrinogen and PAI-1
Elevated thrombin–antithrombin complexes
Decreased antithrombin III, protein C and S levels
Increased LpA
Increased small, dense LDL cholesterol products
Decreased plasminogen activators

Attenuation of clot formation is modulated by specific factors that inhibit one or more of the clotting factors (i.e. ATIII, protein C and S) and by the fibrinolytic system, both of which are abnormal in diabetes and hypertension [2, 4, 48–50]. ATIII, which inhibits thrombin, Xa, IXa and XIIa, has been observed to be deficient in diabetes, particularly when control of blood glucose levels is poor [48]. Protein C antigenic levels have also been reported to be low in diabetic patients with poor metabolic control and the normalization of protein C following glycometabolic control has been observed [50]. High PAI-1 levels have been observed in patients with diabetes mellitus [4, 50]. Furthermore, elevated PAI-1 levels have been reported in non-treated hypertensive people and in men with myocardial infarction at risk for reinfarction [51]. Elevated levels of PAI-1 also appear to be associated with abdominal obesity and elevated serum levels of insulin and triglycerides [4, 50]. Thus, it appears that hyperinsulinaemia, and associated insulin resistance, in hypertension are independent risk factors, along with diabetes for CAD.

5.6   OTHER METABOLIC ABNORMALITIES ASSOCIATED WITH DIABETES MELLITUS AND HYPERTENSION

Additional metabolic abnormalities may be present in patients with diabetes and hypertension [2, 4, 52]. Plasma levels of lipoprotein A (LpA) have been noted to be elevated in diabetic individuals, particularly those diabetic subjects with poor glycaemic control [52]. By inhibiting fibrinolysis, possibly via fibrin binding attributable to structural homology with apolipoprotein A, LpA may delay thrombolysis and thus contribute to plaque progression. Augmented lipoprotein oxidation has also been observed in diabetic states [2, 53, 54]. The generation of reactive oxygen species or free radicals by vascular intimal macrophages and VSMCs results in oxidative modification of lipids and vascular proteins. Oxidation modifies not only the phospholipid content of LDL, but also the amino acid side chains of apolipoprotein B (ApoB), analogous to the modification produced by acetylation [54] (Table 5.4). As a result, oxidized LDL (Ox-LDL) is no longer recognized by the classical LDL receptor, but by the so-called macrophage scavenger receptors. Foam-cell uptake of LDL via the scavenger pathway is enhanced by oxidative modification of LDL. Once taken up by the foam cell, however, Ox-LDL degradation is impaired, which leads to further accumulation in the cell. Ox-LDL is toxic to endothelial cells, altering both structure and function. Ox-LDL increases the adhesion of circulating monocytes to damaged endothelium, increasing their migration into the vascular intima. Ox-LDL also stimulates the production of chemoattractants that enhance this migration. Finally, antibodies to Ox-LDL may be involved in the later stages of atheroma formation.

Glycosylation, the non-enzymatic linkage of glucose to proteins, has also been found to alter LDL particles *in vivo* [54] (Table 5.4). Importantly, ApoB, which regulates receptor-mediated uptake of LDL, can undergo glycosylation, thereby facilitating its atherogenicity in diabetic individuals. Glycooxidized LDL can enhance foam-cell formation and is less well recognized by the native LDL receptor. This modified LDL is also immunogenic, forming antibody–lipoprotein complexes that stimulate foam-cell formation and enhance

Table 5.4 Metabolic consequences of glycooxidation of LDL in diabetes and hypertension

---

Glycation of apolipoprotein B (ApoB) is enhanced in diabetes
Glycation of ApoB decreases recognition by classical LDL receptor
Enhanced uptake and decreased degradation by macrophages, facilitating foam cell formation
Increased sequestration/covalent binding in vessel walls
Stimulation of immune complex formation
Increased cytotoxicity to vascular cells
Increased susceptibility to oxidative damage

---

platelet aggregation. Compared to normal LDL, glycooxidized LDL sequestered in the arterial intima has greater propensity to become bound by glucose-mediated cross-links to local matrix proteins. Once this occurs, the LDL particles may undergo even more extensive glycative and oxidative modification [54].

5.7 ABNORMALITIES OF NON-ESTERIFIED FATTY ACID METABOLISM IN DIABETES AND HYPERTENSION

There is accumulating evidence that abnormalities of non-esterified fatty acid (NEFA) metabolism may contribute to insulin resistance and hypertension [55–58]. NEFA are elevated in persons with central obesity, insulin resistance and hypertension [22–24]. A strong relationship between abnormalities in NEFA metabolism and blood pressure in obese persons has been reported [58]. Further, when NEFAs are elevated locally in normotensive non-obese persons to levels reported in obese hypertensive persons, enhanced vascular constriction is observed [56–58]. Some of these studies implicate an interaction between NEFA and the sympathetic nervous system may be responsible for the increase in vasoconstriction and elevations in blood pressure [56, 57]. The vasoconstrictive effects of NEFA have also been linked to alterations in arachidonic acid

products [59–61]. NEFA, particularly linoleic acid, can increase arachidonic acid which may then be metabolized by enzymes of the cyclooxygenase, lipooxygenase, and cytochrome *P*-450 pathways to several vasoactive products. Indeed, in persons with hypertension, increased activity of enzyme activity mediating changes in essential FA to eicosanoid precursors have been observed [61].

5.8 ENDOTHELIAL DYSFUNCTION IN DIABETES AND HYPERTENSION

Anatomic and functional abnormalities of the vascular endothelium are associated with both diabetes mellitus and hypertension [62] (Table 5.5). Hyperglycaemia and dyslipidaemia also both contribute to endothelial dysfunction [62–64]. Hyperglycaemia activates protein kinase C in endothelial cells, which in turn may account for increased production of vasoconstrictor prostaglandins, endothelin, glycated proteins and platelet and vascular growth factors, which directly and indirectly enhance vasomotor reactivity and vascular remodelling and growth [62–64]. Furthermore, hyperglycaemia alters endothelial cell matrix production, which may contribute to

Table 5.5 Alterations in vascular endothelium associated with diabetes mellitus and hypertension

---

Elevated plasma levels of von Willebrand factor
Elevated expression, synthesis and plasma levels of endothelin-1
Diminished prostacyclin release
Increased destruction of endothelium-derived relaxing factor (NO) and reduced responsiveness to NO
Impaired fibrinolytic activity
Increased endothelial cell procoagulant activity
Increased endothelial cell surface thrombomodulin
Impaired plasmin degradation of glycosylated fibrin
Increased levels of advanced glycosylated end products

---

basement membrane thickening. Hyperglycaemia increases endothelial cell collagen IV and fibronectin synthesis and increases the activity of enzymes involved in collagen synthesis [53]. Hyperglycaemia also delays cell replication and increases endothelial cell death in part by enhancing oxidation and glycation [53, 54].

Hypercholesterolaemia and perhaps hypertriglyceridaemia impair endothelium-dependent relaxation [63]. Both insulin and IGF have potentially important effects on endothelial cells [61]. Insulin appears to have a modulating influence on glucose stimulation of protein kinase C and diacylglycerol in endothelial cells [65]. One hypothesis for endothelial dysfunction in diabetes relates to elevated protein kinase C levels which are induced by hyperglycaemia; insulin treatment that achieves euglycaemia can prevent the increase in diacylglycerol levels and protein kinase C activity [62, 65]. These results suggest that impaired insulin action, as exists in type 2 diabetes and hypertension, may contribute to the endothelial dysfunction seen in these disorders. However, a recent report suggests that when hypertension is not associated with impaired carbohydrate metabolism or dyslipidaemia, endothelium-dependent vasodilation is preserved [66]. This study provides additional support of the concept that the metabolic abnormalities that often accompany hypertension and diabetes mellitus play a pivotal role in the development of endothelial dysfunction.

5.9 KIDNEY DISEASE, DIABETES AND HYPERTENSION: ANALOGY BETWEEN GLOMERULOSCLEROSIS AND ATHEROSCLEROSIS

There are many similarities between renal glomerular and vascular structure and function. Endothelial cells line both glomeruli and vessels, and mesangial cells are VSMC [38]. Endothelial and mesangial cells together account for about 85% of the total number of cells that make up the glomerulus, and these cells are distinguished by their biological characteristics and function. Both produce a variety of mitogens and cytokines known to have autocrine and paracrine activity. Their ability to produce growth factors is relevant given the anatomic relationship of the cells to each other. Anatomically, the glomerular basement membrane incompletely surrounds the endothelial surface, leaving an area of direct contact between the mesangial cells and the endothelium [62]. This simulates the anatomical and functional relationship between endothelial cells and VSMC in the vasculature [38].

Abnormalities in both endothelial and mesangial cell function have been described in diabetes mellitus. Specifically, there is decreased production and release of endothelial-derived relaxing factor or nitric acid (NO) and prostaglandins (PGs) in diabetic states [11, 36,62]. Both these endothelial-derived relaxing factors are known to attenuate the effects of various mitogens such as IGF-1, whereas IGF-1 directly affects growth of both endothelial and mesangial cells in normal and hyperglycaemic states [36, 38]. Consequently, IGF-1, along with other growth factors, interacts with these cells to change their fundamental biological responses to a variety of stimuli [36, 38].

Pathophysiological changes of diabetic nephropathy are histologically different from those of other types of renal disease [2, 36, 38, 67, 68]. In humans, mesangial expansion leads to the earliest lesions seen in type 1 diabetes [67]. In experimental studies, the earliest pathological change is an increase in the thickness of the glomerular basement membrane; usually the volume of the glomerulus is increased compared with that of non-diabetic subjects. Subsequently, the quantity of matrix in the mesangium increases, and in some individuals this mesangial expansion can progress to diffuse or nodular glomerulosclerosis [38]. Basement membranes are specialized regions of extracellular matrix composed of type IV collagen, laminin, entactin/nidogen, and proteoglycans, which together form a complex mesh-like structure [68]. Sieve-like permselectivity is one integral function of basement membrane that may be gradually lost in diabetes mellitus, with associated progressively increasing proteinuria [68]. Non-enzymatic glycosylation of long-lived proteins, such as the basement membrane components type IV collagen and laminin, and cross-link formation of these components may lead to modification of basement membrane ultrastructure and loss of permselectivity [68]. Advanced glycation end-products (AGE) can also have important influences on renal mesangium. AGE binding to mesangial cells can promote a significant increase in fibronectin and several other mesangial structural proteins. AGE binding to mesangial AGE receptors can also lead to an increase in basement membrane collagen. Thus, hyperglycaemia clearly contributes to the pathogenesis of diabetic nephropathy.

Mesangial cells share many properties with VSMCs. They contract in response to vasoactive agents such as angiotensin II (AII), and endothelin-1 [2, 38, 68, 69]. Contraction of mesangial cells is important because the mesangium bind together capillary loops; contraction of the mesangium thus can alter capillary flow, pressures, or both. The mesangial cell synthesizes several growth factors that act in an autocrine/paracrine fashion. These include IGF-1, platelet-derived growth factor, platelet-activating factor, endothelin, prostanoids and interleukin-1. Thus, the mesangial cell has supportive, filtrative and synthetic functions. The glomerular endothelial cell is separated from the mesangial cell of the kidney only by its basement membrane; passage of substances between these two cells is easily accomplished. Substances elaborated by the endothelium affect mesangial cell growth contraction and protein synthesis. For example, endothelin-1 increases growth and extracellular matrix production by mesangial cells. Endothelium-derived relaxing factor

and vasodilator prostaglandins inhibit mesangial cell growth and contraction [69]. Furthermore, increased local production of growth factors by stimulated endothelial and inflammatory cells can result in mesangial expansion. For example, endothelial damage can result in platelet activation, with release of platelet-derived growth factor and other growth factors that can also enhance mesangial cell proliferation and matrix overproduction [38, 69, 70].

Mesangial cell abnormalities typically appear after five to 15 years of known diabetes in individuals with type 1 disease [38, 67, 68]. The most common abnormality observed by light microscopy is diffuse intercapillary sclerosis due to expansion of the mesangium. Nodular intercapillary sclerosis is seen in approximately 25% of patients with diabetic nephropathy [38]. The pathophysiological alterations that occur with glomerulosclerosis are similar to those that occur in vascular atherosclerosis, with mesangial cell changes paralleling those in VSMCs, including proliferation, hypertrophy, foam cell accumulation, appearance of extracellular matrix material, deposits of amorphous debris and evolving sclerosis. The observed mesangial expansion is primarily related to mesangial cell matrix. A number of hormones have been demonstrated to alter mesangial cell growth *in vitro*, but only AII and vasopressin have been clearly demonstrated to promote hypertrophy [38, 67, 69, 70] which is more prominent in glomerulosclerosis than is proliferation. This may help explain why ACE inhibitors have been shown to slow the progression of glomerulosclerosis in both type 1 and type 2 diabetic patients [1, 2].

Diabetic nephropathy has become the leading cause of end-stage renal disease in the USA [1, 2, 71]. Hypertension is acknowledged to be a major risk factor in the progression of diabetic renal disease [2, 71]. Diabetic nephropathy, defined as the appearance of proteinuria, elevated arterial BP and diminished glomerular filtration rate (GFR), will develop in as many as 40% of type 1 diabetic persons [2]. In patients with the onset of diabetes at an early age, renal disease is an important contributor to mortality, accounting for up to 31% of all deaths [2, 71]. Renal disease also complicates type 2 diabetes and contributes significantly to morbidity and mortality in this group [2, 71]. A smaller percentage of patients with type 2 diabetes develop renal disease, and the incidence of end-stage renal disease is strongly related to the duration of diabetes. However, more than 50% of diabetic end-stage renal disease is associated with type 2 diabetes because this form of diabetes constitutes more than 90% of diabetic patients [2, 71].

In both types of diabetes mellitus the appearance of clinically detectable proteinuria (>200 mg/min of urinary albumin excretion) signals the onset of the relentless progression of diabetic nephropathy, which is typically followed by deterioration to end-stage renal disease [2, 67, 68]. Currently, it is believed that diabetic nephropathy develops as a result of the interplay of the metabolic abnormalities inherent to diabetes (e.g. hyperglycaemia) and haemodynamic abnormalities of the microvasculature [36, 38].

5.10 TREATMENT OF HYPERTENSION IN PATIENTS WITH DIABETES MELLITUS

5.10.1 GOALS OF THERAPY

No prospective population-based, randomized trials of hypertension treatment in diabetic patients have been conducted. Nevertheless, as proposed by a consensus statement [1], the goal of treating hypertension in diabetic patients should be to prevent death and disability associated with high blood pressure (BP). In addition, other reversible risk factors for cardiovascular disease need to be addressed. The diagnosis of hypertension should be based on multiple BP measurements obtained in a standardized fashion on at least three occasions. Supine, sitting and standing BPs should be measured in all diabetic patients. Automated ambulatory BP monitoring may be especially helpful in the diabetic patient for evaluating BP control over 24 hours to document the absence of the usual nocturnal fall in BP in diabetes (especially with autonomic dysfunction or nephropathy). In type 2 diabetic patients, who often do not have a normal nocturnal drop in BP [72], a loss of circadian variation of BP is closely related to vascular complications in non-diabetic subjects. Our findings may indicate an important relationship between non-dipping of BP and the high morbidity and mortality rate in diabetic patients with increased urinary albumen excretion rate [72]. Ambulatory BP monitoring may also be useful in documenting episodic hypertension, orthostatic hypotension or resistant hypertension, which are relatively common in diabetic individuals with accompanying hypertension. Although the optimal BP level during antihypertensive treatment in patients with diabetic nephropathy has not been defined, a review of the relationship between the rate of fall in GFR and the BP level during antihypertensive treatments suggests that we should strive for lower goal BP than recommended for other patients with hypertension (i.e. 130/85) [1] (Figure 5.1).

5.10.2 NON-PHARMACOLOGICAL THERAPY IN DIABETIC HYPERTENSIVE PATIENTS

Hygienic measures may serve as definitive therapy for mild hypertension in diabetic patients or as an adjunct to pharmacological therapy to lower the number and dose of antihypertensive drugs. The diet recommended by the American Diabetes Association, which is low in calories and fat, high in carbohydrate and soluble fibre, and moderately low in protein, has been reported to lower BP in diabetic patients [1, 2, 71]. Moderate salt restriction reduces systolic BP, which is often inordinately elevated in diabetic

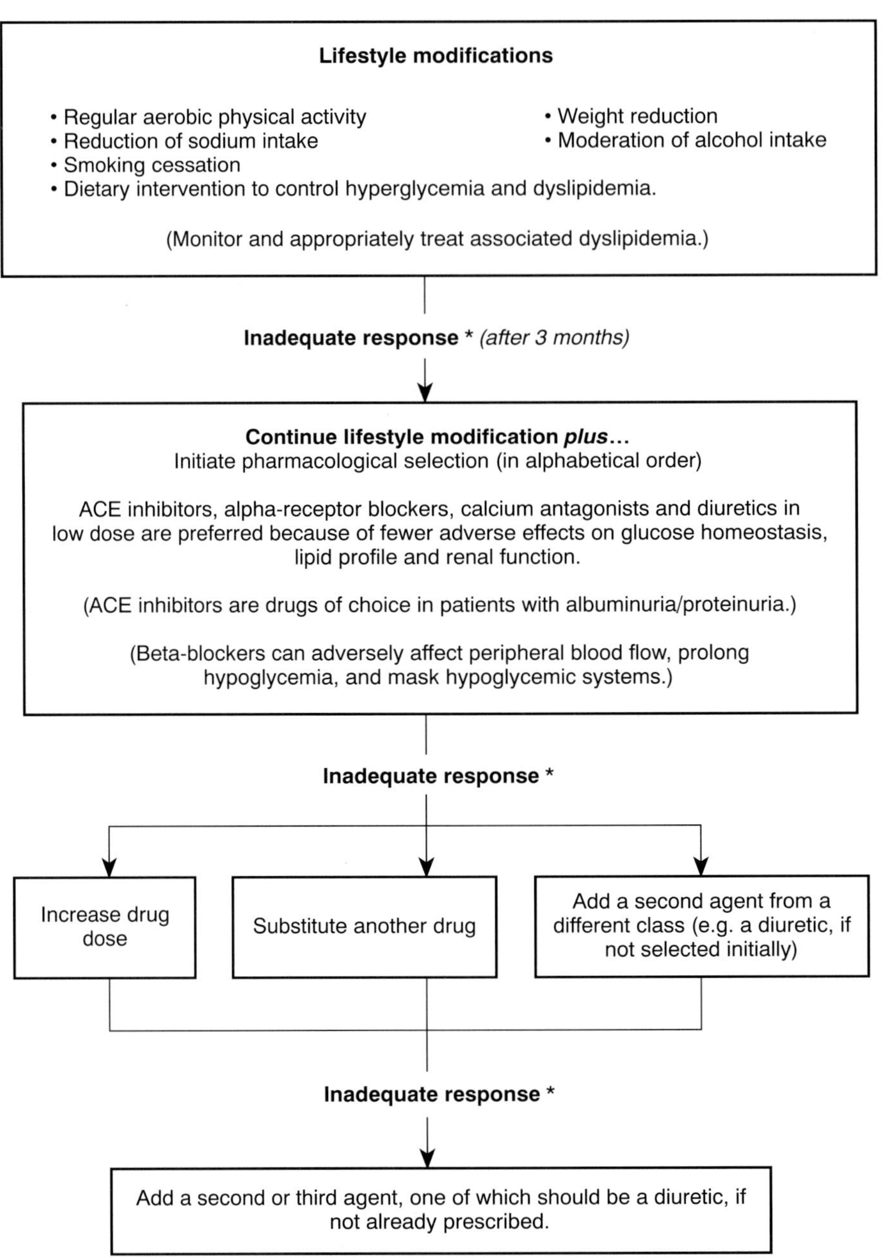

Figure 5.1 Suggested approach to hypertension therapy in diabetic individuals. Treatment goal is to maintain BP at less than 130/85 mmHg. Diabetic renal disease, autonomic dysfunction and adverse effects on glucose and lipid metabolism must be considered before the·course of therapeutic intervention is chosen. (Adapted from [1] with modification.)

patients [2]. Weight reduction is important, particularly in type 2 diabetes and improves glucose tolerance as well as reducing BP [1, 2]. For example, for each 10 lb (4.5 kg) weight reduction, systolic and diastolic pressures can be expected to decrease by 10 and 5 mmHg, respectively [8, 10]. Moderate but regular aerobic exercise improves glycaemic and lipaemic control and helps with weight reduction. Results of the Diabetes Control and Complications Trial (DCCT) [73], a seven-year study of more than 1440 patients with type 1 diabetes, demonstrated that intensive insulin therapy reduced the occurrence of microalbuminuria by 39% and that of albuminuria by 54%. In addition, intensified therapy patients had lower rates of serious retinopathy requiring photocoagulation, lower rates of decreased visual acuity and fewer cases of nephropathy. Similar results were reported from a study designed to test the hypothesis that optimized glycaemic control in type 1 diabetic recipients of renal allografts will prevent or delay diabetic renal lesions in the allograft [74]. These data suggest that aggressive control of blood sugar in the very early stages of this disease process can provide significant protection against its development.

In type 2 diabetes mellitus, oral hypoglycaemic agents are increasingly used in the treatment of hyperglycaemia. These agents have different metabolic effects and have recently been recognized to have disparate effects on blood pressure. In both human and animal studies, chlorpropamide and glyburide (first- and a second-generation sulphonylureas, respectively) have been observed to aggravate pre-existing hypertension [75, 76]. In contrast, thiazolidinediones (pioglitazone, ciglitazone and troglitazone) have been shown recently to significantly lower blood pressure in obese normotensive humans [77] and attenuate hypertension in animal models with high BP [77]. Metformin and thiazolidinediones have been shown to attenuate VSMC inward Ca^{2+} currents [78–80]. In addition, long-term administration of the biguanide metformin has been shown to completely normalize arterial pressure in one group of hypertensive patients [81].

Sulphonylureas are widely recognized for their ability to inhibit adenosine triphosphate (ATP)-sensitive potassium (K) channels in various tissues [76]. Agents which open these channels (e.g. crmakalim) are thought to reduce vascular contractility largely by direct, rapid relaxation of the smooth muscle in the arterial wall. Thus, sulphonylureas may increase vascular tone by inhibiting ATP-sensitive K channels in VSMC. It has been reported that acute administration of thiazolinediones attenuates inward current through voltage-gated calcium channels in isolated aortic and tail arterial VSMC [78, 79]. Additionally, thioglitazones inhibit potassium-induced (membrane depolarization related) contractions in rat aortic rings. Recently, metformin has shown to attenuate agonist-stimulated calcium transients in VSMC [81]. Thus sulphonylareas, metformin and thioglitazones exert different effects on arterial contractile responsiveness simply because of their disparate effects on ion channels in the VSMC membrane.

5.10.3 PHARMACOLOGICAL THERAPY

Four major classes of antihypertensive drugs used in the USA for the diabetic hypertensive patient are discussed below.

Thiazide diuretics

Thiazide diuretics, in relatively low doses (i.e. 25 mg or less hydrochlorothiazide or chlorthalidone daily) appear to be effective and safe antihypertensive agents in patients with diabetes [1, 2, 82] (Figure 5.1). In the SHEP study, elderly men with type 2 diabetes derived as much benefit, in terms of stroke and ischaemic heart disease reduction, as those without diabetes. Diuretics are also useful antihypertensive drugs when used in conjunction with ACE inhibitors; this combination is often synergistic in lowering BP and minimizes the metabolic side effects of diuretics [1, 2].

ACE inhibitors

Experimental studies have provided a theoretic framework for anticipating that ACE inhibition may preferentially retard the progression of diabetic renal disease. In this regard, a sustained increase in glomerular capillary pressure evoked in response to loss of renal mass produces a destructive sclerosing reaction [83]. Administration of ACE inhibitors decreases glomerular capillary pressure with a resultant reduction of glomerular sclerosis, suggesting that ACE inhibitor therapy may protect the injured kidney from haemodynamically mediated glomerular damage [83] in addition to their effects on pathological processes other than glomerular hypertension.. Indeed, ACE inhibitors may selectively affect the mesangial cell, a pivotal cell in the development of glomerulosclerosis. In agreement with this concept, the ACE inhibitor captopril has been shown to be more effective in slowing the progression of diabetic nephropathy than are agents that act primarily by reducing blood pressure in type 1 diabetic patients [84]. A recent long-term five-year clinical trial in 94 type 2 patients was conducted evaluating the effects of ACE inhibition on proteinuria and on the rate of decline in renal function in normotensive type 2 patients with microalbuminuria [85]. It was reported that ACE inhibition during the early stages of diabetic nephropathy resulted in long-term stabilization of plasma creatinine levels and of the degree of urinary loss of albumin. A three-year prospective, double-blind, placebo-controlled trial in type 2 patients demonstrated that an antihypertensive regimen, which included the ACE inhibitor enalapril, preserved renal function to a greater extent than did therapy with antihypertensive agents excluding ACE inhibitors [86]. These investigators suggested that ACE inhibitors should be used as initial treatment for hypertensive type 2 diabetic patients with or without microalbuminuria and not held in reserve until clinical albuminuria or proteinuria develops.

Despite these promising results, several caveats are in order. ACE inhibitors are not free of side effects. An infrequent but important risk with ACE inhibitors is an acceleration of renal insufficiency, particularly in patients with bilateral renal artery stenosis [1, 2]. Close monitoring of renal function and serum potassium should be performed in the first few weeks after initiation of therapy if cardiac failure is present or bilateral renal artery disease is suspected. Importantly ACE inhibitors may provoke hyperkalaemia, particularly in those individuals with decrements in GFR or hyporeninaemic hypoaldosteronism [1, 2]. Finally care must be exercised in initiating ACE inhibitor therapy in patients receiving diuretics because there may be a profound drop in blood pressure and a decline in renal function.

Calcium antagonists

Calcium antagonists preferentially dilate afferent arterioles but their reduction in systemic pressure probably produces a negligible increase in glomerular pressure despite afferent arteriolar vasodilation [87, 88]. Additionally, calcium antagonists have properties that contribute to their ability to afford renal protection under diverse experimental conditions and perhaps in clinical disorders [87, 88]. These include the ability to lessen injury by retarding renal growth, to attenuate mesangial entrapment of macromolecules and to countervail the mitogenic effect of diverse mediators including platelet-derived growth factor and platelet-activating factor [2, 11, 38, 70]. An additional mechanism by which calcium antagonists might exert protective effects is by amelioration of mitochondrial calcium overload with consequent mitochondrial malfunction and eventual cell death [38, 87]. Indeed, a number of studies in animal models of diabetes have suggested that calcium antagonists may be renoprotective in retarding progression of diabetic nephropathy [2, 38, 87, 88]. Studies regarding calcium antagonists and diabetic renal disease have been widely divergent in their design as well as in their findings [88, 89]. Several studies [89–92], including a long-term prospective trial [92], have suggested that calcium antagonists may also be efficacious in ameliorating diabetic proteinuria. Many of the studies have sought to compare calcium antagonists to ACE inhibitor therapy in conferring beneficial effects on glomerular permeability to proteins and, in a few instances, in attenuating progression in patients with established diabetic glomerular disease. The results of these reports have been widely divergent. Although calcium antagonist therapy has been found to diminish proteinuria significantly in some studies [89–91], others have shown either no effect or an actual worsening of the proteinuria [89]. A number of flaws of design in several of the studies have confounded their interpretation [88].

ACE inhibitors versus calcium antagonists

In contrast to the relatively short studies previously described, one study [93] compared the effects of the long-acting dihydropyridine, nisoldipine, with those of an ACE inhibitor, lisinopril, on proteinuria and on the decline of GFR in hypertensive type 2 diabetic subjects. There was a striking dissociation between the antiproteinuric effects and the effects on GFR. Albuminuria was reduced by 47% in the lisinopril group compared with no decrement in the nisoldipine group. In marked contrast, the decline in GFR appeared to be less steep in the nisoldipine group compared with the lisinopril group. These observations clearly demonstrate that a dihydropyridine, presumably operating through mechanisms independent of any renal microcirculatory effect, is renoprotective. In summary, the available results are consistent with the formulation that ACE inhibitors and calcium antagonists act in a complementary manner to attenuate the progression of chronic renal failure.

During the past two years, other studies have been published comparing the effects of an ACE inhibitor with that of dihydropyridine-type calcium antagonist in type 2 diabetic patients [94, 95]. Most studies were of short duration; we will comment only on those studies that were at least of one-year's duration. Chan *et al.* [94] conducted a one-year double-blind study of hypertensive type 2 diabetic patients assigned to either enalapril or nifedipine with matching placebos for the alternative drug. Creatinine clearance fell similarly in both groups but plasma creatinine concentration was increased by 20% in the enalapril group compared with 8% in the nifedipine group. Although enalapril reduced proteinuria significantly more than nifedipine in the microalbuminuric and macroalbuminuric patients, it was more likely to increase plasma creatinine concentrations. Another group [95] compared the effects of enalapril and nifedipine on renal function, proteinuria and BP in type 2 diabetic patients with proteinuria. Both drugs induced a similar hypotensive effect. Enalapril produced an antiproteinuric effect whereas proteinuria persisted in the nifedipine group.

In summary, the available data suggest that the level of pre-existing renal function may be an important determinant of the ultimate renal response to calcium antagonist administration, i.e. patients with renal insufficiency may manifest a worsening of renal function with nifedipine, whereas patients with normal renal function do not. Additional studies will be required to elucidate the determinants of these varying responses. Whether worsening of renal function is attributable only to specific calcium antagonists or represents a class effect remains to be established.

Beta-blockers

Beta-blockers without intrinsic sympathomimetic activity (ISA) have been shown to reduce cardiovascular morbidity and mortality in large, population-based, randomized trials [1, 2]. In addition, they prevent recurrent myocardial infarction and sudden death, and reduce total cardiovascular mortality for up to 18 months after an acute myocardial infarction. Nevertheless, several concerns limit the usefulness of beta-blockers in treating people with diabetes. (a) These agents may have adverse effects on glucose and lipid metabolism. (b) Most troublesome for the insulin-treated diabetic subject is the observation that beta-blockers can interfere with awareness of hypoglycaemia in patients with diabetes and perhaps also prolong the recovery from hypoglycaemia [1, 2]. (c) Beta-blockers can reduce peripheral blood flow and worsen claudication and vasospasm in patients who already have a compromised peripheral vascular system [1, 2]. (d) Finally, when beta-blockers are added to diuretics, an aggravation of the hyperglycaemic effect of the latter may occur [96]. A recently reported study by Bakris *et al.* [97] showed that therapy with the calcium antagonist, verapamil, resulted in a slower rate of decline in renal function and a greater reduction in proteinuria than therapy with the beta-blocker, atenolol (54 months of therapy) in African Americans with type 2 diabetes mellitus. Thus, except under special circumstances (e.g. in the presence of angina pectoris and post-myocardial infarction), beta-blockers should no longer be used as first-line antihypertensive medications in these patients.

Combination of a calcium antagonist and ACE-inhibitor

In addition, it has been proposed that the combination of a calcium antagonist with an ACE inhibitor should result in a greater reduction in urinary protein excretion and slower morphological progression of nephropathy [11, 72]. One study compared the renal haemodynamic and antiproteinuric effects of a calcium antagonist, verapamil, and an ACE inhibitor, lisinopril, alone and in combination in three groups of subjects with type 2 diabetes and documented nephrotic range proteinuria, hypertension and renal insufficiency [98]. Patients treated with the combination of a calcium antagonist and an ACE inhibitor manifested the greatest reduction in albuminuria. In addition, the decline in GFR was the lowest in this group. A six-year follow-up study in these patients with nephropathy from type 2 diabetes supports the observation that combination therapy with ACE inhibitors and calcium antagonists reduces nephrotic-range proteinuria more than either agent alone [99]. This benefit occurred in the absence of additional antihypertensive effects of the combination therapy [99]. While such an approach is extremely attractive, additional studies will be required to confirm and extend these initial observations.

REFERENCES

1. The National High Blood Pressure Education Program Working Group. National high blood pressure education program working group report on hypertension in diabetes. *Hypertension*, 1994, **23**, 145–58.
2. Sowers, J.R. and Epstein, M. Diabetes mellitus and associated hypertension, vascular disease and nephropathy: an update. *Hypertension*, 1995, **26**, 869–79.
3. Zavaroni, I., Bonora, E., Pagliara, M., Dall'Aglio, E., Luchetti, L., Giuseppe, B., Bonati, P.A., Bergonzani, M., Gnudi, L., Passeri, M. and Reaven, G. Risk factors for coronary artery disease in healthy persons with hyperinsulinemia and normal glucose tolerance. *N. Engl. J. Med.*, 1989, **320**, 702–6.
4. Landin, K., Tengborn, L. and Smith, U. Elevated fibrinogen and plasminogen activator inhibitor (PAI-1) in hypertensive are related to metabolic risk factors for cardiovascular disease. *J. Intern. Med.*, 1990, **227**, 273–8.

5. Monolio, T.A., Savage, P.J. and Burke, G.L. Association of fasting insulin with blood pressure and lipids in young adults: the Cardia Study. *Atherosclerosis,* 1990, **10,** 430–6.

6. Spiegelman, D., Issail, R.G., Bouchard, C. and Willett, W.C. Absolute fat mass, percent body fat, and body-fat distribution: which is the real determinant of blood pressure and serum glucose? *Am. J. Clin. Nutr.,* 1992, **55,** 1033–44.

7. Sowers, J.R., Standley, P.R., Ram, J.L., Jacober, S.J., Simpson, L. and Rose, K. Hyperinsulinemia, insulin resistance, and hyperglycemia: contributing factors in the pathogenesis of hypertension and atherosclerosis. *Am J. Hypertens.,* 1993, **6,** 260S–70S.

8. Jacobs, D.B., Sowers, J.R., Hmeidan, A., Niyogi, T., Simpson, L. and Standley, P.R. Effects of weight reduction and cellular cation metabolism and vascular resistance. *Hypertension,* 1993, **21,** 308–14.

9. Walsh, M.F., Dominguez, L.J. and Sowers, J.R. Metabolic abnormalities in cardiac ischemia. *Cardiol. Clin.,* 1995, **13,** 529–38.

10. Ikeda, T., Gomi, T., Hirawa, N., Sakurai, J. and Yoshikawa, N. Improvement of insulin sensitivity contributes to blood pressure reduction after weight loss in hypertensive subjects with obesity. *Hypertension,* 1996, **27,** 1180–6.

11. Bakris, G.L., Weir, M.R. and Sowers, J.R. Therapeutic challenges in the obese diabetic patient with hypertension. *Am. J. Med.,* 1996, **101**(3A), 33S–46S.

12. Pyorala, K. Relationship of glucose tolerance and plasma insulin to the incidence of coronary heart disease: results from two population studies in Finland. *Diabetes Care,* 1979, **2,** 131–41.

13. Ducimentiere, P., Eschwege, E., Papoz, L., Richard, J.L., Claude, J.R. and Rosselin, G. Relationship of plasma insulin level to the incidence of myocardial infarction and coronary heart disease. *Diabetologia,* 1980, **19,** 205–10.

14. Fontbonne, A., Charles, M.A., Thibult, N., Richard, J.L., Claude, J.R., Warnet, J.M., Rosselin, G.E. and Eschwége, E. Hyperinsulinemia as a predictor of coronary heart disease mortality in a healthy population: the Paris Prospective Study, 15-year follow-up. *Diabetologia,* 1991, **34,** 356–61.

15. Després, J.P., Lamarche, B., Mauriege, P., Cantin, B., Dagenais, G.R., Moorjani, S. and Lupien, P.J. Hyperinsulinemia as an independent risk factor for ischemic heart disease. *N. Engl. J. Med.,* 1996, **334,** 952–7.

16. Ferrara, L.A., Mancini, M., Celentano, A., Galderisi, M., Iannuzi, R., Marotta, T. and Gaeta, I. Early changes of the arterial carotid wall in hyperinsulinemia, hypertriglyceridemia versus hypercholesterolemia. *Arterioscler. Thromb.,* 1993, **13,** 367–70.

17. Folsom, A.R., Eckfeldt, J.H., Weitzman, S., Ma, J., Chambless, L.E., Barnes, R.W., Cram, K.B. and Hutchinson, R.G. Atherosclerosis Risk in Communities (ARIC) Study Investigators. Relation of carotid artery wall thickness in diabetes mellitus, fasting glucose and insulin, body size, and physical activity. *Stroke,* 1994, **25,** 66–73.

18. Salomaa, V., Riley, W., Kaark, J.D., Nardo, C. and Folsom, A.R. Non-insulin dependent diabetes mellitus and fasting glucose and insulin concentrations are associated with arterial stiffness index, the ARIC study. *Circulation,* 1995, **91,** 1432–43.

19. Agewall, S., Fagerberg, B., Attvall, S., Wendelhag, I., Urbanavicius, V. and Wikstrand, J. Carotid artery wall intima-media thickness is associated with insulin-mediated glucose disposal in men at high and low coronary risk. *Stroke,* 1995, **26,** 956–60.

20. Shinozaki, K., Naritomi, H., Shimizu, T., Suzuki, M., Ikebuchi, M., Sawada, T. and Harano, Y. Role of insulin resistance associated with compensatory hyperinsulinemia in ischemic stroke. *Stroke,* 1996, **27,** 37–43.

21. Sowers, J.R., Sowers, P.S. and Peuler, J.D. Role of insulin resistance and hyperinsulinemia in development of hypertension and atherosclerosis. *J. Lab. Clin. Med.,* 1994, **123,** 647–52.

22. Landin, D., Krotkiewski, M. and Smith, U. Importance of obesity for the metabolic abnormalities associated with an abdominal fat distribution. *Metabolism,* 1989, **38,** 572–6.

23. Jensen, M., Haymond, M., Rizza, R., Cryer, P. and Moles, J. Influence of body fat distribution on free fatty acid metabolism in obesity. *J. Clin. Invest.,* 1989, **83,** 1168–73.

24. Dowse, G.K., Zimmet, P.Z. and Gareeboo, H. Abdominal obesity and physical inactivity as risk factors for NIDDM and impaired glucose intolerance in Indian, Creole, and Chinese Mauritians. *Diabetes Care,* 1991, **14,** 271–82.

25. Colditz, G.A., Willet, W.C., Rotsnitzky, A. and Manson, J.E. Weight gain as a risk factor for

clinical diabetes in women. *Ann. Intern. Med.,* 1995, **122**, 481–6.

26. Sowers, J.R. Modest weight gain and the development of diabetes: another perspective. *Ann. Intern. Med.,* 1995, **122**, 548–9.

27. Portaluppi, F., Pansini, F., Manfredini, R. and Mollica, G. Relative influence of menopausal status, age and body mass index on blood pressure. *Hypertension,* 1997, **29**, 976–9.

28. Klein, R., Klein, B.E.K. and Moss, S.E. Is obesity related to microvascular complications in diabetes? *Arch. Intern. Med.,* 1997, **157**, 650–6.

29. Ferraro, R.T., Eckel, R.H., Larson, D.E., Fontvielle, A.M., Rising, R., Jensen, D.R. and Ravussin, E. Relationship between skeletal muscle lipoprotein lipase activity and 24-hour macronutrient oxidation. *J. Clin. Invest.,* 1993, **92**, 441–5.

30. Ferrannini, E., Buzzigoli, G., Bonadonna, R., Giorico, M.A., Oleggini, M., Graziadei, L., Pedrinelli, R., Brandi, L. and Bevilacqua, S. Insulin resistance in essential hypertension. *N. Engl. J. Med.,* 1987, **317**, 350–7.

31. Hunt, S.C., Hassedt, S.J. and Kuida, H. Genetic heritability and common environmental components of resting and stressed blood pressures, lipids, and body mass index in Utah pedigrees and twins. *Am. J. Epidemiol.,* 1989, **129**, 625–38.

32. Williams, R.R., Hunt, S.C. and Hasstedt, S.J. Are there interactions and relations between genetic and environmental factors predisposing to high blood pressure? *Hypertension,* 1991, (suppl 1), I29–I37.

33. Shinozaki, K., Suzuki, M., Ikebuchi, M., Takaki, H., Hara, Y., Tsushima, M. and Harano, Y. Insulin resistance associated with compensatory hyperinsulinemia as an independent risk factor for vasospastic angina. *Circulation,* 1995, **92**, 1749–57.

34. Welborn, T.A. and Wearne, K. Coronary heart disease incidence and cardiovascular mortality in Busselton with reference to glucose and insulin concentrations. *Diabetes Care,* 1979, **2**, 154–60.

35. Taittonen, L., Uhari, M., Nuutinen, M., Turtinen, J., Pokka, T. and Akerblom, H.K. Insulin and blood pressure among healthy children; cardiovascular risk in young Finns. *Am J. Hypertens.,* 1996, **9**, 193–9.

36. Sowers, J.R. Insulin and insulin-like growth factor in normal and pathological cardiovascular physiology. *Hypertension,* 1997, **29**, 691–9.

37. King, G.L., Goodman, A.D., Buzney, S. and Moses, A. Receptors and insulin-like growth factors on cells from bovine retinal capillaries and aorta. *J. Clin. Invest.,* 1985, **75**, 1028–36.

38. Bakris, G.L., Palant, C.E., Walsh, M.F. and Sowers, J.R. Analogy between endothelial/mesangial cell and endothelial/vascular smooth muscle cell interactions: role of growth factors and mechanotransduction. In *Endocrinology of the Vasculature,* (ed. J.R. Sowers), Humana Press, Totowa, NJ, 1996, pp. 341–55.

39. Davi, G., Catalons, I., Averna, M. *et al.* Thromboxane biosynthesis and platelet function in type II diabetes mellitus. *N. Engl. J. Med.,* 1990, **322**, 1768–74.

40. Standley, P.R., Ali, S., Bapna, C. and Sowers, J.R. Increased platelet cytosolic calcium responses to low density lipoprotein in type II diabetes with and without hypertension. *Am J. Hypertens.,* 1993, **6**, 938–43.

41. Levy, J., Gavin, J.R. III and Sowers, J.R. Diabetes mellitus: a disease of abnormal cellular calcium metabolism? *Am. J. Med.,* 1994, **96**, 260–70.

42. Winocour, P.D., Bryszewska, M., Watula, C. *et al.* Reduced membrane fluidity in platelets from diabetic patients. *Diabetes,* 1990, **39**, 241–4.

43. Sampretro, T., Lenzi, S., Cicchetti, P. *et al.* Non-enzymatic glycation of human platelet membrane proteins *in vitro* and *in vivo. Clin. Chem.,* 1986, **32**, 1328–31.

44. Aviram, M. Modified forms of low density lipoproteins affect platelet aggregation in vitro. *Thromb. Res.,* 1989, **53**, 561–7.

45. GarcRa Frade, L.J., de la Calle, H., Alava, I., Navarro, J.L., Creight, L.J. and Gaffney, L.J. Diabetes mellitus as an hypercoagulable state: its relationship with fibrin fragments and vascular damage. *Thromb. Res.,* 1987, **47**, 533–40.

46. Ford, I., Singh, T.P., Kitchen, S., Makris, M., Ward, J.D. and Preston, F.E. Activation of coagulation in diabetes mellitus in relation to the presence of vascular complications. *Diabetic Med.,* 1991, **8**, 322–9.

47. Carmassi, F., Morale, M., Puccetti, R. *et al.* Coagulation and fibrinolytic system impairment in insulin dependent diabetes mellitus. *Thromb. Res.,* 1992, **67**, 643–54.

48. Sowers, J.R., Tuck, M.L. and Sowers, D.K. Plasma antithrombin III and thrombin generation time: correlation with hemoglobin A1 and fasting serum glucose in young diabetic women. *Diabetes Care,* 1980, **3,** 655–8.

49. Ceriello, A., Quatraro, A., Dello Russo, P. *et al.* Protein C deficiency in insulin dependent diabetes: a hyperglycemia-related phenomenon. *Thromb. Haemost.,* 1990, **64,** 104–7.

50. Vukovich, T.C., Proidl, S., Knöbl, P., Teufelsbauer, H., Schnack, C. and Schernthaner, G. The effect of insulin treatment on the balance between tissue plasminogen activator and plasminogen activator inhibitor-1 in type 2 diabetic patients. *Thromb. Haemost.,* 1992, **68,** 253–6.

51. Hamsten, A., de Faire, U., Walldius, G. *et al.* Plasminogen activator inhibitor in plasma: risk factor for recurrent myocardial infarction. *Lancet,* 1987, **ii,** 3–9.

52. Ramirez, L.C., Arauz-Pacheco, C., Lackner, C. *et al.* Lipoprotein (a) levels in diabetes mellitus: Relationship to metabolic control. *Ann. Intern. Med.,* 1992, **117,** 42–7.

53. Cagliero, E., Roth, T., Roy, S. and Lorenzi, M. Characteristics and mechanisms of high-glucose-induced over-expression of basement membrane components in cultured human endothelial cells. *Diabetes,* 1991, **40,** 102–10.

54. Bucala, R., Makita, Z., Koschinsky, T., Cerami, A. and Vlassara, H. Lipid advanced glycosylation: pathway for lipid oxidation *in vivo. Proc. Natl Acad. Sci. USA,* 1993, **90,** 6434–8.

55. Grekin, R.J., Vollmer, A.P. and Sider, R.S. Pressor effects of portal venous oleate infusion: a proposed mechanism for obesity hypertension. *Hypertension,* 1995, **26,** 193–8.

56. Stepniakowski, K.T., Goodfriend, T.L. and Egan, B.M. Fatty Acids enhance vascular α-adrenergic sensitivity. *Hypertension,* 1995, **25,** 774–8.

57. Stepniakowski, K.T., Sallee, F.R., Goodfriend, T.L., Zhang, Z. and Egan, B.M. Fatty acids enhance neurovascular reflex responses by effects on α1-adrenoceptors. *Am. J. Physiol.,* 1996, **270,** R1340–6.

58. Egan, B.M., Hennes, M.M.I., O'Shaughnessy, I.M., Stepniakowski, K.T., Kissebah, A.H. and Goodfriend, T.L. Obesity hypertension is more closely related to impairment of insulin's fatty acid than glucose lowering action. *Hypertension,* 1996, **27,** 723–8.

59. Simon, J.A., Fong, J. and Bernert, J.T. Serum fatty acids and blood pressure. *Hypertension,* 1996, **27,** 303–7.

60. Egan, B.M. and Stepniakowski, K.T. Evidence linking fatty acids, the risk factor cluster, and vascular pathophysiology: implications for the diabetic hypertensive patient. In *Endocrinology of the Vasculature,* (ed. J.R. Sowers), Humana Press, Totowa, NJ, 1996, pp. 157–72.

61. Golub, M.S., Hori, M.T. and Tuck, M.L. Arachidonic acid metabolites in the vasculature. In *Endocrinology of the Vasculature,* (ed. J.R. Sowers), Humana Press, Totowa, NJ, 1996, pp. 357–72.

62. Hsueh, W.A. and Anderson, P.W. Hypertension, the endothelial cell, and the vascular complications of diabetes mellitus. *Hypertension,* 1992, **20,** 253–63.

63. Creager, M.A., Cooke, J.P., Mendelsohn, M., Gallagher, S.J., Coleman, S.M., Loscalzo, J. and Dzau, V.J. Impaired vasodilation of forearm resistance vessels in hypercholesterolemic humans. *J. Clin. Invest.,* 1990, **86,** 228–34.

64. Tesfamariam, B., Brown, M.L. and Cohen, R.A. Elevated glucose impaired endothelium-dependent relaxation by activating protein kinase C. *J. Clin. Invest.,* 1991, **87,** 1643–8.

65. Inoguchi, T., Xia, P., Kunisaki, M., Higashi, S., Feener, E.P. and King, G.L. Insulin's effect on protein kinase C and diacylglycerol induced by diabetes and glucose in vascular tissues. *Am. J. Physiol.,* 1994, **267,** E369–79.

66. Cockcroft, J.R., Chowienczyk, P.G., Benjamin, N. and Ritter, J.M. Preserved endothelium-dependent vasodilation in patients with essential hypertension. *N. Engl. J. Med.,* 1994, **330,** 1036–40.

67. Chavers, B.M., Bilous, R.W., Ellis, E.N., Steffes, M.W. and Mauer, S.M. Glomerular lesions and urinary albumin excretion in type I diabetes without overt proteinuria. *N. Engl. J. Med.,* 1989, **320,** 966–70.

68. Myers, B.D. Pathophysiology of proteinuria in diabetic glomerular disease. *J. Hypertens.,* 1990, **8,** S41–6.

69. Shultz, P.J., Schorer, A.E. and Raij, L. Effects of endothelium-derived relaxing factor and nitric oxide on rat mesangial cells. *Am. J. Physiol.,* 1990, **258,** F162–F167.

70. Bakris, G.L., Fairbanks, R. and Traish, A.M. Arginine vasopressin stimulates human mesangial cell production of endothelin. *J. Clin. Invest.,* 1991, **87,** 1158–64.

71. Sowers, J.R. and Epstein, M. Diabetes mellitus and hypertension, emerging therapeutic perspectives. *Cardiovasc. Drug Rev.*, 1995, **13**, 149–210.

72. Equiluz-Bruck, Schnack, C., Kopp, H.P. and Schernthaner, G. Nondipping of nocturnal blood pressure is related to urinary albumen excretion rate in patients with type 2 diabetes mellitus. *Am J. Hypertens.*, 1996, **9**, 1139–43.

73. The Diabetes Control and Complications Trial Health Research Group. The effect of intensive treatment of diabetes on the development and progression of long term complications in insulin dependent diabetes mellitus. *N. Engl. J. Med.*, **329**, 977–86.

74. Barbosa, J., Steffes, M.W., Sutherland, D.E.R., Connett, J.E., Rao, K.V. and Mauer, M.S. Effect of glycemic control on early diabetic renal lesions: a 5-year randomized controlled clinical trial of insulin-dependent diabetic kidney transplant recipients. *J. Am. Med. Assoc.*, 1994, **272**, 600–6.

75. Peuler, J.D., Johnson, B.A.B., Phare, S.M. and Sowers, J.R. Sex-specific effects of an insulin secretagogue in stroke-prone hypertensive rats. *Hypertension*, 1993, **22**, 214–20.

76. Schmitt, J.K. and Moore, J.R. Hypertension secondary to chlorpropamide with amelioration by changing to insulin. *Am J. Hypertens.*, 1993, **6**, 317–19.

77. Nolan, J.J., Ludvik, B., Beerdsen, P., Joyce, M. and Olefsky, J. Improvement in glucose tolerance and insulin resistance in obese subjects treated with troglitazone. *N. Engl. J. Med.*, 1994, **331**, 1188–93.

78. Zhang, F., Sowers, J.R., Ram, J.L., Standley, P.R. and Peuler, J.D. Effects of pioglitazone on L-type calcium channels in vascular smooth muscle. *Hypertension*, 1994, **24**, 170–5.

79. Song, J., Walsh, M.F., Igwe, R., Ram, J.L., Barazi, M., Dominguez, L.J. and Sowers, J.R. Troglitazone reduces contraction by inhibition of vascular smooth muscle cells Ca^{2+} currents and not endothelial nitric oxide production. *Diabetes*, 1997, **46**, 659–64.

80. Dominguez, L.J., Davidoff, A.J., Srinivas, P.R., Standley, P.R., Walsh, M.F. and Sowers, J.R. Effects of metformin on tyrosine kinase activity, glucose transport, and intracellular calcium in rat vascular smooth muscle. *Endocrinology*, 1996, **137**, 113–21.

81. Landin, K., Tengborn, L. and Smith, U. Treating insulin resistance in hypertension with metformin reduces both blood pressure and metabolic risk factors. *J. Intern. Med.*, 1991, **229**, 181–7.

82. Curb, J.D., Pressel, S.L., Cutler, J.A. *et al.* Effect of diuretic-based anti-hypertensive treatment on cardiovascular disease risk in older diabetic patients with isolated systolic hypertension. *J. Am. Med. Assoc.*, 1996, **276**, 1886–92.

83. Meyer, T.W., Anderson, S., Rennke, H.G. and Brenner, B.M. Reversing glomerular hypertension stabilizes established glomerular injury. *Kidney Int.*, 1987, **31**, 752–9.

84. Lewis, E.J., Hunsicker, L.G., Bain, R.P. and Rohde, R.D. for the Collaborative Study Group. The effect of angiotensin-converting enzyme therapy on diabetic nephropathy. *N. Engl. J. Med.*, 1993, **329**, 1456–62.

85. Ravid, M., Savin, H., Jutrin, I., Bental, T., Katz, B. and Lishner, M. Long-term stabilizing effect of angiotensin-converting enzyme inhibition on plasma creatinine and on proteinuria in normotensive type II diabetic patients. *Ann. Intern. Med.*, 1993, **118**, 577–81.

86. Lebovitz, H.E., Wiegmann, T.B., Cnaan, A., Shahinfar, S., Sica, D.A., Broadstone, V., Schwartz, S.L., Mengel, M.C., Segal, R., Versaggi, J.A. and Bolton, W.K. Renal protective effects of enalapril in hypertensive NIDDM: role of baseline albuminuria. *Kidney Int.*, 1994, **45** (suppl 45), S150–5.

87. Epstein, M. Calcium antagonists and renal protection: Current status and future perspectives. *Arch. Intern. Med.*, 1992, **152**, 1573–84.

88. Epstein, M. Calcium antagonists and diabetic nephropathy. *Arch. Intern. Med.*, 1991, **151**, 2361–4.

89. Demarie, B.K. and Bakris, G.L. Effects of different calcium antagonists on proteinuria associated with diabetes mellitus. *Ann. Intern. Med.*, 1990, **113**, 987–8.

90. Baba, T., Ishizaki, T., Ido, Y., Aoyagi, K., Murabayashi, S. and Takebe, K. Renal effects of nicardipine, a calcium entry blocker, in hypertensive type II diabetic patients with nephropathy. *Diabetes*, 1986, **35**, 1206–14.

91. Bakris, G.L. Effects of diltiazem or lisinopril on massive proteinuria associated with diabetes mellitus. *Ann. Intern. Med.*, 1990, **112**, 701–2.

92. Doyle, A.E. Comparison between perindopril and nifedipine in hypertensive and normotensive diabetics with microalbuminuria. Mel-

bourne Diabetic Nephropathy Study Group. *Br. Med. J.*, 1991, **302** (6770), 210–15.

93. Rossing, P., Tarnow, L., Boelskifter, S., Jensen, B.R., Nielsen, F.S. and Parving, H.H. Differences between nisoldipine and lisinopril on glomerular filtration rates and albuminuria in hypertensive IDDM patients with diabetic nephropathy during the first year of treatment. *Diabetes*, 1997, **46**, 481–7.

94. Chan, J.C., Cockram, C.S., Nicholls, M.G., Cheung, C.K. and Swaminathan, R. Comparison of enalapril and nifedipine in treating non-insulin dependent diabetes associated with hypertension: one year analysis. *Br. Med. J.*, 1992, **305**, 981–5.

95. Ferder, L., Daccordi, H.A. and Mariello, M. Angiotensin converting enzyme inhibitors versus calcium antagonists in the treatment of diabetic hypertensive patients. *Hypertension*, 1992, **19** (suppl 2), 237–42.

96. Dornhorst, A., Powell, S.H. and Pensky, J. Aggravation by propranolol of hyperglycaemic effect of hydrochlorothiazide in type II diabetics without alterations of insulin secretion. *Lancet*, 1985, **i**, 123–6.

97. Bakris, G.L., Mangrum, A., Copley, J.B., Vicknair, N. and Sadler, R. Effect of calcium channel or β-blockade on the progression of diabetic nephropathy in African Americans. *Hypertension*, 1997, **29**, 744–50.

98. Bakris, G.L., Barnhill, B.W. and Sadler, R. Treatment of arterial hypertension in diabetic man: Importance of therapeutic selection. *Kidney Int.*, 1992, **41**, 912–19.

99. Bakris, G.L., Copley, J.B., Vicknair, N., Sadler, R. and Leurgans, S. Calcium channel blockers versus other antihypertensive therapies on progression of NIDDM associated nephropathy: Results of a six year study. *Kidney Int.*, 1996, **50**, 1641–50.

RISK FACTORS FOR ARTERIAL DISEASE IN DIABETES: DYSLIPIDAEMIA

D. John Betteridge

6.1 INTRODUCTION

Lipid and lipoprotein abnormalities are common in patients with diabetes particularly patients with non-insulin-dependent diabetes (NIDDM). Furthermore, these abnormalities are apparent prior to the development of impaired glucose tolerance and appear to be related to insulin resistance. In addition, insulin deficiency may also contribute to quantitative and qualitative lipoprotein abnormalities through effects on key regulatory points in lipoprotein metabolism.

Although marked diabetic lipaemia can produce a severe clinical picture including pancreatitis, this is rare and the major interest in lipid abnormalities in diabetic subjects relates to the increased risk of atherosclerotic vascular disease. Coronary heart disease (CHD) and the other manifestations of macrovascular disease are common in the diabetic state and account for significant morbidity and mortality. Plainly the aetiology of atherosclerosis is multifactorial. However, lipid and lipoprotein abnormalities no doubt play a prominent role and are open to therapeutic manipulation. Furthermore, there are now data, albeit from subgroup analysis from major clinical trials, showing benefit of lowering cholesterol for vascular disease in diabetic patients.

This chapter discusses the burden of macrovascular disease in the diabetic population, together with a brief overview of lipid and lipoprotein physiology and the relationship of lipoproteins to atherosclerosis. The abnormalities, both quantitative and qualitative, in lipoproteins in diabetes are described. Finally, an approach to the management of diabetic dyslipidaemia is outlined.

Perhaps in the past, diabetologists have been reluctant to embrace the non-glycaemic metabolic abnormalities of the condition. The physician responsible for the care of diabetic patients is entrusted not only with ensuring symptom relief with minimal hypoglycaemia but also with prevention of long-term complications. The Diabetes Control and Complications Trial (DCCT) has shown without question the importance of attention to glycaemic control in preventing the onset and progression of retinopathy, neuropathy and nephropathy [1]. Furthermore the benefits of treatment of hypertension on progression of nephropathy, particularly with the angiotensin converting enzymes, is now clear [2]. Yet little has been achieved in the reduction of macrovascular disease. It is almost as though CHD has been accepted as an inevitable consequence of diabetes. This should not be the case and, as the authors of the St Vincent document pointed out, what is needed is a vigorous approach to the prevention of CHD particularly through the reduction of known risk factors [3]. Lipid and lipoprotein abnormalities in diabetes are open to therapeutic intervention and their control is likely to make a significant impact on atherosclerosis-related disease.

6.2 ATHEROSCLEROSIS-RELATED DISEASE IN DIABETES

Atherosclerosis-related disease remains the commonest cause of death and up to three-quarters of the diabetic population will die from cardiovascular events [4]. All manifestations of atherosclerosis-related disease are increased; CHD by two- to threefold with a similar increase in cerebrovascular disease. Peripheral arterial disease is even more frequent in the diabetic population. An indication of the size of the problem comes from the National Hospital Discharge Survey in the USA. In this survey, 77% of hospitalizations due to diabetic complications were related to cardiovascular disease [5].

Although the possibility of a specific diabetic large vessel disease has been raised in the past, it is likely that the major factor is premature and extensive atherosclerosis. In the International Atherosclerosis Project, the prevalence of fatty streaks and more advanced lesions was increased in diabetic subjects compared to non-diabetic subjects across the 13 different participating countries with varying rates of background atherosclerosis [6].

In a cohort of insulin-dependent diabetes (IDDM) patients followed at the Joslin Diabetes Center, the cumulative mortality from CHD at age 55 years was about one-third. This represents a sixfold excess when compared to the control population [7]. It is interesting to note that proteinuria confers a massive increased risk for CHD even at the early stage of microalbuminuria [8].

In NIDDM patients, many studies have pointed to the threefold increased CHD risk compared with non-diabetic subjects. Some studies such as that from Framingham have also pointed to the high prevalence of CHD at the time that NIDDM is diagnosed [9]. Most but not all studies have shown that diabetic women are at particular high risk when compared to non-diabetic women and diabetes appears to remove the usual cardioprotective effect of the premenopausal state [9–11].

The prognosis for diabetic patients with established CHD is much worse than the non-diabetic population. The time to recurrent myocardial infarction or fatal event was 5.3 years in diabetic men compared with 7.1 years in non-diabetic men in the Framingham study [12]. Similar findings were seen for women. In a five-year follow-up of patients with myocardial infarction from Goteborg, Sweden, the in-hospital mortality for diabetic patients was 12% versus 8% for controls, five-year mortality was 55% versus 30% and the reinfarction rate was 42% versus 25%; and it appeared that diabetes was an independent determinant for mortality and reinfarction [13].

Diabetic patients do less well following surgical intervention for CHD. In a large survey of coronary artery bypass graft patients in the USA, the five-year survival for diabetic subjects was 0.8% versus 0.91% ($p<$ 0.0001) [14]. In the recent Bypass Angioplasty Revascularisation Investigation, the five-year survival post-coronary artery bypass graft was 80.6% in the diabetic subgroup compared with 89.3% in non-diabetic patients. In individuals undergoing percutaneous transluminal coronary angioplasty (PTCA), the five-year survival was markedly reduced in the diabetic patients at 65.5% compared with 86.3% [15]. This finding may have important implications for the choice of therapy in patients with multivessel disease. However in the EAST study [16], the marked reduction in survival post-PTCA in diabetic patients was not observed albeit in a smaller population. More information is needed in this regard, particularly now that coronary stenting is used more widely.

6.3 THE PHYSIOLOGY OF LIPID AND LIPOPROTEIN TRANSPORT

A simplified overview of lipid and lipoprotein metabolism is given here and the reader is referred to several recent, more comprehensive reviews [17–20]. The major plasma lipids, cholesterol and triglyceride, are insoluble in the aequeous environment of plasma and are transported in lipoproteins. Lipoproteins are multi-molecular aggregates consisting of a hydrophobic lipid core containing cholesterol ester and triglyceride and at the interface with the plasma, more polar substances such as phospholipid, free cholesterol and apoproteins (see Figure 6.1). Apoproteins not only serve to stabilize the lipid component of the lipoproteins but also act as ligands for important receptors in lipoprotein metabolism and also important activators or inhibitors of various enzymes.

There is a family of lipoproteins in plasma which vary in size and composition from the large chylomicrons to small, high-density lipoprotein (HDL) particles (see Figure 6.2). The generally accepted convention for lipoprotein nomenclature comes from separation of lipoproteins by hydrated density by ultracentrifugation. To simplify the description of lipoprotein metabolism it is usual to separate exogenous lipoprotein metabolism from endogenous lipoprotein metabolism and also to consider reverse cholesterol transport (Figure 6.3).

6.3.1   EXOGENOUS PATHWAY

The daily intake of triglyceride in the typical Western diet is approximately 80–140 grams together with 0.5 to 1.5 grams of cholesterol. Following digestion of dietary fat, triglycerides are re-esterified in the enterocyte and free cholesterol is esterified to cholesterol ester. These dietary-derived lipids are incorporated into the lipid core of chylomicrons. Chylomicrons are the largest of the lipoprotein species and serve to transport dietary fat from the intestine via the intestinal lymphatic system, entering the circulation through the thoracic duct. The major apoproteins of chylomicrons are apoprotein B48, A-I, A-II and A-

IV. Apoprotein B48 is necessary for chylomicron formation and secretion and is composed of the N-terminal portion of hepatic apoprotein B100. Apoprotein B48 lacks the binding site for the low density lipoprotein (LDL) receptor.

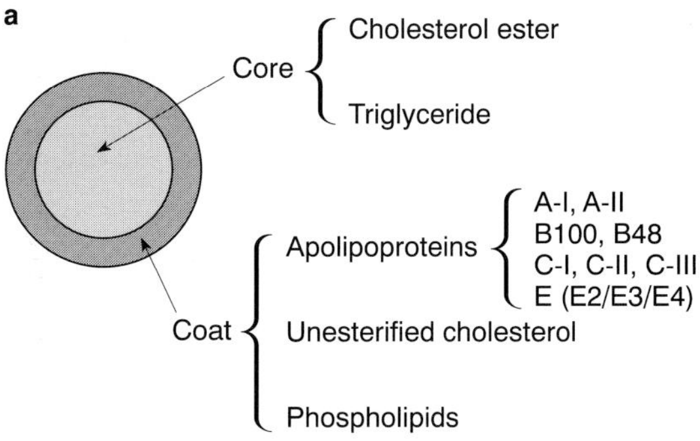

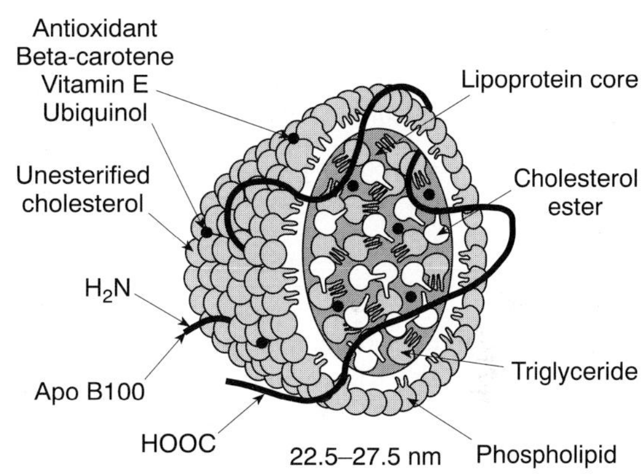

Figure 6.1 Lipoprotein structure. (a) Generalized schematic of lipoprotein showing the central core of insoluble lipid and the outer layer of amphipathic compounds, phospholipid, free cholesterol and apoproteins. The lipid and apoprotein content will vary depending on the particular lipoprotein. (b) Structure of low density lipoprotein (LDL), the major cholesterol-carrying lipoprotein, demonstrating how the single apoprotein, apoprotein B100, is thought to be present at the interface of the surface monolayer with the plasma environment. [Source: *Atlas of Heart Diseases*, ed. E. Brunwald, Vol. 10. *Atherosclerosis: Risk Factors and Treatment.* Current Medicine, Philadelphia, 1996]

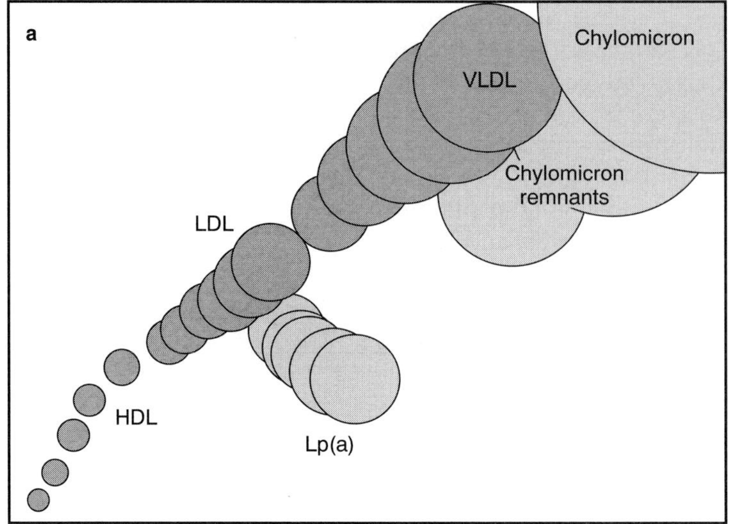

b

				Chemical composition (% of dry mass)				
Class	*Diameter (nm)*	*Density (g/ml)*	*Electro- phoretic mobility*	*Trigly- cerides*	*Cholesteryl esters*	*Chol- esterol*	*Phospho- lipids*	*Proteins*
Chylomicrons	80–500	0.930	α_2	86	3	2	7	2
VLDL	30–80	0.960–1.006	Pre-β	55	12	7	18	8
IDL	25–35	1.006–1.019	Slow pre-β	23	29	9	19	19
LDL	21.6	1.019–1.063	β	6	42	8	22	22
HDL$_2$	10	1.063–1.125	α_t	5	17	5	33	40
HDL$_3$	7.5	1.125–1.210	α_1	3	13	4	25	55
Lipoprotein (a)	30	1.055–1.085	Slow pre-β	3	33	9	22	33

Figure 6.2 The lipoprotein family. (a) The lipoprotein family differs in size and density from the large less dense, triglyceride-rich chylomicrons and very low density lipoprotein (VLDL) to the smaller, more dense cholesterol-carrying particles, low density lipoprotein (LDL) and high density lipoprotein (HDL). (b) The physical and chemical characteristics of the individual lipoproteins.

In the circulation, apoproteins of the C family and apoprotein E transfer from HDL to chylomicrons. Apoprotein C-II is an important activator of the enzyme lipoprotein lipase, which is bound to capillary endothelium in adipose tissue and muscle, whereas apoprotein C-III can inhibit this enzyme. Chylomicron triglyceride is hydrolysed by lipoprotein lipase to free fatty acids and glycerol. The fatty acids are used as fuel or re-esterified to triglyceride for storage in adipose tissue. During this process redundant surface components of chylomicrons, particularly apoproteins, phospholipid and free cholesterol, transfer to HDL.

Chylomicron remnant particles which are formed following the progressive hydrolysis of triglyceride are removed rapidly by the liver. This process involves a receptor process which recognizes apoprotein E. LDL receptor-related protein is a likely candidate for the remnant receptor, and glycosaminoglycans and liberated lipoprotein lipase enzyme protein are important in facilitating the interaction of the remnant particle with the receptor.

a
FFA + MG
TG
B48+A
Golgi
INTESTINAL MUCOSAL CELL
HDL
A
E
A
C
B-48
A
CHYLOMICRON
Blood Capillary
Lyso-some
B-48
E
C
REMNANT
B100 E Receptors
C
B-48
A
E
Lipoprotein Lipase
FFA-Albumin
FFA
LIVER CELL

b
B100+E+C
Golgi
TG
B100
E
C
VLDL
HDL
A
E
A
C
Lipoprotein Lipase
B100
E
C
REMNANT
Lyso-some
B100
C
B-48...
B100 E Receptors
C
B100
LDL
FFA Albumin
FFA
LIVER CELL
Blood Capillary
PERIPHERAL CELLS
B100 E Receptors
Lyso-some

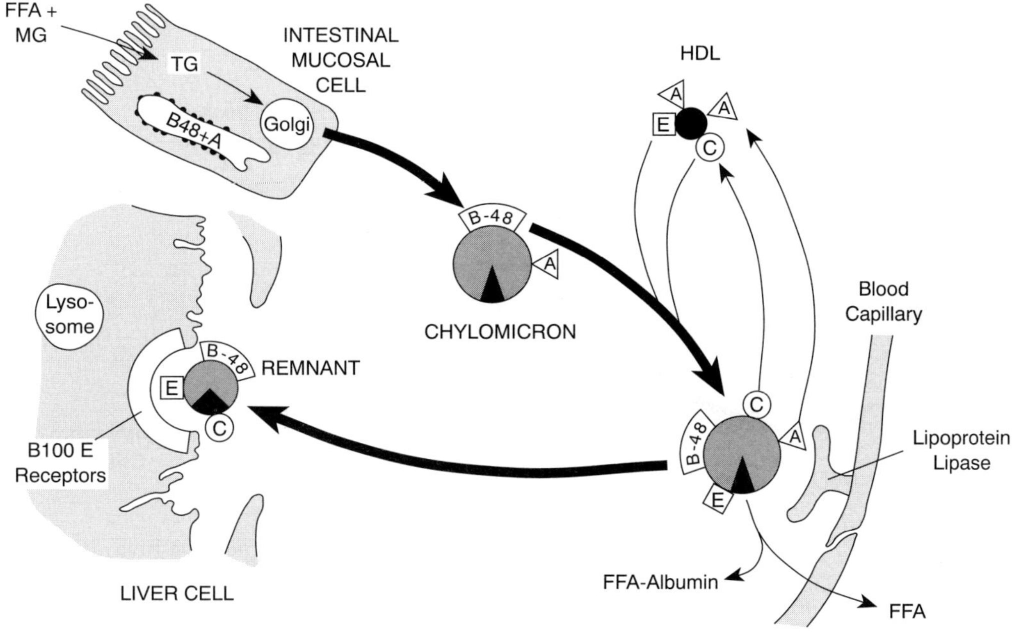

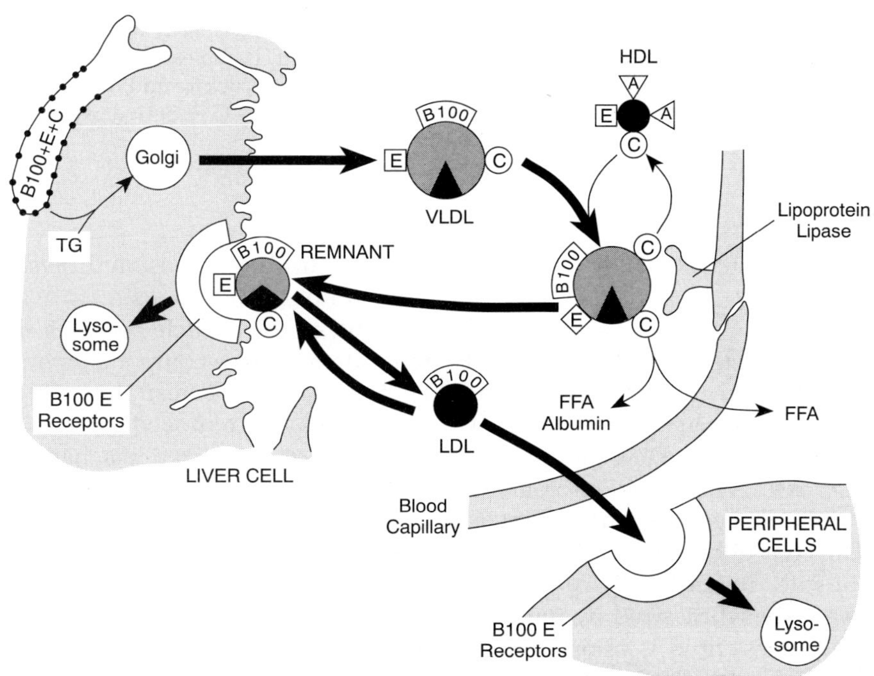

Figure 6.3

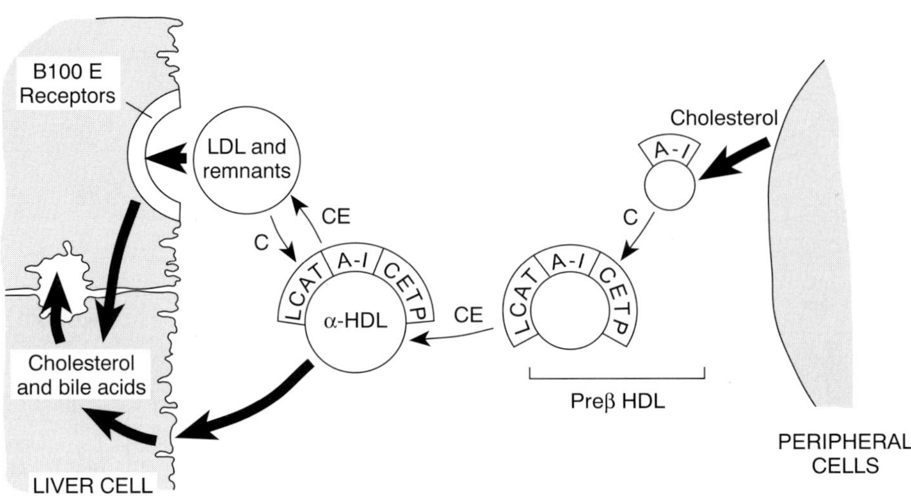

Figure 6.3 Overview of lipoprotein metabolism. (a) The exogenous lipoprotein pathway. Chylomicron triglyceride is hydrolysed by lipoprotein lipase producing chylomicron remnants which are taken up by the liver through receptors which recognize apoprotein E. (b) The endogenous lipoprotein pathway. VLDL triglyceride is hydrolysed by lipoprotein lipase, producing VLDL remnants which can be removed directly by the liver or further hydrolysed by hepatic lipase to LDL. LDL can be taken up by peripheral cells or the liver via LDL receptors which recognize apoproteins B100 and E. (c) Reverse cholesterol transport. Cholesterol is returned from peripheral cells to the liver either directly via HDL or indirectly following transfer of cholesterol from HDL to other lipoproteins. FFA, free fatty acids; MG, monoglycerides; TG, triglycerides; LCAT, lecithin cholesterol acyltransferase; CETP, cholesterol ester transfer protein; C, cholesterol; CE, cholesterol ester. [Source: R.J. Havel and J.P. Kane. Structure and metabolism of plasma lipoproteins. In *The Metabolic and Molecular Bases of Inherited Disease* (eds C.R. Scriver, A. L. Beaudet, W.S. Sly and D. Valle), McGraw Hill, New York, 1995]

6.3.2   ENDOGENOUS LIPOPROTEIN PATHWAY

Endogenously synthesized triglyceride and cholesterol are secreted by the liver in the form of very low density lipoprotein (VLDL). The major apoprotein of VLDL is apoprotein B100 but VLDL also contains apoproteins of the C family and apoprotein E which transfer from HDL. The control of hepatic VLDL production is not fully understood. Apoprotein B100 is continuously synthesized by the liver but is degraded unless lipid is transferred to it. Microsomal lipid transfer protein is important in this process.

VLDL triglyceride is hydrolysed by lipoprotein lipase and, in a similar way to chylomicrons, as the particle becomes smaller then redundant surface components transfer to the HDL fraction. The resulting VLDL remnant particle may be removed directly by the liver or further metabolized via hepatic lipase to LDL. VLDL remnants which can accumulate in various disease states have intermediate density and are referred to as intermediate density lipoproteins (or IDL).

LDL is the end product of VLDL breakdown. It is cholesterol-rich and has one molecule of apoprotein B100 per lipoprotein particle. It serves to transport cholesterol to

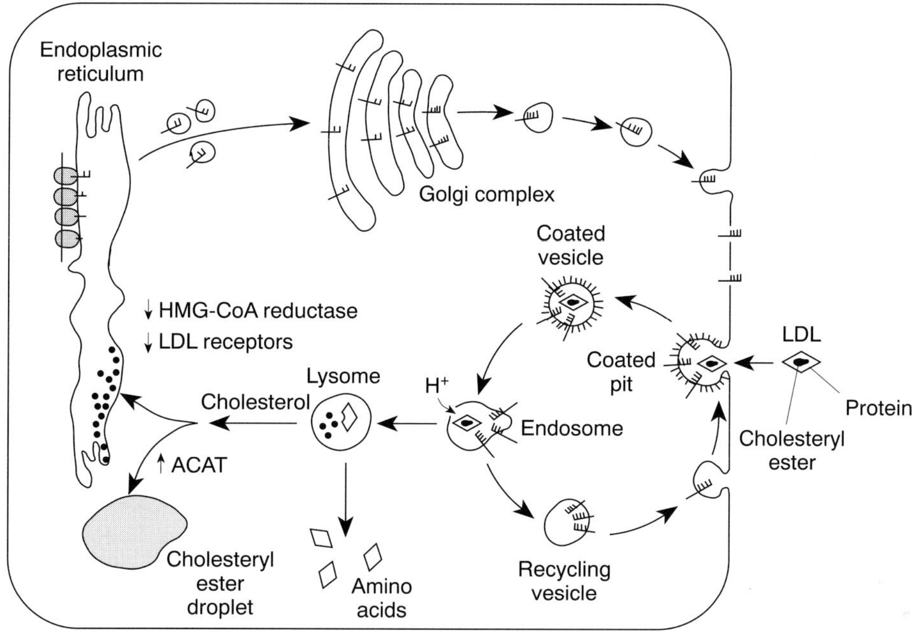

Figure 6.4 LDL receptor pathway. LDL binds to a specific, high affinity receptor located in the coated pit regions of the cell membrane. The complex is internalized by endocytosis, the endosome fuses with lysosomes where cholesterol ester is hydrolysed to free cholesterol. Increasing free cholesterol suppresses HMG-CoA reductase activity and LDL receptor synthesis and stimulates ACAT activity. [Source: M.S. Brown and J.L. Goldstein. *Curr. Top. Cell Regul.* 1985, **27**, 3.]

peripheral cells for membrane synthesis and, in some tissues, hormone synthesis. It is taken up by a specific, high affinity LDL receptor. Excess LDL is removed via the same receptor on liver. The LDL receptor is a glycoprotein of 839 amino acids and is coded for by a well characterized gene located on the short arm of chromosome 19. LDL receptor structure and function has been well characterized through analysis of different receptor mutations found in familial hypercholesterolaemia. LDL receptors are located in a specialized area to the cell membrane known as coated pits. These cellular organelles are concerned with internalization of macromolecules.

LDL bound to its receptor is internalized through endocytosis, and cholesterol entering the cells through LDL has important regulatory functions on cellular cholesterol homeostasis (Figure 6.4). The receptor recognizes apoprotein B100 and apoprotein E as

ligands. Bound LDL is taken up by absorptive endocytosis and the endocytotic vesicle fuses with cellular lysosomes. Cholesterol ester is hydrolysed to free cholesterol and the protein component is hydrolysed by proteases to amino acids. Accumulating cellular cholesterol inhibits the rate-determining enzyme in cholesterol synthesis, HMG-CoA reductase, with consequent reduction in cellular cholesterol synthesis, and cholesterol acyl-CoA acyltransferase (ACAT) is stimulated, facilitating re-esterification of cholesterol to cholesterol ester for storage within the cell. In addition, cellular LDL receptor expression is suppressed.

6.3.3　HIGH DENSITY LIPOPROTEIN AND REVERSE CHOLESTEROL TRANSPORT

HDL is the most heterogeneous of all the lipoprotein species, resulting in part from complex metabolic interactions with other lipoproteins, as discussed earlier. New HDL particles are synthesized by liver and intestine, appearing as bilayer discs containing phospholipid and apoprotein A-I. These discs are modified and become spherical as they accept free cholesterol from other lipoproteins or peripheral cells and esterify it to cholesterol ester which forms a hydrophobic lipid core. Cholesterol esterification results from the activity of the enzyme lecithin cholesterol acyltransferase which circulates with HDL and apoprotein A-I, the major apoprotein of HDL, is an important activator of this enzyme.

Cholesterol ester can transfer from HDL to other particles of lower density such as VLDL and LDL through the action of cholesterol ester transfer protein. This protein facilitates a mole for mole exchange of triglyceride for cholesterol ester. As previously described, redundant surface components of triglyceride-rich lipoproteins transfer to the HDL fraction and this leads to the formation of larger, more buoyant HDL particles, namely HDL_2. Under certain circumstances HDL_2 can be a substrate for hepatic lipase and as a result smaller, denser HDL_3 are formed.

Because of its ability to accept free cholesterol, HDL is involved in reverse cholesterol transport, i.e. removal of cholesterol from the periphery including arterial wall, back to the liver which is the major site of excretion of cholesterol.

6.3.4 LIPIDS, LIPOPROTEINS AND ATHEROSCLEROSIS

LDL cholesterol can be considered to be causally related to atherosclerosis because of the following factors: the strength of the relationship; its independence from other risk factors; the consistency of the data both within and between populations; its dose–response relationship; and the existence of plausible mechanisms to explain the association. Indeed, cholesterol has been called the one essential CHD risk factor. Support for this statement comes from between-population comparisons. In the Japanese, for instance, CHD prevalence is low despite a high smoking rate and a high prevalence of hypertension. However the average plasma cholesterol level in the Japanese is low [21], so it appears that a certain level of cholesterol is required for the other important risk factors to make an impact on CHD.

The largest epidemiological study relating cholesterol to CHD incidence comes from the follow-up of the middle-aged men screened to take part in the Multiple Risk Factor Intervention Trial (MRFIT) [22]. A total of 361 662 men aged 35–57 years and free of CHD were followed up and the incidence of cardiovascular disease linked to baseline cholesterol concentrations. The relationship between serum cholesterol and CHD death was continuous, graded and strong across the whole age range and was independent of cigarette smoking and hypertension. Studies in rural China [23] where mean cholesterol levels are low (≈ 3 mmol/l) still show a gradient of risk between cholesterol and CHD so there does not appear to be a threshold for cholesterol above which CHD risk develops.

The association between cholesterol and CHD risk has been underestimated due to regression dilution bias and surrogate dilution effect [24]. After correction for these factors it has been calculated that most (>80%) of the international variation in CHD can be explained by differences in plasma cholesterol. From cohort studies it has been calculated that a difference in serum cholesterol of 0.6 mmol/l is associated with a difference in CHD mortality of 54% at the age of 40 years [24].

It is increasingly understood how LDL cholesterol interacts with cells of the arterial wall to produce foam cells which accumulate under the arterial endothelium leading to fatty streak formation [25]. Studies in experimental atherosclerotic animals pointed to a central role for the monocyte in foam cell formation. Scanning electron micrographs of arterial endothelium in primates fed a high fat, high cholesterol diet have shown the adhesion of circulating monocytes to endothelium as an early event. At a later stage these cells penetrate through the endothelium and accumulate in the subendothelial space. The cells take on the characteristics of macrophages and become laden with cholesterol ester.

Accumulation of these cells is toxic to the overlying endothelium which is disrupted, thus allowing platelets to adhere and aggregate. Aggregating platelets can release powerful mitogens which lead to smooth muscle proliferation and progression of the plaque. Native LDL is not taken up by monocyte macrophage experimentally. However, if LDL is altered, monocytes do recognize it and take it up through receptors distinct from the LDL receptor. These so-called scavenger receptors are, unlike the LDL receptor, not downregulated by increasing cellular cholesterol concentration. The fact that altered LDL could be taken up in this manner was first shown by Brown and Goldstein using acetylated LDL [26]. However, *in vivo* it is likely that LDL is modified by oxidative mechanisms.

Through the work of Steinberg *et al.* and others it has become clear that oxidatively modified LDL is involved in several processes which contribute to atherogenesis [27]. In addition to being taken up by monocytes and producing foam cells, oxidatively modified LDL is known to be cytotoxic to endothelium and to stimulate monocyte adhesion through inducing the expression of adhesion molecules. Furthermore, oxidatively modified LDL inhibits monocyte chemotaxis such that the monocytes are less likely to leave the subendothelial space.

Since the development of the powerful HMG-CoA reductase inhibitors, or statins which lead to marked reductions in LDL cholesterol, it has been possible to show that atherosclerotic risk can be reduced dramatically by lowering plasma cholesterol concentrations [28, 29]. This reversibility of CHD risk by cholesterol lowering is further confirmation for the causal role of LDL cholesterol in atherogenesis.

HDL is the other important cholesterol-carrying lipoprotein. In plasma it transports 20–30% of plasma cholesterol and is strongly and independently linked to CHD risk. However, unlike LDL, the relationship is inverse; in other words as HDL cholesterol increases then risk of CHD declines. Conversely, low HDL cholesterol is an important additional risk factor for the development of CHD [30]. From Framingham and other prospective population studies it has become clear that the total cholesterol:HDL ratio is a very useful determinant of vascular risk [31].

How HDL cholesterol protects against atherosclerosis is yet to be fully worked out [32]. Certainly its role in reverse cholesterol transport is an attractive hypothesis. However HDL may act in other ways to restrict the progression of atheroma. An alternative hypothesis postulates that the primary abnormality of lipoprotein metabolism leading to increased coronary risk is decreased efficiency of clearance of triglyceride-rich particles. Low HDL cholesterol levels merely reflect this process as surface components transfer from triglyceride-rich particles to HDL during their catabolism. If this process was inefficient this would contribute to low HDL levels. HDL may also be involved in other processes; it may act as an antioxidant, it may impair uptake of LDL cholesterol and it may have antiplatelet activity.

HDL cholesterol concentrations can be altered by various factors. It increases following weight reduction and increased physical activity. In addition, drugs such as fibrates and nicotinic acid will increase HDL levels. As yet there have been no clinical trials specifically designed to look at whether increasing HDL cholesterol levels reduce CHD risk. However, attempts have been made to assess the relative contribution of HDL cholesterol changes to reduction of CHD in some of the lipid-lowering trials. In the Helsinki Heart

Study, for instance, there was a 34% reduction in CHD risk. From the 9.3% reduction in LDL cholesterol with gemfibrozil treatment, it would be predicted from other studies that CHD would be reduced at 15.3%. However, the actual reduction in CHD risk observed was 34%. It has been proposed that this additional benefit was conferred by the 8.9% increase in HDL cholesterol during that study [33]. From these and other data, it has been calculated that a 1 mg/dl increase in HDL cholesterol would be associated with a 2–3% reduction in CHD risk. HDL cholesterol levels, in addition to LDL cholesterol levels, have also been shown to be related to the progression and regression of coronary atherosclerotic plaques in the angiographic studies [34].

Controversy still remains about the relationship of plasma triglycerides to atherosclerosis. There is no doubt that plasma triglycerides are related to CHD risk in univariate analysis. However, on multivariate analysis the relationship with triglyceride is weakened and in many analyses disappears [35]. Hypertriglyceridaemia is often associated with low HDL and it has been proposed that it is the low HDL cholesterol that is the predictor of risk in such individuals.

It is now increasingly recognized that, because triglycerides show such inherent biological variability, they come out less strongly in mathematical models compared with measurements which are less variable, such as cholesterol and HDL cholesterol. Furthermore, it is probably inappropriate to separate triglyceride and HDL cholesterol in multivariate analysis as they are intimately related metabolically, as previously discussed. Approximately 50% of HDL comes from the transfer of redundant surface components during the hydrolysis of triglyceride-rich particles.

Several authors have analysed the relationship between triglycerides and vascular risk in a different way. Data from the Framingham study pointed to the importance of triglyceride as a risk factor when HDL cholesterol concentrations were low [36]; and, in the placebo group of the Helsinki Heart Study [33] and in the PROCAM study [37], increasing triglyceride was associated with vascular risk when LDL:HDL cholesterol ratio was >5. A recent extensive analysis of population-based prospective studies has suggested an independent role for plasma triglycerides in CHD risk [38]. However, it is unlikely that epidemiological studies will give the final verdict on triglycerides and what is needed is a better understanding of the mechanisms whereby triglyceride predicts risk.

Some triglyceride-rich particles, namely the VLDL remnants (IDL), are atherogenic. These accumulate in type III hyperlipidaemia which is associated with premature and extensive vascular disease [39]. Furthermore, hypertriglyceridaemia is associated with important alterations in other lipoproteins. As previously discussed, it is associated with a low HDL cholesterol and more recently there has been much interest focused on the effects of increasing triglyceride concentrations on LDL. LDL is not homogeneous and it has been recognized for several years that there are distinct subspecies which vary in size, density and lipid content [40]. As the density of LDL increases then particle diameter, the relative content of total and polar lipids and flotation rate all decrease. In healthy subjects LDL_2 is the most abundant subspecies and women tend to have proportionately more LDL_1 than men who have proportionately more LDL_3 (Figure 6.5).

LDL fractions are separated optimally by density gradient ultracentrifugation but the technique is difficult to apply in large studies; non-denaturing gradient gel electrophoresis, which determines particle size, is perhaps the most commonly used technique for studying LDL heterogeneity. Using this technique, two distinct LDL subclasses have been defined which have been designated pattern A, with a

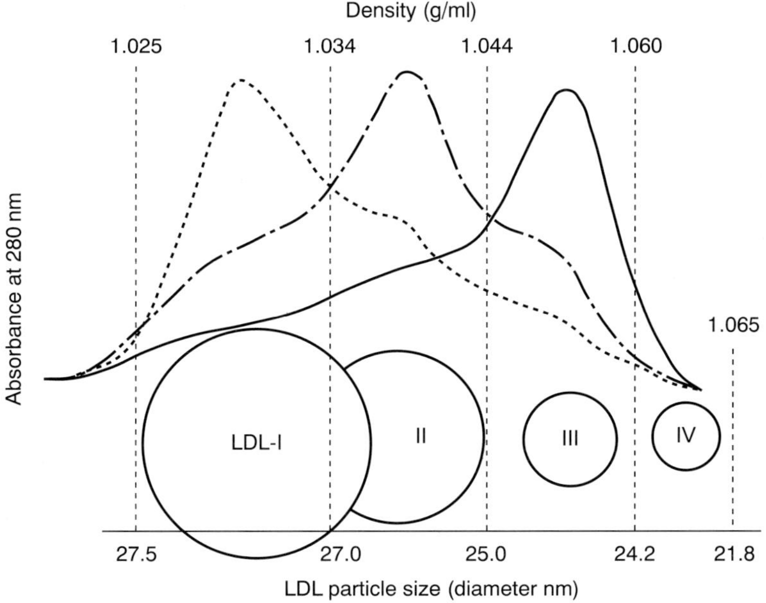

Figure 6.5 LDL subfractions by density and particle. Top: LDL subclass density profiles obtained by density gradient ultracentrifugation and representative of a normal healthy female (—·—), male (———) and coronary heart disease patient (—). Bottom: LDL particle size as determined by 2–16% gradient gel electrophoresis. [Source: B.A. Griffin. Dyslipidaemia, *Ballière's Clin. Endocrinol. Metab.*, 1995, **9**, 687–703]

major peak diameter >25.5 nm and pattern B with a major peak diameter of <25.5 nm. Pattern B LDL has been shown to be associated with a threefold increased risk of myocardial infarction independent of age, gender and body weight but dependent on HDL cholesterol and plasma triglyceride [41]. Furthermore, small dense LDL has been shown to be related to reduced coronary artery diameter in the angiographic regression studies [42]. The clustering of lipid abnormalities characterized by a predominance of small dense LDL, low HDL and hypertriglyceridaemia has been termed the atherogenic lipoprotein profile.

LDL subclass distribution is influenced by many factors but plasma triglyceride is the major determinant, accounting for approximately 70% of the variability of the LDL distribution [43]. Other important factors are the activity of cholesterol ester transfer protein, hepatic lipase activity, body weight, gender and apoprotein E phenotype. A probable mechanism to explain the relationship of hypertriglyceridaemia to the accumulation of small dense LDL involves the stimulation of neutral lipid exchange by high concentrations of triglyceride-rich lipoprotein. LDL becomes enriched transiently with triglyceride in exchange for cholesterol ester and the triglyceride-enriched particle becomes a substrate for hepatic lipase which hydrolyses the triglyceride producing a protein-rich lipid-poor particle with a density resembling LDL_3. From kinetic studies it has been shown that it is the larger $VLDL_1$ particles which give rise to the LDL_3 particles whereas smaller $VLDL_2$ particles which are present in normotriglyceridaemic individuals give rise to LDL_2 particles [44].

There are several mechanisms whereby small dense LDL may be atherogenic. These include increased infiltration into the arterial wall, increased binding to arterial proteoglycans and increased susceptibility to oxidation [45].

Hypertriglyceridaemia is known to be associated with abnormalities of coagulation and fibrinolysis. Plasminogen activator inhibitor I levels are increased in hypertriglyceridaemic individuals [46]. This will lead to decreased fibrinolysis. Furthermore, the serine protease factor VII, an important component of the extrinsic coagulation system is also positively associated with increasing triglycerides [47].

6.3.5   LIPOPROTEIN(a)

There has been considerable recent interest in this lipoprotein. It consists of LDL to which is attached an additional apoprotein, apoprotein(a), via a disulphide bond. Apoprotein(a) has striking homology with plasminogen [48]. It consists of the serum protease domain together with kringle 5 and a highly variable number of kringle 4 repeats of plasminogen. It is likely that apoprotein(a) is secreted directly by the liver and associates with LDL in the plasma. Although lipoprotein (a) binds to the LDL receptor, it is unlikely that this is the major route of catabolism and it appears that its rate of production is a primary determinant of its plasma concentration.

There is immense variation in lipoprotein(a) concentrations both within and between populations, and concentrations remain reasonably stable throughout life. Much of the variation in concentration is determined by the apoprotein(a) gene locus [49].

Numerous case control studies have pointed to an association between lipoprotein (a) levels and CHD risk; some prospective studies have not shown an association. However, there is no doubt that lipoprotein(a) is present in atheromatous lesions and that, in patients with familial hypercholesterolaemia, the concentration of Lp(a) is high in those with established CHD [50].

6.4   LIPID AND LIPOPROTEIN METABOLISM IN DIABETES

Quantitative abnormalities of both total serum lipids and lipoproteins are common in the diabetic population, particularly in those with NIDDM [51–56]. There are many contributory factors including the degree of glycaemic control, insulin resistance, body mass index and the presence of any nephropathy. In addition, other secondary causes of dyslipidaemia can co-exist in the diabetic patient, as can primary dyslipidaemias. Diabetes mellitus is also associated with important qualitative changes in lipoproteins which may contribute to increased atherosclerotic risk.

6.4.1   NIDDM PATIENTS

The most apparent lipid abnormalities in NIDDM patients are increased total serum triglycerides, often associated with a low level of HDL cholesterol. Importantly, these lipid abnormalities are also found in patients at the pre-diabetic stage of impaired glucose tolerance. Total and LDL cholesterol concentrations tend to be similar to those of control populations. In a population-based study from the USA, the frequency of hypertriglyceridaemia was increased two- to threefold in diabetic subjects compared with non-diabetic subjects [57]. The atherogenic lipoprotein profile characterized by mixed hyperlipidaemia and low HDL cholesterol was two- to threefold more prevalent in middle-aged NIDDM patients in the PROCAM study from Northern Germany [58].

In addition to low HDL cholesterol, apoprotein A-I, the major apoprotein of HDL, is low in NIDDM patients. It appears that it is the HDL$_2$ subfraction that is reduced in diabetes and these abnormalities often persist in patients well established on conventional treatment. The increase in total triglycerides and triglyceride-rich lipoproteins is related to insulin resistance in NIDDM patients. There is increased VLDL secretion by the liver. This is secondary to a direct effect on the liver and also increased flux of free fatty acids, the major precursor of VLDL triglyceride to the liver, because of impaired insulin-mediated suppression of hormone-sensitive lipase.

Postprandial triglyceride metabolism is also abnormal in NIDDM and abnormalities can be demonstrated even in individuals whose fasting triglyceride levels are within the usually defined normal range. Postprandially hepatic VLDL production continues unsuppressed and there is therefore competition with chylomicrons for lipoprotein lipase. Saturation of this clearance mechanism leads

to prolonged postprandial lipaemia (Figure 6.6).

Hypertriglyceridaemia has an important impact on HDL metabolism and also LDL metabolism. It is likely that the reduced HDL concentration in NIDDM is explained by increased catabolism of HDL because of qualitative effects secondary to the hypertriglyceridaemia. Because of increased neutral lipid transfer, HDL becomes triglyceride-enriched and is then a substrate for hepatic lipase which has increased activity in NIDDM. The action of this enzyme leads to a small, denser HDL particle which is more rapidly catabolized. In a similar way, hypertriglyceridaemia is associated with the production of small, dense LDL so that the important features of the lipid abnormalities associated with NIDDM and the insulin-resistant state are hypertriglyceridaemia, low HDL cholesterol and small dense LDL. Important contributors to these abnormalities are the increased

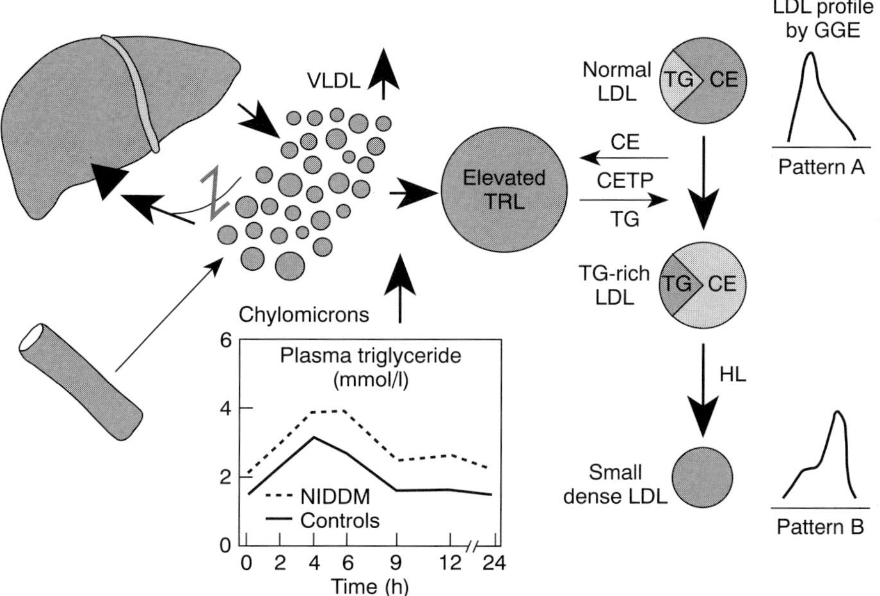

Figure 6.6 Lipid metabolism in type 2 diabetes. TG, triglyceride; CETP, cholesterol ester transfer protein; CE, cholesterol ester; LDL, low density lipoprotein; VLDL, very low density lipoprotein; HDL, high density lipoprotein. [Source: M.-R. Taskinen. *Lancet*, 1997, **350** (suppl. 1), S120–3]

hepatic VLDL output, increased neutral lipid transfer through increased activity of cholesterol ester transfer protein and increased hepatic lipase activity (Figure 6.6).

6.4.2   IDDM PATIENTS

In IDDM patients with good glycaemic control, lipid and lipoprotein concentrations are similar to non-diabetic patients. Indeed, in some studies lower concentrations of VLDL and LDL and higher concentrations of HDL have been observed. In those with poor glycaemic control there tends to be increased concentrations of VLDL due to increased hepatic output and, in addition, decreased clearance through decreased activity of lipoprotein lipase which is an insulin-sensitive enzyme. Occasionally severe diabetic lipaemia is seen in insulin-deficient patients; it resolves rapidly with adequate insulinization.

In nephropathic patients, lipid abnormalities develop with increases in total and LDL cholesterol and total and VLDL triglycerides. Apoprotein B, the major protein of the VLDL cascade, is also increased and HDL cholesterol is reduced particularly HDL_2. Abnormalities are already apparent at the microalbuminuric stage. The mechanism of these disturbances in nephropathic individuals is not fully understood. HDL can be lost in the urine in nephropathic patients and this may contribute to reduce serum HDL levels.

An important qualitative abnormality that is likely to be important for IDDM as well as NIDDM patients is glycation of lipoproteins, particularly LDL [59]. Glycosylated LDL is not recognized as well by the LDL receptor. Furthermore, glycosylated LDL can interact with macrophages leading to increased cholesterol ester synthesis. These findings suggest that LDL may be potentially more atherogenic in diabetic subjects. Furthermore, HDL can be glycosylated and this may interfere with HDL receptor-mediated efflux of cholesterol from cells.

6.4.3   LIPID AND LIPOPROTEIN LEVELS IN RELATION TO DIABETIC MACROVASCULAR DISEASE

Serum cholesterol

Many cross-sectional studies have shown that total serum cholesterol is an important predictor of macrovascular disease in diabetic subjects, just as it is in non-diabetic subjects. There are extensive data from the Framingham Study in the USA [60] and also Finnish [61] and British populations [62]. In the men screened for the Multiple Risk Factor Intervention Trial there were 5163 known diabetic subjects [63]. In this study the risk of vascular disease for any given level of cholesterol was increased threefold in the diabetic patients. However, as cholesterol increased so did the cardiovascular death rate and the absolute risk was steeper in the diabetic men.

As might be expected, it is LDL cholesterol that correlates positively with the presence of macrovascular disease in cross-sectional studies and this is also true for apoprotein B, the major protein of LDL. HDL cholesterol, as expected, is found to be inversely related to the presence of vascular disease, but this was particularly true in NIDDM patients. HDL measured by ultracentrifugation was the most powerful lipoprotein determinant for CHD in a Finnish study of 313 NIDDM patients. Low HDL increased risk of CHD death fourfold [64]. The findings for HDL in IDDM patients have shown variable results. Some studies have found lower HDL and apoprotein A-I cholesterol concentrations in CHD patients whereas others have not.

Triglyceride

Both cross-sectional and prospective studies have shown that serum triglycerides are associated with either the presence or development of macrovascular disease in diabetic patients. Often, in these large studies HDL cholesterol was not measured and therefore it is not possible to assess the independent nature of the association with triglyceride. Nevertheless it is clear from many studies that the relationship with triglyceride appears to be strong. In a substudy of the WHO Multinational Study, for instance, triglyceride levels were significantly higher among subjects with major Q wave abnormalities on the electrocardiogram. This association remained significant after adjustment for age, cholesterol and systolic blood pressure [65]. HDL cholesterol was not measured.

In a large study from Germany, serum triglyceride levels were higher in patients who had undergone a major cardiovascular event and in women only they remained significant after adjustment for blood pressure and duration of diabetes [66]. In a large study from Finland in NIDDM patients, triglyceride was significantly related to myocardial infarction in men and women but the relationship did not persist after multivariate analysis [67]. In IDDM patients, significant associations between triglyceride and CHD have been seen in populations from Finland and the USA [68, 69]. In the Paris Prospective Study, triglyceride was found to predict CHD events in men with either impaired glucose tolerance or diabetes after 11 years of follow-up. The relationship with triglyceride persisted after adjustment for total cholesterol, systolic blood pressure, body mass index and cigarette smoking. HDL cholesterol was again not measured in this study [70].

Lipoprotein(a)

More information is required on the relationship of lipoprotein(a) to the presence of macrovascular disease in diabetic patients. Although a positive association was seen in NIDDM patients between lipoprotein(a) concentrations and those with previous myocardial infarction [71], this has not been confirmed in other studies of NIDDM and IDDM patients [72, 73]. So far there is only one prospective study as part of the Wisconsin Epidemiology Survey and no association was found between lipoprotein(a) and CHD risk [74].

6.5 MANAGEMENT OF DYSLIPIDAEMIA IN DIABETIC PATIENTS

6.5.1 SCREENING

A plasma lipid profile is an important part of the annual assessment of all diabetic patients. The measurement of fasting cholesterol, triglyceride and HDL cholesterol is generally sufficient for most clinical purposes. It is best to obtain a fasting sample to allow more accurate determination of HDL cholesterol and also to ensure that exogenous-derived triglyceride is cleared from the plasma prior to the test. However, this can be inconvenient clinically. Non-fasting samples allow reasonable measurement of total cholesterol and it is likely that if non-fasting triglyceride is below 2.5 mmol/l then fasting triglyceride is going to be satisfactory.

LDL can be calculated by the Friedewald equation [75]:

$$\text{LDL cholesterol} = \text{Total cholesterol} - \text{HDL cholesterol} - ([\text{triglyceride}]/[\,2.19])$$

where all concentrations are in mmol/l.

This equation gives a reasonable estimate of LDL cholesterol provided that total triglycerides are below 4.5 mmol/l. However, the accuracy of the Friedewald equation has been questioned in NIDDM because of qualitative changes in VLDL which alter the proportion of cholesterol to triglyceride in the particles [76].

When significant dyslipidaemia is found it is important to bear in mind the possibility of other primary or secondary causes (see Tables 6.1 and 6.2). The possibility of hypothyroidism, which is common in the diabetic population, should always be considered. In addition, many NIDDM patients are likely to be treated for hypertension and it is important to remember the potential adverse effect of some antihypertensive agents on dyslipidaemia (see Table 6.3). Severe abnormalities

Table 6.1 Primary dyslipidaemias

Disease	WHO phenotype	Typical lipid levels (mmol/l)	Lipoproteins	CHD risk	Pancreatic risk	Possible clinical signs
Polygenic hypercholesterolaemia	IIa	C 6.5–9, TG < 2.3	LDL ↑	+	–	Xanthelasma, corneal arcus
Familial hypercholesterolaemia	IIa	C 7.5–16, TG < 2.3	LDL ↑	+++	–	Tendon xanthoma, arcus, xanthelasma
Familial defective apoprotein B100	IIa	C 7.5–16, TG < 2.3	LDL ↑	+++	–	Tendon xanthoma, arcus, xanthelasma
Familial combined hyperlipidaemia	IIa, IIb, IV or V	C 6.5–10, TG 2.3–12	LDL ↑ VLDL ↑ HDL ↓	++	–	Arcus, xanthelasma
Remnant particle disease	III	C 9–14, TG 9–14	IDL ↑	+++	±	Palmar striae, tuberoeruptive xanthomata
Familial hypertriglyceridaemia	IV, V	C 6.5–12, TG 10–30	VLDL ↑ Chylomicrons ↑	?	++	Eruptive xanthomata, lipaemia retinalis, hepatosplenomegaly
Lipoprotein lipase deficiency	I	C < 6.5, TG 10–30	Chylomicrons ↑	–	+++	Eruptive xanthomata, lipaemia retinalis, hepatosplenomegaly
High HDL	–	HDL cholesterol > 2.0	HDL ↑	–	–	–

TG, triglycerides; C, cholesterol; CE, cholesterol ester; LDL, low density lipoprotein; VLDL, very low density lipoprotein; HDL, high density lipoprotein; IDL, intermediate density lipoprotein.

Table 6.2 Other secondary dyslipidaemias

Increased LDL cholesterol	Increased triglycerides	Decreased HDL
Hypothyroidism	Obesity	Hypertriglyceridaemia
Nephrotic syndrome	Lack of exercise	Obesity
Obstructive liver disease	Alcohol intake	Cigarette smoking
Progestins	Renal insufficiency	Lack of exercise
Anabolic steroids	Oestrogens	Beta blockers
	Beta blockers	Progestins
		Anabolic steroids

Table 6.3 Effects of antihypertensive drugs on lipid and lipoprotein levels

Drugs	Total cholesterol	LDL cholesterol	HDL cholesterol	Triglycerides
Beta blockers	↓	↓	↑	↓
Vasodilators				
Calcium antagonists	→	→	→	→
ACE inhibitors				
Diuretics	↑	↑	→↓	↑
Beta blockers				
B$_1$- and non-selective	→	→	↓	↑
Intrinsic sympathomimetic activity	→	→	→↑	↑
Vasodilatory properties	→	→	→	→

in either cholesterol or triglyceride are unlikely to be due to the diabetic state *per se*, and other causes should be sought.

6.5.2 TREATMENT TARGETS

Various national and international consensus committees have published guidelines for lipid and lipoprotein values in NIDDM. The European Working Group on NIDDM suggests that, in mmol/l, optimum total cholesterol should be below 5.2, triglycerides below 1.7 and HDL cholesterol greater than 1.1 [77]. However, this document did not give any clear guidance as to when to introduce pharmacological therapy if attention to glycaemic control and diet and other measures fail to achieve these optimum levels. Recently, the American Diabetes Association has updated its recommendations [78, 79] (Table 6.4). It can

be seen that the American Diabetes Association advocates a low threshold for pharmacological intervention based on LDL cholesterol concentrations. The National Cholesterol Education Program in the USA [80] also advocates aggressive treatment for NIDDM patients because of their very high risk of vascular disease. It has provided similar guidelines for LDL cholesterol along the lines proposed for individuals with clinical coronary heart disease; that is, hypolipidaemic drug therapy for persisting LDL cholesterol concentrations greater than 3.4 mmol/l with the goal of therapy less than 2.6 mmol/l.

Guidelines for hypertriglyceridaemia have also been provided. However, it should be borne in mind that there is little clinical trial intervention data on which to base guidelines for the treatment of hypertriglyceridaemia. The American Diabetes Association suggests

Table 6.4 Subgroup analysis of diabetic patients included in 4S

	Placebo (n=97)	Simvastatin (n=105)	Relative risk ↓
Overall deaths	24 (24.7%)	15	43% (−70 → +8%) $p=0.087$
CHD deaths	17 (17.5%)	12	36% (−69% → +35%) $p=0.242$
Major CHD events	44 (45.4%)	24	55% (−73% → −26%) $p=0.002$
Non-diabetics			32%

CHD, coronary heart disease.

that therapy with a fibrate is indicated for total serum triglyceride concentrations greater than 4.5 mmol/l [79]. The National Cholesterol Education Program suggests that pharmacological therapy may be indicated in borderline hypertriglyceridaemia (2.3–4.5 mmol/l) in dyslipidaemias associated with increased CHD risk such as diabetic dyslipidaemia [80].

Because of the potential atherogenicity of cholesterol in triglyceride-rich particles in diabetes, together with the less reliable calculation of LDL cholesterol using the Friedewald formula, Garg and Grundy have proposed non-HDL cholesterol as a target for therapy. They suggest that a minimum goal of therapy should be non-HDL cholesterol of 4.1 mmol/l with an ideal goal of less than 3.4 mmol/l [81].

6.5.3   TREATMENT

Glycaemic control

Improved glycaemic control in IDDM patients is associated with beneficial effects on lipid and lipoprotein concentrations, with reduction in total and VLDL triglyceride and LDL cholesterol. In the DCCT trial, intensive insulin therapy was associated with a significant reduction in the number of individuals with an LDL cholesterol greater than 4.14 mmol/l [82]. HDL cholesterol concentrations also rise with improved glycaemic control. In NIDDM patients plasma triglyceride concentrations fall with improved glycaemic control with some studies showing increases in HDL cholesterol particularly when insulin therapy is used. LDL cholesterol concentrations tend to stay the same. However, in surveys of diabetic patients established on treatment, dyslipidaemia remains very common in diabetic populations. This implies that, in clinical practice, best endeavours at glycaemic control are not always sufficient to correct diabetic dyslipidaemia [83].

Early studies with sulphonylureas implicated them in reducing HDL cholesterol concentrations. However, these findings have not been confirmed and it is likely that such treatment does not adversely affect HDL cholesterol concentrations. Metformin has been shown to have small but potentially beneficial reductions in cholesterol and LDL cholesterol, fasting triglyceride and postprandial triglyceride concentrations [84–86].

Lifestyle measures

The most important lifestyle measures in the treatment of diabetic dyslipidaemia are weight reduction and exercise. Weight reduction leads to improvement not only in lipid and lipoprotein profile but also in glycaemic control and insulin sensitivity. The major impact is on plasma triglycerides with more modest reductions in LDL cholesterol. Slight increases in HDL cholesterol might be observed. Exercise appears to confer additional benefit [87] to the weight reduction. However, the feasibility of undertaking physical training at the level required to produce beneficial effects on lipid profile in diabetic patients is low because of associated problems of cardiovascular disease, age and obesity [88]. Furthermore, long-term motivation and compliance to exercise regimes has been reported to be poor [89]. Despite these problems there is no doubt of the strength of the epidemiological evidence linking regular exercise and physical fitness to decreased CHD risk in non-diabetic populations. Similar benefits are likely to accrue to diabetic patients. In IDDM patients, the level of physical activity may be associated with a reduction in overall mortality [90].

Dietary therapy should be individualized for the particular patient. The American Diabetes Association recommends the adoption of a diet which is low in saturated fat and cholesterol with replacement of calories by increased carbohydrate content [91]. This should be accompanied by a high fibre intake which improves glycaemic control and has a modest cholesterol-lowering effect [92]. An alternative is to substitute saturated fat with an increased intake of cis-monounsaturated fat. This approach has been shown to have beneficial effects both on plasma glucose, insulin sensitivity and lipoprotein levels [93–97]. This approach may be more acceptable to many patients. Furthermore there are potential disadvantages of a very high carbohydrate diet unaccompanied by a high fibre intake; postprandial lipaemia may be exacerbated in NIDDM patients [98] and in non-diabetic patients there may be a shift in LDL subfraction distribution towards small dense particles [99].

Hypolipidaemic drugs

Hypolipidaemic drug therapy should be considered in all diabetic patients with significant dyslipidaemia which persists despite attention to glycaemic control, diet and exercise programmes. Diabetic patients with established CHD should be treated with lipid-lowering agents, and beneficial effects have been observed in subgroup analysis of two major secondary prevention trials [100, 101] (Tables 6.4 and 6.5). It can be seen that diabetic subjects appear to show similar benefit to non-diabetic subjects. These studies were performed with HMG-CoA reductase inhibitors and less information is available on the treatment of hypertriglyceridaemia with low HDL. In the Helsinki Heart Study, a primary prevention trial performed with gemfibrozil, the small group of diabetic subjects did show a reduction in events with the fibrate drug but, probably because of small numbers, the reduction did not reach statistical significance [102] (Figure 6.7).

More information should be available from ongoing studies on the potential benefits of treating dyslipidaemia. The Diabetes Atherosclerosis Intervention Study (DAIS) is a double-blind, randomized placebo-controlled trial in men and women (aged 40–65 years) with NIDDM [103]. Its primary objective is to determine changes in regression or progression of coronary atherosclerotic plaques with

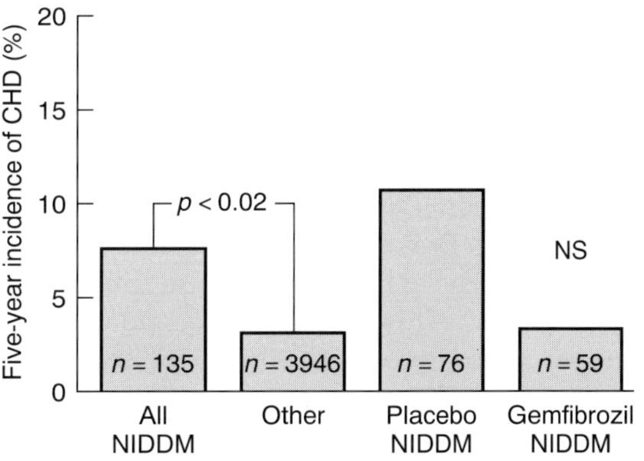

Figure 6.7 Subgroup analysis of diabetic patients in the Helsinki Heart Study. CHD, coronary heart disease; NIDDM, non-insulin dependent diabetes.

Table 6.5 Subgroup analysis of diabetic patients in CARE study ($n=586$)

	Placebo	Pravastatin	Relative risk ↓
Non-fatal MI or PTCA or CABG or death from CHD	37%	29%	25% (0–43) $p=0.05$

MI, myocardial infarction; PTCA, percutaneous transluminal coronary angioplasty; CABG, coronary artery bypass graft; CHD, coronary heart disease.

quantitative angiography. Baseline lipid criteria are total triglyceride ≤5.2 mmol/l with LDL cholesterol between 3.5 and 4.5 mmol/l or total triglyceride between 1.7 and 5.2 mmol/l and LDL cholesterol ≤4.5 mmol/l together with a total cholesterol to HDL cholesterol ratio ≥4. The trial drug is micronized fenofibrate, 200 mg daily, and the treatment period is three years after the last patient is randomized.

Further information on the benefits of treating dyslipidaemia in diabetic subjects with established CHD will come from the Bezafibrate Infarction Prevention Study being performed in Israel. Of the 3122 patients with previous myocardial infarction or angina pectoris in this ongoing study, approximately 10% have diabetes. The study has been set up to determine the effects of lowering triglyceride with concomitant increase in HDL cholesterol using the fibrate Bezafibrate in a dose of 400 mg daily. The baseline total cholesterol concentrations lie between 4.6 and 6.5 mmol/l, with HDL cholesterol concentrations <1.1 mmol/l. The median follow-up period will be 6.25 years [104].

Ongoing trials of statin therapy, including diabetic patients, include the Longterm Intervention with Pravastatin in Ischaemic Disease (LIPID) study which should be published shortly [105]. This is a large secondary prevention trial involving 9014 patients (aged 31–75 years; 17% women) with previous myocardial infarction or angina pectoris. Baseline total cholesterol concentrations are 4 to 7 mmol/l. Approximately 9% of the patients are known to have diabetes. The Heart Protection Study currently underway in the UK and co-ordinated from Oxford is a large trial of cholesterol-lowering in approximately 20 000 high-risk individuals using simvastatin 40 mg daily. This trial involves both primary and secondary prevention of CHD and the predicted number of diabetic subjects to be included in the study is approximately 7000, of whom approximately 15 000 will have established CHD [106]. Atorvastatin is the HMG-CoA reductase inhibitor in a primary prevention trial in NIDDM patients in progress in the UK called the Collaborative Atorvastatin Diabeties Study (CARDS).

6.5.4 CHOICE OF LIPID-LOWERING DRUGS

The choice of lipid-lowering drugs for the treatment of dyslipidaemia in diabetes will depend on the nature of the underlying dyslipidaemia together with the presence or absence of concomitant complications, particularly whether significant nephropathy is present. Optimally the hypolipidaemic agent chosen should not adversely affect glycaemic control.

The individual classes of lipid-lowering drugs will be described briefly together with an overview of the effects likely to be seen in diabetic patients. Finally, an approach to drug therapy in diabetic patients will be outlined.

Bile acid sequestrant resins

The basic anion-exchange resins cholestyramine (a copolymer of styrene and divinylbenzine) and colestipol (a copolymer of diethylpentamine and epichlorohydrin) have been available for many years. They remain unabsorbed after ingestion and combine with bile salts in the intestine to interrupt the enterohepatic circulation. In response, there is increased hepatic synthesis of bile acid which results in upregulation of hepatic LDL receptors. Part of the cholesterol-lowering ability of these compounds is offset by increased hepatic synthesis of cholesterol. However, in high dose they can lower LDL cholesterol by up to 30%.

A major advantage of the resins is that they are not absorbed and therefore will not produce systemic side effects. However, they commonly produce gastrointestinal effects, including bloating and constipation, resulting in poor compliance. Their use in diabetes has been limited particularly because they tend to increase triglycerides. Furthermore they can interfere with the absorption of other drugs. Decreased absorption of fat-soluble vitamins and folic acid can occur with high-dose resin therapy but this is not usually a clinical problem. These drugs are particularly useful in women of child-bearing age and children, and may be useful for the treatment of moderate hypercholesterolaemia in diabetic patients where triglyceride levels are normal [107].

Fish-oil

In some countries, fish-oil liquid or capsules which are high in the omega-3 fatty acids, eicosapentanoic acid and docosahexanoic acid, have received licences for the treatment of hypertriglyceridaemia. They can substantially lower total and VLDL triglyceride in individuals with severe hypertriglyceridaemia associated with increased hepatic output of VLDL. In these individuals there tends to be a slight increase in LDL cholesterol during therapy with fish-oil and little or no change in HDL cholesterol. There are several studies that have shown that fish-oil supplements can exacerbate hyperglycaemia [108] and for this reason they are less useful in diabetic dyslipidaemia. If they are used then glycaemic control should be monitored and therapy altered accordingly.

Fibrates

There are many fibrate preparations available for clinical use. However, some countries have not licensed all of them and other countries such as the USA have only a small number available. They have been available for clinical use since the early 1960s when the first of the class, clofibrate, was introduced. This drug is now obsolete because of its limited efficacy and also its ability to increase the lithogenicity of bile and precipitate gallstones. Newer fibrates have much less impact on the lithogenicity of bile.

The best known effects of the fibrates include increased activity of lipoprotein lipase, which results in enhanced hydrolysis of triglyceride-rich particles. There is also a reduction in hepatic VLDL secretion secondary to decreased fatty acid flux to the liver. The fibrates also appear to increase the catabolism of LDL, probably through effects on the LDL size distribution rather than direct effects on the LDL receptor.

The major effect of fibrate therapy is to reduce triglyceride by up to 60% and along with this HDL cholesterol concentrations tend to rise. Effects on total cholesterol and LDL cholesterol vary considerably depending on the lipid phenotype of the individual being treated. In hypertriglyceridaemic individuals there may be a slight increase in LDL cholesterol. The clinical significance of this is not known and certainly the LDL in these individuals tends to reflect a move from small, dense particles to larger, more buoyant particles. Some fibrates also lower fibrinogen which is an important risk factor for vascular disease. The drugs are generally well tolerated with little in the way of side effects. The fibrate drugs should not be used if renal impairment is present and care needs to be exercised in patients taking anticoagulants as the fibrates are highly protein-bound.

HMG-CoA reductase inhibitors (statins)

The introduction of this class of drugs into clinical practice in 1987 represented a substantial advance on previously available therapies. They were discovered in the 1970s following isolation from the culture broths of various fungus species. They are specific competitive inhibitors of the enzyme HMG-CoA reductase, which is the rate-limiting enzyme in cholesterol synthesis. Inhibition of cholesterol synthesis at this site leads to a decrease in cholesterol synthesis and upregulation of the hepatic LDL receptors. In addition, the more potent of these compounds appear to have an effect in reducing VLDL secretion by the liver. They are the most potent drugs available for reducing LDL cholesterol, with reductions of up to 60% recorded. They also produce moderate reductions in triglyceride and slight increases in HDL cholesterol.

The statins are generally well-tolerated and significant adverse effects are rare. Occasionally there are minor gastrointestinal disturbances but the most important side effect is a myositis. Fortunately this is extremely rare, but patients should be warned to stop the drugs if there is severe muscle pain and tenderness. Occasionally, modest abnormalities of liver function are observed but discontinuation of the drugs for this reason is rare. Care should be exercised when these drugs are used in combination with fibrates or nicotinic acid, which in themselves can cause myositis. Other compounds which may interact with statins resulting in increased risk of side effects include the antifungal azoles (itraconazole and ketoconazole), macrolide antibiotics (erythromycin and clarithromycin) and the antidepressant netazodone. The drugs are mainly excreted through the liver and abnormal liver function or very high alcohol intake are relative contraindications. The drugs can be used in moderate renal impairment as they do not undergo significant renal excretion. However, care should be exercised in the presence of severe renal insufficiency.

6.5.5   CHOICE OF LIPID-LOWERING THERAPY

It will be clear from the above description of the individual drug classes that the use of nicotinic acid and the anion-exchange resins is not so appropriate in the diabetic population as in the non-diabetic population. Furthermore, fish-oil supplements, which might be useful in lowering high triglyceride concentrations, are relatively contraindicated in diabetes. The major choice of drugs in diabetes rests between the fibrates and the statins and the choice will depend on the lipoprotein phenotype in the individual patient [78, 81].

There is no doubt that the statins are the drugs of choice for lowering total and LDL cholesterol and there is reasonable experience of their use in diabetes. Marked reductions in total cholesterol, LDL cholesterol and apoprotein B have been observed with no significant adverse effects on glycaemic control. The statins have also been studied in patients with diabetic nephropathy and similar reductions in cholesterol and LDL cholesterol have been observed with no apparent adverse effect on glomerular function.

Considerable variation is apparent in the literature regarding the effects of the fibrate drugs on cholesterol and LDL cholesterol in diabetic patients. Effects appear to depend largely on the baseline triglyceride concentrations in the population studied. Certainly, if triglycerides are raised then LDL cholesterol does not fall with fibrate therapy and increases have been observed. When baseline triglycerides are lower, then moderate total and LDL cholesterol reductions have been observed. There is considerable variation in the reported studies on concurrent effects on glycaemic control with either no change, deterioration or improvement observed.

As described earlier, there is reasonable information from secondary prevention trials that lowering LDL cholesterol with statins will have a beneficial effect in patients with diabetes and less information is available with the fibrates. However, ongoing studies will provide further evidence on their potential use in diabetic populations.

If LDL cholesterol concentrations are within the accepted range but triglycerides are elevated with a low HDL, then the fibrate drugs may be indicated in high-risk patients and it is likely that substantial reductions in triglycerides will be observed together with increases in HDL cholesterol. These findings have been observed in many clinical studies. In this situation LDL cholesterol concentrations may rise, and the clinical significance of this is not known. Obviously controlled clinical trial data with hard end-points is required. However the increase in LDL cholesterol does represent a shift in particle distribution to larger, more buoyant LDL particles which are thought to be less atherogenic. The recent BECAIT and LOCAT studies imply that lowering triglyceride and increasing HDL may have beneficial effects in non-diabetic subjects [109, 110]. These angiographic studies observed similar changes in lack of progression of coronary plaques to those changes seen in the regression trials using statin therapy. An interesting clinical trial has just started in the UK, co-ordinated from Oxford, which will compare the effects on clinical end-points in NIDDM of a statin, cerivastatin, a fibrate, fenofibrate, and a combination of the two.

6.5.6   AN APPROACH TO LIPID-LOWERING THERAPY IN DIABETIC PATIENTS

On currently available evidence, diabetic patients with established CHD should be treated in a similar way to non-diabetic patients. This is supported by subgroup analysis of recent important end-point trials and the bulk of currently available evidence

points to the use of statin drugs. In diabetic individuals with established CHD and low LDL cholesterol but raised triglycerides and low HDL cholesterol, a fibrate drug is indicated.

In the primary prevention of CHD, it is important to bear in mind that many diabetic subjects will fill the risk criteria for introduction of drug therapy. It is important to assess the individual risk of the patient, taking into account the presence of other risk factors such as hypertension, cigarette smoking, proteinuria, the presence of retinopathy and family history. Again, the choice of lipid-lowering drug will depend on the lipoprotein phenotype present. For hypercholesterolaemia, the drug of choice will be a statin and for hypertriglyceridaemia associated with low HDL and an acceptable LDL cholesterol, the drug of choice will be a fibrate. Hopefully, current ongoing primary prevention trials involving statins and fibrates will further clarify the best clinical practice.

REFERENCES

1. The DCCT Research Group. Lipid and lipoprotein levels in patients with IDDM: Diabetes Control and Complications Trial experience. *Diabetes Care*, 1992, **15,** 886–94.
2. Lewis, E.J., Hunsicker, L.G., Bain, R.P. and Rhode, R.D. The effect of angiotensin-converting enzyme inhibition on diabetic nephropathy. *N. Engl. J. Med.*, 1993, **329,** 1456–62.
3. Krans, H.M.J. *et al.* (eds) *The St. Vincent Declaration. Diabetes Care and Research in Europe,* World Health Organisation, Geneva, 1992.
4. Pyörälä, K., Laakso, M. and Uusitupa, M. Diabetes and atherosclerosis: an epidemiologic view. *Diabetes Metab. Rev.,* 1987, **3,** 463–524.
5. Centre for Economic Studies in Medicine. *Direct and Indirect Costs of Diabetes in the United States in 1987,* American Diabetes Association, Alexandria, 1988.
6. Robertson, W.B. and Strong, J.P. Atherosclerosis in persons with hypertension and diabetes mellitus. *Lab.Invest.,* 1968, **18,** 538–51.

7. Krowlewski, A.S., Kosinski, E.J., Warram, J.H. *et al.* Magnitude and determinants of coronary artery disease in juvenile onset insulin dependent diabetes mellitus. *Am. J. Cardiol.,* 1987, **59**, 750–5.

8. Deckert, T., Feldt-Rasmussen, B.M. and Borch-Johnsen, K. Proteinuria, an indicator of malignant angiopathy. *Diabetic Complications: Early Diagnosis and Treatment,* (eds D. Andreaani, G. Crepaldi and V. DiMario), John Wiley & Sons, Chichester, 1987, pp. 257–61.

9. Margolis, J.R., Kannel, W.B., Feinlieb, M., Dawber, T.R. and McNamara, P.M. Clinical features of unrecognized myocardial infarction; silent and symptomatic. Eighteen year follow-up. The Framingham Study. *Am. J. Cardiol.,* 1973, **32**, 1–7.

10. Barrett-Connor, E. and Wingard, D.L. Sex differential in ischaemic heart disease mortality in diabetics: a prospective population-based study. *Am. J. Epidemiol.,* 1983, **118**, 489–96.

11. Heyden, S., Heiss, G., Bartel, A.G. and Hames, C.G. Sex differences in coronary mortality among diabetics in Evans County, Georgia. *J. Chronic Dis.,* 1980, **33**, 265–73.

12. Abbott, R.D., Donahue, R.P., Kannel, W.B. and Wilson, P.W.F. The impact of diabetes on survival following myocardial infarction in men vs women. The Framingham Study. *J. Am. Med. Assoc.,* 1988, **260**, 3456–60.

13. Herlitz, J., Malmberg, K., Karlsson, B., Ryden, L. and Hjalmarsson, A. Mortality and morbidity during a five year follow up of diabetics with myocardial infarction. *Acta Med. Scand.,* 1988, **24**, 31–8.

14. Mossis, J.J., Smith, L.R., Jones, R.H. *et al.* Influence of diabetes mammary artery grafting on survival after coronary bypass. *Circulation,* 1991, **84** (suppl 3), 275–84.

15. The Bypass Angioplasty Revascularization Investigation (BARI) Investigators. Comparison of coronary bypass surgery with angioplasty in patients with multivessel disease. *N. Engl. J. Med.,* 1996, **335**, 217–25.

16. Kosinski, A.S., Barnhart, H.X., Weintraub, W.S. *et al.* Five year outcome after coronary surgery or coronary angioplasty: results from the Emory Angioplasty vs Surgery Trial (EAST). *Circulation,* 1995, **91** (suppl 1), 1–543 (abstract).

17. Betteridge, D.J. ed. *Baillière's Clinical Endocrinology and Metabolism,* Vol. 9, No. 5. *Dyslipidaemia.* Baillière Tindall, London, 1995.

18. Durrington, P.M. *Hperlipidaemia: Diagnosis and Management,* 2nd edn, Butterworth Heinemann, Oxford, 1995.

19. Betteridge, D.J. (ed.) *Lipids: Current Perspectives,* Martin Dunitz, London, 1996.

20. Brown, W.V. and Braunwald, E. *Atlas of Heart Diseases: Atherosclerosis: Risk Factors and Treatment,* Vol. 10, Current Medicine, Philadelphia, 1996.

21. Keys, A. *Seven Countries: a Multinational Analysis of Death and Coronary Heart Disease,* Harvard University Press, 1980.

22. Martin, M.J., Hulley, S.B., Browner, W.S., Kuller, L.H. and Wentworth, D. Serum cholesterol, blood pressure and mortality: implications from a cohort of 361 662 men. *Lancet,* 1986, **ii**, 933–6.

23. Chen, Z., Peto, R., Collin, R. *et al.* Serum cholesterol concentration and coronary heart disease in a population with low cholesterol concentrations. *BMJ,* 1991, **303**, 276–82.

24. Law, M.R., Wald, N.J., Wu, T., Hackshaw, A. and Bailey, A. Systematic underestimation of association between serum cholesterol concentration and ischaemic heart disease in observational studies: data from the BUPA study. *BMJ,* 1994, **308**, 363–6.

25. Ross, R. The pathogenesis of atherosclerosis: a perspective for the 1990s. *Nature,* 1993, **362**, 801–9.

26. Brown, M.S. and Goldstein, J.L. Lipoprotein metabolism in the macrophage. *Annu. Rev. Biochem.,* 1983, **52**, 223–61.

27. Steinberg, D., Parthasarathy, S., Carew, T.E. *et al.* Beyond cholesterol: modifications of low density lipoprotein that increase its atherogenicity. *N. Engl. J. Med.,* 1989, **320**, 915–24.

28. Scandinavian Simvastatin Survival Group Study. Randomised trial of cholesterol-lowering in 4444 patients with coronary heart disease: the Scandinavian simvastatin survival study (4S). *Lancet,* 1994, **344**, 1383–9.

29. Shepherd, J., Cobbe, S.M., Ford, I. *et al.* Prevention of coronary disease with pravastatin in men with hypercholesteorlaemia. *N. Engl. J. Med.,* 1995, **333**, 1301–7.

30. Gordon, D.J., Probstfield, J.L., Garrison, R.J. *et al.* High density lipoprotein cholesterol and cardiovascular disease: four prospective American studies. *Circulation,* 1989, **79**, 8–15.

31. Castelli, W.P., Garrison, R.J., Wilson, P.W.F., Abbott, R.D., Kalousdran, S. and Kannel, W.B.

Incidence of coronary heart disease and lipoprotein cholesterol levels: the Framingham study. *J. Am. Med. Assoc.*, 1986, **256**, 2835–8.

32. Miller, N.E. HDL vs triglycerides: which is important in cardiovascular disease? In *Atherosclerosis, X*, (eds F.P.Woodford, J. Davignon and A.Sniderman), Elsevier Science, Amsterdam, 1995, pp. 743–8.

33. Manninen, V., Tenkanen, H., Koskinen, P. *et al.* Joint effects of triglycerides and LDL cholesterol and HDL cholesterol concentrations on coronary heart disease risk in the Helsinki Heart Study. Implications for treatment. *Circulation*, 1992, **85**, 37–45.

34. Brown, G.B., Xue-Qiao, Z., Sacco, D.E. and Alberti, J.J. Lipid lowering and plaque regression. New insights into prevention of plaque disruption and clinical events in coronary disease. *Circulation*, 1993, **87**, 1781–91.

35. Hulley, S.B., Rosenman, R.H., Bawal, R.D. *et al.* Epidemiology as a guide to clinical decisions: the association between triglyceride and coronary heart disease. *N. Engl. J. Med.*, 1980, **302**, 1383–9.

36. Castelli, W.P. The triglyceride issue: a view from Framingham. *Am. Heart J.*, 1986, **112**, 432–7.

37. Assmann, G. and Schulte, H. Relation of high density lipoprotein cholesterol and triglycerides to incidence of atherosclerotic coronary artery disease (the PROCAM experience). *Am. J. Cardiol.*, 1992, **70**, 733–7.

38. Hokanson, J. and Austin, M.A. Plasma triglyceride level is a risk factor for cardiovascular disease independent of high density lipoprotein cholesterol level: a metaanalysis of population-based prospective studies. *J. Cardiovasc. Risk*, 1996, **3**, 213–9.

39. Mahley, R.W. and Rall, S.C. Jr. Type III hyperlipoproteinaemia (dysbetalipoproteinaemia): the role of apolipoprotein E in normal and abnormal lipoprotein metabolism. In *The Metabolic and Molecular Basis of Inherited Disease*, (eds C.R. Scriver, A.L. Beaudet, W.D. Sly and D. Valle), 7th edn, McGraw Hill, New York, 1995, pp. 1953–80.

40. Krauss, R.M. and Burke, D.J. Identification of multiple subclasses of plasma low density lipoproteins in normal humans. *J. Lipid Res.*, 1982, **23**, 97–104.

41. Austin, M.A., Breslow, J.L., Hennekens, C.H., Buring, J.E., Willott, W.C. and Krauss, R.M. Low density lipoprotein subclass patterns and risk of myocardial infarction. *J. Am. Med. Assoc.*, 1988, **260**, 1917–21.

42. Watts, G.F., Mandalia, S., Brunt, J.N.H. *et al.* Independent associations between plasma lipoprotein subfraction levels and the course of coronary artery disease in the St Thomas' Atherosclerosis Regression Study. *Metabolism*, 1993, **42**, 1461–7.

43. McNamara, J.R., Campos, H., Ordouas, J.M. *et al.* Effect of gender, age and lipid status on low density lipoprotein subfraction distribution. Results from the Framingham Offspring Study. *Arterioscler. Thromb.*, 1987, **7**, 483–90.

44. Packard, C.J. Plasma lipid and lipoprotein metabolism in the 1990s: what we know and what we need to know. In *Lipids: Current Perspectives*, (ed D.J. Betteridge), Martin Dunitz, London, 1996, pp. 1–20.

45. Griffin, B.A. Low density lipoprotein heterogeneity. In *Baillière's Clinical Endocrinology and Metabolism*, Vol. 9, No. 5. *Dyslipidaemia*, (ed D.J. Betteridge), Baillière Tindall, London, 1995, pp. 687–703.

46. Hamsten, A., Wiman, B., de Faire, U. and Blomback, M. Increased plasma levels of a rapid inhibitor of tissue plasminogen activator in young survivors of myocardial infarction. *N. Engl. J. Med.*, 1985, **313**, 1557–63.

47. Hamsten, A. and Karpe, F. Triglyerides and coronary heart disease – has epidemiology given us the right answer? In *Lipids: Current Perspectives*, (ed D.J. Betteridge), Martin Dunitz, London, 1996, pp. 43–68.

48. Eaton, D.L., Fless, G.M., Kohr, W.J. *et al.* Partial amino acid sequence of apolipoprotein(a) is homologous to plasminogen. *Proc. Natl Acad. Sci. USA*, 1987, **34**, 3224–8.

49. Boerwinkle, E., Leffert, C.C., Lin, J., Lackner, C., Chiesa, G. and Hobbs, H.H. Apolipoprotein(a) gene accounts for greater than 90% of the variation in plasma lipoprotein(a) concentrations. *J. Clin Invest.*, 1992, **90**, 52–60.

50. Seed, M., Hopplicher, F., Reaveley, D. *et al.* Relation of serum lipoprotein(a) concentration and apolipoprotein(a) phenotype to coronary heart disease in patients with familial hypercholesterolaemia. *N. Engl. J. Med.*, 1990, **322**, 1494–9.

51. Betteridge, D.J. Lipids, diabetes and vascular disease: the time to act. *Diabet. Med.*, 1989, **6**, 195–218.

52. Stern, M.P. and Haffner, S.M. Dyslipidaemia in type II diabetes. *Diabetes Care*, 1991, **14**, 1144–59.
53. Ginsberg, H.N. Diabetic dyslipidaemia: basic mechanisms underlying the common hypertriglyceridaemia and low HDL cholesterol levels. *Diabetes*, 1996, **45** (suppl 3), S27–30.
54. Syvanne, M. and Taskinen, M.R. Lipids and lipoproteins as coronary risk factors in non insulin dependent diabetes mellitus. *Lancet*, 1997, **350** (suppl 1), S120–3.
55. Betteridge, D.J. Diabetic dyslipidaemia – implications for vascular risk. In *Lipids: Current Perspectives*, (ed D.J. Betteridge), Martin Dunitz, London, 1996, pp. 135–57.
56. Laakso, M.L. and Lehto, S. Epidemiology of macrovascular disease. *Diabetes Rev.*, 1997, **5**, 294–315.
57. Barrett-Connor, E., Grundy, S.M. and Holdbrook, M.J. Plasma lipids and diabetes mellitus in an adult community. *Am. J. Epidemiol.*, 1982, **115**, 657–63.
58. Assmann, G. and Schulte, H. The prospective cardiovascular Munster (PROCAM) study: prevalence of hyperlipidaemia in persons with hypertension and/or diabetes mellitus and the relationship to coronary heart disease. *Am. Heart J.*, 1988, **116**, 1713–24.
59. Lyons, T.J. and Jenkins, A.J. Glycation, oxidation, and lipoxidation in the development of the complications of diabetes: a carbonyl stress hypothesis. *Diabetes Rev.*, 1997, **5**, 365–91.
60. Kannel, W.B. and McGee, D.L. Diabetes and cardiovascular risk factors: the Framingham Study. *Circulation*, 1979, **59**, 8–13.
61. Rönnemaa, T., Laakso, M., Kallio, V. *et al.* Serum lipids, lipoproteins and apolipoproteins and the excessive occurrence of coronary hearet disease in non insulin dependent diabetic patients. *Am. J. Epidemiol.*, 1989, **130**, 632–45.
62. Jarrett, R.J. and Shipley, M.J. The Whitehall Study: comparative mortality rates and indicators of risks in diabetics. *Acta Endocrinol.*, 1985, **10** (suppl 272), 21–6.
63. Stamler, J., Vaccaro, O., Neaton, J.D. and Wentworth, D. for the Multiple Risk Factor Intervention Trial Resarch Group. Diabetes, other risk factors and 12 year cardiovascular mortality for men screened in the Multiple Risk Factor Intervention Trial. *Diabetes Care*, 1993, **16**, 434–44.
64. Laakso, M., Lehto, S., Penttila, I. and Pyörälä, K. Lipids and lipoproteins predicting coronary heart disease mortality and morbidity in patients with non insulin dependent diabetes. *Circulation*, 1993, **88**, 1421–30.
65. West, K.M., Ahuja, M.M.S., Bennett, P.H. *et al.* The role of circulating glucose and triglyceride concentrations and their interactions with other 'risk factors' as determinants of arterial disease in nine diabetic population samples from the WHO multinational study. *Diabetes Care*, 1983, **6**, 361–9.
66. Janka, H.V. Five year incidence of macrovascular complications in diabetes mellitus. *Horm. Metab. Res.*, 1985, **15** (suppl), 15–19.
67. Rönnemaa, T., Laakso, M., Kallio, V. *et al.* Serum lipids, lipoproteins and apolipoproteins and the excessive occurrence of coronary heart disease in non-insulin dependent diabetic patients. *Am. J. Epidemiol.*, 1989, **130**, 632–45.
68. Laakso, M., Pyörälä, K., Sarlund, H. and Voutilainen, E. Lipid and lipoprotein abnormalities associated with coronary heart disease in patients with insulin dependent diabetes mellitus. *Arteriosclerosis*, 1986, **6**, 679–84.
69. Maser, R.E., Wolfson, S.K. Jr., Ellis, D., Stein, E.A., Drash, A.L., Becker, D.J., Dorman, J.S. and Orchard, T.H.J. Cardiovascular disease and arterial calcificaton in insulin dependent diabetes mellitus interrelation and risk factor profiles. *Atheroscler. Thromb.*, 1991, **11**, 958–65.
70. Fontbonne, E., Eschwege, E., Cambien, F. *et al.* Hypertriglyceridaemia as a risk factor for coronary heart disease mortality in subjects with impaired glucose tolerance or diabetes. *Diabetologia*, 1989, **32**, 300–4.
71. Velho, G., Erlich, D., Turpin, E., Neel, D., Cohen, D., Froguel, P. and Passa, P. Lipoprotein(a) in diabetic patients and normoglycaemic relatives in familial NIDDM. *Diabetes Care*, 1993, **16**, 742–7.
72. Heller, F.R., Jamart, J., Honore, P., Derue, G., Novik, V., Galante, L., Parfonry, A., Hondekujn, J.C. and Buysschaert, M. Serum lipoprotein(a) in patients with diabetes mellitus. *Diabetes Care*, 1993, **16**, 819–23.
73. Maser, R.E., Usher, D., Becker, D.J., Drash, A.L., Kuller, L.H. and Orchard, T.J. Lipoprotein(a) concentration shows little relationship to IDDM complications in the Pittsburgh

Epidemiology of Diabetes Complications Study Cohort. *Diabetes Care,* 1993, **16,** 755–8.

74. Haffner, S.M., Valdez, R.A., Hazuda, H.P., Mitchell, B.D., Morales, P.A. and Stern, M.P. Prospective analysis of the insulin resistance syndrome (syndrome X). *Diabetes,* 1992, **41,** 715–22.

75. Friedewald, W.T., Levy, R. and Frederickson, D.S. Estimation of the concentration of low density lipoprotein in plasma without use of the preparative ultracentrifuge. *Clin. Chem.,* 1972, **18,** 499–502.

76. Rubies-Prat, J., Reverter, J.L., Senti, M., Pedro-Botet, J., Salinas, I., Lucas, A., Nogues, X. and Sanmarti, A. Calculated low density lipoprotein cholesterol should not be used for management of lipoprotein abnormalities in patients with diabetes mellitus. *Diabetes Care,* 1993, **16,** 1081–6.

77. Alberti, K.G.M.M. and Gries, F.A. Management of non-insulin-dependent diabetes mellitus in Europe: a consensus view. *Diabet. Med.,* 1988, **5,** 275–81.

78. Haffner, S.M. Management of dyslipidaemia in adults with diabetes. *Diabetes Care,* 1988, **21,** 160–78.

79. American Diabetes Association. Management of dyslipidaemia in adults with diabetes. *Diabetes Care,* 1998, **21,** 179–82.

80. National Cholesterol Education Program. Second Report of the Expert Panel on Detection, Evaluation and Treatment of High Blood Cholesterol in Adults (Adult Treatment Panel II). *Circulation,* 1994, **19,** 1329–445.

81. Garg, A. and Grundy, S.M. Diabetic dyslipidaemia and its therapy. *Diabetes Rev.,* 1997, **5,** 425–33.

82. Diabetes Control and Complications Trial Research Group. Effect of intensive treatment of diabetes on the development and progression of longterm complications in insulin dependent diabetes mellitus. *N. Engl. J. Med.,* 1993, **329,** 977–86.

83. Stern, M.P., Mitchell, B.D., Haffner, S.M. and Hazuda, H.P. Does glycaemic control of type II diabetes suffice to control diabetic dyslipidaemia? A community perspective. *Diabetes Care,* 1992, **15,** 638–44.

84. Wu, M.S., Johnston, P., Sheu, W.H.H., Hollenbeck, C.B., Jeng, C.Y., Goldfine, I.D., Chen, Y.D.I. and Reaven, G.M. Effect of metformin on carbohydrate and lipoprotein metabolism in NIDDM patients. *Diabetes Care,* 1990, **13,** 1–8.

85. Nagi, D.K. and Yudkin, J.S. Effects of metformin on insulin resistance, risk factors for cardiovascular disease and plasminogen activator inhibitor in NIDDM subjects. *Diabetes Care,* 1993, **16,** 621–9.

86. Jeffersen, J., Zhou, M.Y., Che, Y.D.I., Reaven, G.M. Effect of metformin on postprandial lipaemia in patients with fairly to poorly controlled NIDDM. *Diabetes Care,* 1994, **17,** 1093–9.

87. American Diabetes Association. Guidelines for prescribing exercise for type II diabetes. *Diabetes Care,* 1990, **13,** 639–44.

88. Schneider, S.H. and Ruderman, N.B. Exercise and NIDDM, Technical review. *Diabetes Care,* 1990, **13,** 785–9.

89. Skarfors, E.T., Wegener, T.A., Lithell, H. and Selinus, I. Physical training as treatment for type 2 (non insulin dependent) diabetes in elderly men: a feasibility study over 2 years. *Diabetologia,* 1987, **30,** 930–3.

90. Moy, C.S., Songer, T.J., LaPorte, R.E., Dorman, J.S., Kriska, A.M., Orchard, T.J., Becker, D.J. and Drash, A.L. Insulin dependent diabetes mellitus, physical activity and death. *Am. J. Epidemiol.,* 1993, **137,** 74–81.

91. American Diabetes Association. Nutrition recommendations and principles for people with diabetes melitus. *Diabetes Care,* 1994, **17,** 519–22.

92. Garg, A. Efficacy of dietary fibre in lowering serum cholesterol. *Am. J. Med.,* 1994, **97,** 501–3.

93. Garg, A., Bonanome, A., Grundy, S.M., Zhang, Z.J. and Unger, R.H. Comparison of a high-carbohydrate diet with a high monounsaturated-fat diet in patients with non insulin dependent diabetes mellitus. *N. Engl. J. Med.,* 1988, **319,** 829–34.

94. Garg, A., Grundy, S.M. and Unger, R.H. Comparison of effects of high and low carbohydrate diets on plasma lipoproteins and insulin sensitivity in patients with mild NIDDM. *Diabetes,* 1992, **41,** 1278–85.

95. Parillo, M., Rivellese, A.A., Giardullo, A.V., Capaldo, B., Giacco, A., Genovese, S. and Riccardi, G. A high monounsaturated fat/low carbohydrate diet improves peripheral insulin sensitivity in non-insulin-dependent diabetic patients. *Metabolism,* 1992, **41,** 1373–8.

96. Campbell, L.V., Marmot, P.E., Dyer, J.A., Borkman, M. and Storlien, L.H. The high monounsaturated fat diet as a practical alternative for NIDDM. *Diabetes Care,* 1994, **17,** 177–88.

97. Garg, A., Bantle, J.P., Henry, R.R. *et al.* Effects of varying carbohydrate content of diet in patients with non insulin dependent diabetes mellitus. *J. Am. Med. Assoc.,* 1994, **271,** 1421–8.

98. Chen, Y.D.I., Swami, S., Skowronski, R., Coulston, A.M. and Reaven, G.M. Effect of variations in dietary fat and carbohydrate intake on postprandial lipaemia in patients with non insulin dependent diabetes mellitus. *J. Clin. Endocrinol. Metab.,*1993, **76,** 347–51.

99. Dreon, D.M. and Krauss, R.M. Apolipoprotein E isoform phenotypes are associated with differing LDL subclass responses to reduced fat diets. *Circulation,* 1993, **86,** I–406.

100. Pyörälä, K., Pedersen, T.R., Kjeksus, J., Faergerman, O., Olsson, A.G. and Thorgeirsson, G. Cholesterol lowering with simvastatin improves prognosis of diabetic patients with coronary heart disease: a subgroup analysis of the Scandinavian Simvastatin Survival Study (4S). *Diabetes Care,* 1997, **20,** 614–20.

101. Sacks, F.M., Pfeffer, M.A., Moye, L.A. *et al.* for the Cholesterol and Recurrent Events Trial Investigators. The effect of pravastatin on coronary events after myocardial infarction in patients with average cholesterol levels: Cholesterol and Recurrent Events Trial Investigators. *N. Engl. J. Med.,* 1996, **335,** 1001–9.

102. Koskinen, P., Mänttari, M., Manninen, V., Huttinen, J.K., Heinonen, O.P. and Frick, M.H. Coronary heart disease incidence in NIDDM patients in the Helsinki Heart Study. *Diabetes Care,* 1992, **15,** 820–5.

103. Steiner, G. for the DAIS Project Group. The Diabetes Atherosclerosis Intervention Study (DAIS): a study conducted in cooperation with the World Health Organization. *Diabetologia,* 1996, **39,** 1655–61.

104. Goldbourt, U., Behar, S., Reicher-Reiss, H., Agmon, J., Kaplinsky, E., Graff, E., Kishon, Y., Caspi, A., Weisbort, J. and Mandelzweig, L. Rational and design of a secondary prevention trial of increasing serum high density lipoprotein cholesterol and reducing triglycerides in patients with clinically manifest atherosclerotic heart disease (the Bezafibrate Infarction Prevention Trial). *Am. J. Cardiol.,* 1993, **71,** 909–15.

105. Tonkin, A.M. for the LIPID study group. Management of the Long-term Intervention with Pravastatin in Ischaemic Disease (LIPID) study after the Scandinavian Simvastatin Survival Study (4S). *Am. J. Cardiol.,* 1995, **76,** 107C–112C.

106. Medical Research Council/British Heart Foundation. Heart Protection Study: a randomized study of the effects on mortality and morbidity of HMG-CoA reductase inhibitors and of antioxidant vitamin in a wide range of people at high risk of coronary heart disease. Protocol Oxford Heart Protection Study, 1994.

107. Garg, Z. and Grundy, S.M. Cholestyramine therapy for dyslipidaemia in non insulin dependent diabetes mellitus: a short term, double blind, crossover trial. Ann. Intern. Med., 1994, **121,** 416–22.

108. Kasim, S. Dietary marine fish oils and insulin action in type 2 diabetes. *Ann. NY Acad. Sci. USA,* 1993, **683,** 250–7.

109. Ericsson, C.G., Hamsten, A., Nilsson, J. *et al.* Angiographic assessment of effects of bezafibrate on progression of coronary artery disease in young male postinfarction patients. *Lancet,* 1996, **347,** 849–53.

110. Frick, M.H., Syvanne, M., Nieminen, M.S. *et al.* for the Lipid Coronary Angiographic Trial Study Group (LOCAT). Prevention of the angiographic progression of coronary and vein graft atherosclerosis by gemofibrozil after coronary bypass surgery in men with low levels of HDL cholesterol. *Circulation,* 1997, **96,** 2137–43.

RISK FACTORS FOR ARTERIAL DISEASE IN DIABETES: COAGULOPATHY

Peter J. Grant

7.1 INTRODUCTION

Diabetes mellitus is characterized by fasting hyperglycaemia and the chronic development of vascular complications. Although the underlying pathogenesis of insulin-dependent diabetes mellitus (IDDM) and non-insulin-dependent diabetes mellitus (NIDDM) patients is different, both types of diabetes exhibit the manifestations of micro- and macrovascular disorders leading to an enormous burden of morbidity and mortality in this population. The results of the Diabetes Control and Complications Trial (DCCT) study in IDDM subjects have demonstrated that improvements in glycaemic control and protein glycosylation lead to amelioration of the development and progression of micro-vascular complications. There is an under-current of assumption in the diabetes community that the same will be true for macrovascular disease in IDDM and for both micro- and macrovascular complications in NIDDM, although this remains to be sub-stantiated. Whatever the ultimate answer to this is, there remains the question of what mechanisms are involved in translating poor glycaemic control into vascular disorders. There are many candidates for this process including protein glycosylation and advanced glycation endproduct (AGE) formation, oxi-dative stress, lipid abnormalities and changes in haemostasis and coagulation. If the model of insulin resistance, discussed in Chapter 8, is any indication, it is likely that abnormal-ities in all these pathways will have some role in the development of vascular disorders associated with both IDDM and NIDDM. The aim of this chapter is to review some of the information regarding variation in important components of the haemostatic process in relation to IDDM, NIDDM and vascular complications.

7.2 MECHANISMS IN THROMBOSIS

The biochemical processes that regulate the formation and subsequent lysis of a clot are complex and dependent on a wide variety of interrelated metabolic reactions (Figure 7.1).

7.2.1 COAGULATION

The critical reaction in the fluid phase of coagulation concerns the conversion of pro-thrombin to thrombin, which is the pivotal enzyme in coagulation processes. Thrombin acts to convert fibrinogen to soluble fibrin and then to fibrinolysis-resistant cross-linked fibrin, the latter reaction dependent on throm-bin activation of factor XIII. The conversion of prothrombin is governed by the generation of activated factor X, which in turn is regulated by the action of the intrinsic pathway (factors XII, XI, IX, VIII) and the extrinsic pathway (tissue factor, factor VII). With the exception of tissue factor, which is released from

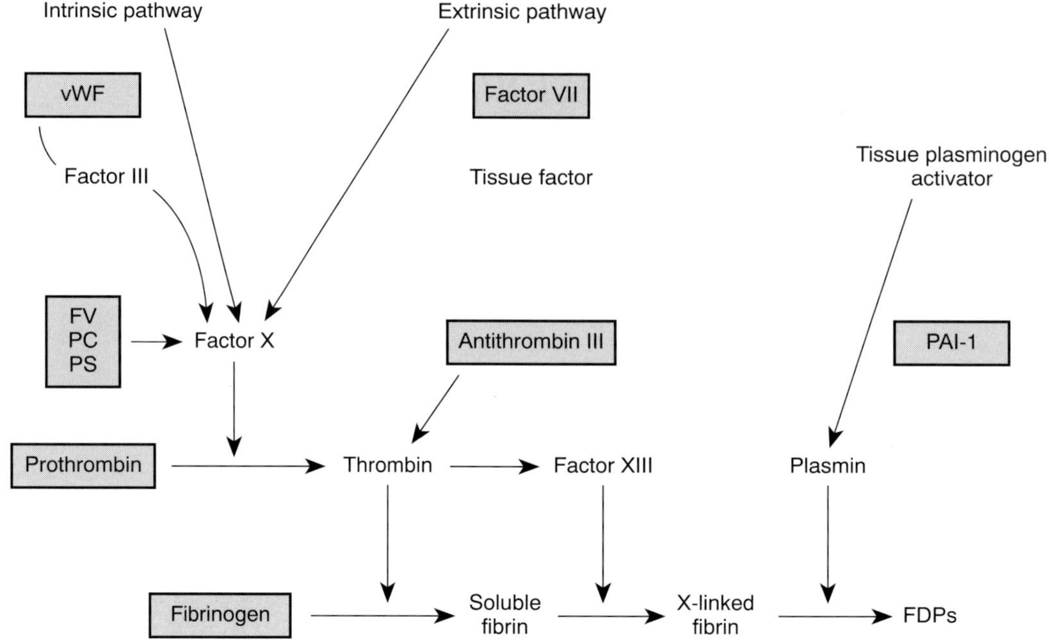

Figure 7.1 The main components of the coagulation and fibrinolytic cascades. The extrinsic pathway consists of tissue factor and factor VII. The intrinsic pathway is contact-activated through factor XII leading to a 'cascade' or 'waterfall' of activation of factors XI, IX, VIII and V. Both pathways converge and lead to activation of factor X which converts prothrombin to thrombin. The tissue factor/VII complex is able to activate the intrinsic pathway by converting factor IX to the active zymogen. The activity of thrombin is substantially diminished by the effects of heparin, antithrombin III and thrombomodulin. The principal components of the fibrinolytic pathway are tissue plasminogen activator which converts plasminogen to plasmin and plasminogen activator inhibitor-1 (PAI-1) which inhibits this reaction by binding to tissue plasminogen activator. Plasmin is inhibited in the circulation by plasmin inhibitor. The urokinase-mediated pathway of plasminogen activation is also inhibited by PAI-1, although this pathway is thought to be less important in maintaining vascular patency. FDPs, fibrin degradation products; FV, Factor V; PC, protein C; PS, protein S; vWF, von Willebrand factor.

damaged cells in its active form, all the coagulation factors circulate in the inactive state and are activated in a coagulation cascade. The coagulation system has a number of inhibitors and anticoagulants including antithrombin III, protein C, protein S and thrombomodulin. These reactions are all localized to the site of damage by binding to specific cell ligands such as tissue factor. It will be appreciated that this is far too large a topic to give adequate coverage here and more comprehensive details can be found in the excellent *Disorders of Hemostasis* [1].

7.2.2　FIBRINOLYSIS

The fibrinolytic cascade consists of a number of activators and inhibitors that regulate the conversion of plasminogen to plasmin which acts to lyse fibrin. The conversion of plasminogen to plasmin is crucial to the development of lytic activity and this reaction is regulated by tissue plasminogen activator (tPA) and urokinase (uPA). Both activators are quenched in the circulation by the binding of their fast-acting inhibitor, plasminogen activator inhibitor-1 (PAI-1) which exists in the circulation in excess. Cross-linked fibrin binds plasminogen, plasmin and tPA and allows these reactions to proceed unhindered by the effects of PAI-1. The net result is that fibrinolysis is localized to the site of thrombus formation and systemic fibrinolysis does not occur under normal circumstances. One benefit of this is that fibrinogen is protected from systemic fibrinogenolysis, the consequences of which are clearly seen in conditions associated with disseminated intravascular coagulation. For a fuller description of fibrinolysis, there are a number of excellent reviews on this subject [2–4].

7.2.3   PLATELETS

Platelets are crucial in the development of both thrombosis and atheroma [1]. The development of endothelial damage exposes epitopes on collagen that permit binding of von Willebrand factor (vWF). vWF binds to the platelet integrin, GpIb/IX which has two effects: the development of platelet adhesion and exposure of the fibrinogen binding integrin GpIIb/IIIa. The latter reaction is dependent on factor XIII cross-linking and leads to the development of platelet aggregation and activation. Platelet activation leads to release of procoagulant factors such as platelet factor 4, β-thromboglobulin and PAI-1. It is likely that these reactions play a role in the development of atherothrombotic vascular disorders as all the major components (platelets, vWF, fibrinogen and PAI-1) have been related to the development of myocardial infarction.

7.3   DIABETES AS A HYPERCOAGULABLE STATE

7.3.1   INTRODUCTION

The study of haemostatic function in relation to diabetes and its complications has revealed a colossal combination of variations in circulating measures, that defy sensible interpretation. It is often said that diabetes is a 'hypercoagulable state' and this is most commonly based on the variety of changes in coagulation, fibrinolysis and platelet function that extrapolated from first principles might indicate this to be the case. There are problems with this argument as measurement of haemostatic proteins occur *ex vivo* and inevitably involve an element of artefact. Also, to qualify as a hypercoagulable state, there should be a greater tendency to thrombosis *for a given stimulus*. Clear examples of this are congenital antithrombin III deficiency or possession of factor V (Leiden) where there is an increased risk of venous thrombosis under any given set of conditions compared to those subjects who do not possess these abnormalities [5].

There is no doubt that patients with diabetes are at increased risk of myocardial infarction of which thrombosis plays a part. However, they also tend to have more coronary atheroma and other vascular risk factors which make it difficult to be sure that the above criteria are fulfilled. The development of deep vein thrombosis and pulmonary embolus in diabetic subjects is interesting as there might be expected to be an increased incidence if diabetes is accompanied by a procoagulant state. Several studies have partially addressed this issue as part of larger studies into risk factors for thromboembolic disease. In a study of 2103 subjects by self-administered questionnaire, thrombosis and pulmonary embolus were reported as significantly associated with female sex, increasing age and diabetes [6]. In small studies of abdominal surgery [7] and post renal transplant [8], diabetes was found to be a risk factor for the development of venous thrombosis. The FINNVASC study reported on 7533 patients of whom 34 (0.45%) had an episode of thrombosis and reported no relationship to diabetes [9] as did a smaller study of thrombosis following knee arthroplasty [10]. The study in the USA reported on a 16-year follow-up of 112 822 female nurses in whom 125 primary cases of pulmonary embolus occurred [11]. In this study, which is the largest to date, obesity, smoking and hypertension were related to the development of venous thrombosis, but there was no relationship with diabetes.

7.3.2 BIOCHEMICAL EVIDENCE FOR A PRO-COAGULANT STATE IN DIABETES

Diabetes mellitus is characterized by a wide variety of abnormalities in coagulation, fibrinolysis and platelet function. Amongst the most commonly described changes are increases in the coagulant proteins, factor VIII/vWF [12], factor VII and factor X [13] and fibrinogen [13–16] with potentially pro-thrombotic alterations in the coagulation inhibitors protein C and antithrombin III [17, 18]. In NIDDM, profound suppression of the fibrinolytic pathway as reflected by elevated PAI-1 concentrations occurs in association with underlying insulin resistance [19, 20]. Interestingly, as shown in Table 7.1, the development of albuminuria is associated with exaggerated changes in haemostatic function [21, 22] which is taken by some to provide a link between nephropathy and the increased risk of vascular disorders.

None of these observations *per se* indicates the presence of a pro-coagulant state, although elevated factor VIII concentrations

have been shown to increase *ex vivo* thrombin generation in IDDM subjects with nephropathy [23]. As circulating coagulation factors exist in a non-activated state, it is possible to have increased concentrations of a protein without affecting rates of coagulation. The biochemical acid test for a hypercoagulable or pro-coagulant state is the existence of increased levels of activation peptides reflecting cleavage and activation of coagulation proteins. Examples include fibrinopeptide A (FPA) which is cleaved from fibrinogen by the action of thrombin, or prothrombin fragments F_{1+2} which are released during the conversion of prothrombin to thrombin. There is little work in this area involving diabetes; however, two studies from one centre have reported higher levels of FPA in IDDM that are further increased with hyperglycaemia [24] and similarly increased prothrombin F_{1+2} in 40 IDDM subjects compared with controls [25]. Our own studies of FPA in IDDM subjects did not confirm the effects of hyperglycaemia on FPA concentrations [26] although an early study of IDDM subjects with retinopathy reported increases in FPA with hyperglycaemia [27].

Interpretation of some of these data is difficult as the act of venepuncture can lead to local activation of coagulation which may cause artefactual increases in activation peptides. Although there is some evidence of a biochemical hypercoagulable state in diabetic subjects, the clinical data, particularly in relation to venous thrombosis, are inconsistent. A likely scenario for the involvement of a heightened haemostatic response is that it is mediated by interactions with other established risk factors such as dyslipidaemia, abnormal oxidation reactions and the presence of arterial atheroma. In this way the momentum towards atheroma formation and thrombosis is developed and maintained by the metabolic milieu of diabetes mellitus that is composed of multiple interacting cardiovascular risk factors.

Table 7.1 Prothrombotic risk factors elevated in association with microalbuminuria in NIDDM and IDDM subjects (numbers in square brackets are references)

NIDDM	IDDM
Fibrinogen [53]	Fibrinogen [22,33,53,54]
von Willebrand factor [70]	von Willebrand factor [53]
Factor VII [70]	Factor VII [22,33,53]
PAI-1 [70]	PAI-1 [22]
Protein C [53]	Protein C [53]
Plasminogen [72]	Protein S [53,73]
Plasmin inhibitor [72]	ATIII [73]

7.4 DIABETES AND ATHEROTHROMBOTIC RISK

Microvascular complications account for much of the morbidity in the diabetic population, but ultimately it is the macrovascular complications (coronary artery, cerebrovascular and peripheral vascular disease) that lead to early mortality. Although both types of diabetes share a high risk of cardiovascular disorders, most studies have been carried out in NIDDM because of the greater numbers of subjects available for investigation. The metabolic disturbance in subjects with NIDDM is related to decreased glucose uptake and resistance to the action of insulin in skeletal muscle, increased hepatic glucose output and abnormalities in insulin secretion. This pattern of metabolism is more common in the general population than in NIDDM subjects, with estimates of the prevalence of insulin resistance of 25%, depending on the definition employed [28]. Diagnosed NIDDM is thus only the tip of an iceberg which comprises undiagnosed NIDDM, impaired glucose tolerance (IGT) and compensated normal glucose tolerance (NGT).

The original WHO criteria for the diagnosis of diabetes were based on levels of glycaemia associated with the development of microvascular complications. Evidence is accumulating that minor increases in blood glucose, previously thought to be harmless, are associated with subtle alterations in cardiac function and increase in mortality from ischaemic heart disease. In the Honolulu Heart Study, subjects with a one-hour blood glucose above 6.4 mmol/l had an increased 12-year coronary artery disease risk that was further increased in the groups with higher blood glucose levels at one hour [29]. The Bedford study reported increased cardiovascular mortality in subjects with IGT and a two- to threefold increase in 10-year mortality in NIDDM, both being more marked in females [30]. The Framingham study reported that the incidence of cardiovascular disease in diabetes was twice that seen in non-diabetic males and approaching threefold in females [31]. Figures for other vascular conditions reveal a similar extent of morbidity and mortality. The Honolulu Heart Study showed diabetes to be associated with a twofold risk of stroke, and other studies have confirmed that at all ages, men and women have twice the risk of cerebral infarction compared with non-diabetic subjects [32]. Framingham revealed a fourfold increase in peripheral vascular disease associated with diabetes and, again, a relatively greater increase in females.

7.5 COAGULATION

7.5.1 FIBRINOGEN

Fibrinogen in IDDM and NIDDM subjects

The study of coagulation factors in diabetes has produced a huge literature with conflicting results that are often difficult to interpret. An exception to this is fibrinogen, where there is almost universal agreement as to its importance in diabetes and vascular disorders. In IDDM subjects, levels of fibrinogen are reported to be elevated compared to non-diabetic controls [17, 33–35], although generally not to the same extent as in NIDDM. In a study of identical twins discordant for IDDM, the IDDM twin had increased systolic blood pressure and elevated fibrinogen levels compared with the non-diabetic twin [35]. IDDM subjects without complications also have elevated fibrinogen [17] and both these studies suggest that elevated fibrinogen is associated with the diabetic state rather than secondary to the development of vascular complications.

In NIDDM subjects, most studies have reported increased levels of fibrinogen. In 1574 NIDDM patients, 50% had a plasma fibrinogen greater than 3.5 g/l [18] and many others have reported similar findings [36–41]. One major exception to this has come from the Rotterdam study of 2640 subjects without diabetes compared with 331 with NIDDM. In this study there was increased fibrinogen only in insulin-treated NIDDM, but no difference in diabetic subjects as a whole [42]. Racial studies have produced results consistent with most studies in Caucasian subjects, describing increased fibrinogen in diabetic subjects from Japan [43], native Africa [44], China [45] and in American Indians [46]. Interestingly, there is a report that fibrinogen levels in Asian diabetic subjects are lower than in non-Asian diabetic subjects [47], although both diabetes and vascular disorders are more common in the former group.

Determinants of plasma fibrinogen in diabetic subjects

There is evidence that fibrinogen is weakly associated with features of the insulin resistance syndrome [48, 49], and both glycosylated haemoglobin [18] and body mass index [38] have been related to increased fibrinogen concentrations. In NIDDM subjects, body mass index and smoking accounted for 23% of the variance in fibrinogen levels, and low levels of physical activity are associated with higher fibrinogen [38]. The latter findings are similar to those described in non-diabetic subjects [50,51].

Possibly the most important association with elevated fibrinogen concentrations is the presence of diabetic nephropathy. Diabetic subjects with albuminuria with otherwise normal renal function and those with frank renal impairment are at markedly increased risk of myocardial infarction. A number of studies have attempted to tease out the factors involved in this link, with emphasis often placed on associated changes in haemostasis. Several have demonstrated that there are consistent increases in plasma fibrinogen in IDDM and NIDDM subjects with microalbuminuria [18, 33, 52–54]. Similar findings have been reported in American Indians with diabetes [46] and nephropathy where differences in fibrinogen occurred in subjects with and without nephropathy that are associated with a marked increase in cardiovascular disease in caucasian subjects [55]. Although microalbuminuria appears to be associated with increased cardiovascular disease in the non-diabetic population [56], a study of haemostatic changes in hypertensive non-diabetic subjects with microalbuminuria showed weaker relationships with vWF and fibrinogen than would be expected in the diabetic population [57]. These findings imply that microalbuminuria and the associated changes in fibrinogen are not directly related, but rather independently associated with another factor which could be either protein glycosylation and/or ambient glucose concentrations.

Fibrinogen and vascular disorders

Prospective studies have demonstrated a strong relationship between fibrinogen and the development of both cardiovascular and cerebrovascular disease [55], and fibrinogen was more strongly associated with cardiovascular disease than cholesterol in the Northwick Park Heart Study [58]. There have been no prospective studies of fibrinogen in relation to macrovascular disorders in diabetic subjects, although it would be purist to suggest that hyperfibrinogenaemia will not have a role under these conditions. Plasma fibrinogen has been shown to relate to vascular disorders in case control studies [59, 60] and it is held that elevated fibrinogen increases the risk of cardiovascular disease in diabetic subjects [60].

Genetics of fibrinogen and diabetes mellitus

The α, β and γ chains of the fibrinogen molecule are coded for by three genes in close proximity on chromosome 4 position q21–28. Close physical linkage of these was suggested by the high degree of linkage dysequilibrium of polymorphic sites on the coding regions.

The gene coding for the β chain of the fibrinogen molecule is thought to be self-limiting in fibrinogen synthesis and as a result interest has centred on polymorphisms in this region. Evidence indicates a strong genetic component to fibrinogen levels, with as much as 51% of the variation in levels due to genetic factors [61, 62]. The associations of both the β-fibrinogen gene –455 and Bcl-1 polymorphisms with fibrinogen levels appear to be gender-specific [63, 64] and results from our group suggest that this is also the case with the β 448 G/A polymorphism [65]. A study of 100 NIDDM subjects reported that the Bcl-1 site was associated with fibrinogen levels [66]. The Bcl-1 polymorphism is associated with the development of peripheral arterial disease [67] and the rare allele is associated with myocardial infarction [68]. The β 448 G/A polymorphism is associated with cerebrovascular disease in women, and the β –455 G/A polymorphism is independently associated with coronary artery disease in subjects with NIDDM [65, 69].

7.5.2 FACTOR VII

Factor VII in NIDDM and IDDM subjects

Compared to fibrinogen and PAI-1, there have been relatively few reports on factor VII in diabetes. Several studies have reported increased concentrations of factor VII in NIDDM, both without clinical evidence of complications [37, 70–72] and with further increases in the presence of microalbuminuria [70]. In IDDM subjects, factor VII is similarly elevated with microalbuminuria [22], although it is not clear if baseline values for factor VII are increased in non-complicated IDDM. A study of 70 diabetic subjects reported increased factor VII/X complexes but omitted to discuss the clinical categories of diabetes that were studied [73]. The study of identical twins non-discordant for IDDM reported lower levels of factor VII in the IDDM twin [35], the significance of which is not clear.

There appears to be a gender effect, although conflicting results have been obtained. Factor VII has been described as lower in female IDDM [74] and higher in male NIDDM [72, 74]. However, our study in 213 NIDDM subjects, of whom 124 were male, demonstrated levels in females nearly 25% higher than in their male counterparts [75]. In a study of first degree relatives of NIDDM subjects, we also found higher levels of factor VII in the group as a whole with a trend towards increased concentrations of factor VII in the females studied [49]. As factor VII appears to be related to features of the insulin resistance syndrome and is increased in women with the polycystic ovary syndrome, it may be that menopausal status explains the differences between female IDDM and NIDDM and is causing some of the confusion related to levels in NIDDM.

Determinants of factor VII concentrations in diabetes mellitus

The major determinants of factor VII concentrations in diabetes appear to be gender, microalbuminuria and some features of the insulin resistance syndrome. In non-diabetic populations there is evidence that levels of factor VII are related to cholesterol and, to a greater extent, triglyceride [76–79]. These observations may help to explain some of the relationships between factor VII and vascular disease.

In a study of 95 NIDDM patients characterized for features of insulin resistance, factor VII concentrations correlated strongly with total cholesterol, insulin and triglycerides and to a lesser extent with age and body mass index [80]. These findings together with observations in NIDDM first-degree relatives [49] indicate that elevated factor VII clusters with insulin resistance in a manner similar to that described for PAI-1.

Factor VII and vascular disorders

The Northwick Park Heart Study put factor VII on the map as a cardiovascular risk factor when increased concentrations were associated with fatal but not non-fatal myocardial infarction in a prospective study of middle-aged men [58]. These findings have been partially supported in the prospective PROCAM study, although there was only a trend towards an association [81]. Other case control studies have shown associations between factor VII and vascular disease and the PLAT study reported an association between factor VII and carotid intimal thickening [82].

It is, however, difficult to imagine how a protein in such a complex system could be related to fatal but not non-fatal myocardial infarction. Acceptance of these findings at face value requires considerable mental gymnastics, as death from myocardial infarction is related to powerful influences such as site of the lesion, left ventricular function and the development of dysrhythmias. It is unlikely that factor VII would interact with these factors to cause sudden death without increasing, concurrently, non-fatal infarction.

A possible explanation for these findings, apart from the play of chance, is that they reflect weak associations with some features of insulin resistance and other cardiovascular risk such as triglyceride, cholesterol and insulin. This could provide a plausible explanation, as the strongest relationships would be demonstrated in those subjects with the greatest clustering of risk and greatest risk of fatal myocardial infarction. If this were true, however, it remains difficult to see why there is no relationship to non-fatal infarction.

Genetics of factor VII and diabetes

Studies of the factor VII gene have demonstrated two sites in linkage disequilibrium that relate to circulating levels of factor VII, a promoter decanucleotide repeat and a single base change at position R353Q in exon 8 [83].

Several studies have demonstrated a relationship between circulating factor VII and dyslipidaemia. Also, in a study of patients with coronary artery disease, those homozygous for the insertion at the R353Q site had significantly higher levels of factor VII although there was no relationship between possession of a particular genotype or FVII:C levels and either extent of atheroma or a past history of AMI [84]. Similar results were obtained in the ECTIM study [85]. Both studies are flawed, however, if factor VII predisposes to fatal rather than non-fatal infarction as fatal infarcts would not have been identified.

7.6   FIBRINOLYSIS

7.6.1   FIBRINOLYSIS IN NIDDM AND IDDM SUBJECTS

In patients with IDDM, there is no consistent defect in fibrinolysis. Review of the major studies of fibrinolysis [86, 87] suggests an increase in basal fibrinolytic activity and tPA concentrations, with normal or reduced levels of PAI-1 in IDDM patients. In our study uncomplicated IDDM was associated with normal responses to venous occlusion with a rise in tPA while PAI-1 remained unchanged [88]. This response was progressively less with increasing evidence of vascular disease; PAI-1 remaining at a similar level, but tPA activity and antigen failing to rise [88]. Similar results were found in a much smaller study of six IDDM patients [89]. In a study of 31 patients with IDDM, euglobulin clot lysis, tPA and PAI-1 were found to be similar to levels in controls [90]. However with increasing degrees of renal disease there was a progressive reduction in euglobulin clot lysis activity and a significant increase in PAI-1 [90].

Marked differences exist in fibrinolytic activity when subjects with IDDM and NIDDM are compared. Patients with NIDDM have profound suppression of fibrinolysis due to increased levels of PAI-1 [20]. Several studies have noted the strong relationship between features of the metabolic syndrome and elevated PAI-1 levels in NIDDM. In particular, PAI-1 strongly correlates with triglyceride concentrations [20, 91]. Many population studies have shown a relationship between fasting insulin concentrations and PAI-1 in diabetic and non-diabetic subjects and insulin has been shown to enhance PAI-1 synthesis and secretion in cells of hepatic origin [92, 93]. In humans, however, no study has yet demonstrated an increase in PAI-1 in response to insulin [94, 95] and it seems that insulin levels in population studies are probably acting as a surrogate for insulin resistance, which appears to be the major determinant of plasma PAI-1 concentrations.

7.6.2 DETERMINANTS OF FIBRINOLYTIC ACTIVITY IN DIABETES MELLITUS

Changes in levels of blood glucose affect fibrinolytic function in experimental systems and *in vivo*. Endothelial cells express PAI-1 and tPA at about twice the rate in culture medium containing 30 mM compared with 5 mM glucose, though overall fibrinolytic potential fell slightly [96]. These *in vitro* data are consistent with findings in patients. We found that euglobulin clot lysis activity was increased in response both to hyper- and hypoglycaemia in patients with IDDM [26] though there was no change in cross-linked fibrin-fibrinogen degradation products. In a similar study of hypoglycaemia, fibrin plate lysis area increased slightly, as did tPA antigen concentration, while PAI-1 activity fell and fibrin degradation products (FDP) remained unchanged [89].

In NIDDM there has been considerable interest generated by the relationship between features of insulin resistance and elevated PAI-1 concentrations. Insulin increases PAI-1 synthesis and secretion in cells of hepatic origin [92, 93], although there is no *in vivo* work to support these findings [94, 95]. Triglyceride concentrations correlate strongly with PAI-1 [20, 91] and *in vitro* studies have shown that triglyceride interacts with the LDL receptor to release PAI-1, a response that is augmented in the presence of insulin [97]. Furthermore there is molecular evidence described below to support the view that triglyceride is the important determinant of PAI-1 in diabetes.

7.6.3 FIBRINOLYSIS AND VASCULAR DISORDERS

Several large-scale prospective studies have evaluated the role of the fibrinolytic system in vascular disease, although none have specifically investigated diabetic subjects. The Northwick Park Heart Study of middle-aged men reported that global suppression of fibrinolysis was related to subsequent risk of myocardial infarction [58]. Hamsten *et al.* found that levels of PAI-1 activity three months after a first myocardial infarction in young men predicted recurrent myocardial infarction [98]. The Physicians Heart Study described tPA as being independently associated with stroke in a large study of American physicians [99].

7.6.4 GENETICS OF PAI-1 AND DIABETES MELLITUS

A 4G/5G polymorphism 675 Bp 5′ of the start site of transcription in the PAI-1 promoter has been identified that relates to circulating PAI-1 levels. The functional nature of this mutation lies in the fact that the 5G allele binds both a transcription and a repressor factor, whereas the 4G allele only binds the transcription factor [100]. This has been shown to lead to higher PAI-1 gene expression in cells *in vitro* [101] and higher PAI-1 levels in populations homozygous for the 4G allelle [91,100]. Studies in NIDDM diabetic patients have demonstrated a triglyceride/genotype interaction with further increases in PAI-1 in subjects homozygous for the 4G allele compared to 4G/5G or 5G/5G in the presence of hypertriglyceridaemia [102, 103]. Four case control studies have investigated the relationship between genotype at this locus and the development of AMI, three of which have shown an increased frequency of the 4G/4G allele in cases of AMI [100, 104, 105], whereas the ECTIM study showed no relationship [106]. Additionally the large prospective American Physicians Study also found no relationship between PAI-1 genotype and myocardial infarction [107]. PAI-1 and triglyceride levels were not measured in this group and it remains questionable as to whether these data can be applied to the general population.

7.7 PLATELETS AND VON WILLEBRAND FACTOR

7.7.1 PLATELET FUNCTION IN DIABETES MELLITUS

A number of studies have been carried out on platelet function in diabetes [108]. In most, samples from patients with IDDM and NIDDM have not been differentiated and it is not clear whether there is any systematic difference in platelet behaviour. Most investigators have found platelets from diabetic subjects to react abnormally, with a lowered threshold to activation by aggregating agents, increased plasma concentrations of released α-granule proteins and platelet eicosanoids, altered platelet plasma membrane function and reduced platelet survival. In general, abnormalities have been more marked in patients with overt vascular disease. As many of the changes seen in platelets from diabetic patients are similar to those observed in patients with atherosclerotic vascular disease, it is not clear whether they are related mainly to the metabolic disturbances or to the vascular disease in diabetes.

Platelets from diabetic subjects are more likely to aggregate when exposed to a range of platelet agonists. Many workers in the 1970s showed that diabetic platelets aggregated at lower concentrations of adenosine diphosphate (ADP) than controls [109]. Aggregation is similarly induced more readily in response to collagen [110, 111], sodium arachidonate [110–112] and platelet-activating factor [113]. Use of platelet aggregation in whole blood (which avoids artefacts induced by processing) has shown platelets from diabetic subjects to be more susceptible to activation by shaking and stirring [114]. This abnormality was greater in patients with IDDM who had vascular complications. In some studies, improved diabetic control and exposure of platelets to lower levels of plasma glucose restored the pattern of platelet activity towards control values [111] whereas in others it did not [110].

Platelets from patients with diabetes also exhibit more GpIIb/IIIa receptors on their surface [115] and bind greater amounts of fibrinogen [116] than platelets from non-diabetic subjects.

As might be expected, platelets which are more sensitive to agonists which induce aggregation will be more likely to release the contents of the α-granules into plasma. Most observers have found increased levels in diabetic plasma of the released proteins β-thromboglobulin (βTG) [113, 117, 118] and platelet factor 4 (PF4) [113, 118]. Minimal platelet activation and release can lead to increase in plasma βTG during processing, but studies which circumvent this by using the ratio of βTG:PF4 [118] or urinary βTG levels [119] have similarly shown that plasma from diabetic subjects has higher concentrations of platelet release proteins. This is consistent with a low level of intravascular platelet activation in diabetes.

An early observation was that diabetic platelets produced increased amounts of metabolites of arachidonic acid following stimulation [120]. Plasma from patients with diabetes has higher than normal levels of thromboxane B_2 (TXB_2) a metabolite of TXA_2

which activates platelets and induces vaso-constriction [108, 112]. One study using gas chromatography–mass spectrometry to detect a stable metabolite of TXB_2 in urine (although in small numbers of patients) failed to detect any increase in TXB_2 production from plate-lets in patients with IDDM whether or not they had vascular disease [121]. In contrast, using urine extraction and refined immuno-assay, levels of 11-dehydro-TXB_2 were increased in the urine of 50 patients with NIDDM and levels of the metabolite fell after a period of tight metabolic control [111].

Platelets activated by interaction with dam-aged blood vessels, artificial surfaces or other platelets have a shortened life-span in the circulation. A number of studies, using differ-ent techniques to determine platelet survival, has shown that platelets in the circulation of patients with diabetes survive for a shorter time than in healthy controls [108, 120].

There are three broad explanations for the abnormalities of platelet function in diabetes: abnormal platelets are synthesized; platelets become abnormal exposed to the metabolic environment of diabetic plasma; or platelets are affected by interaction with damaged blood vessels. There is little evidence to sug-gest that diabetic platelets are inherently abnormal and it is more plausible that plate-lets become abnormal in diabetic plasma, due to changes induced in platelet plasma-membrane function. Glycation of membrane proteins occurs following chronic exposure of platelets to high blood glucose levels [108, 120]. High concentrations of cholesterol and triglycerides, particularly in NIDDM, can alter the fluidity of platelet membranes, lead-ing to a lowered threshold for platelet activa-tion. Finally, platelets from diabetic patients exist in a circulation in which they are exposed early in the disease to an endothe-lium which has subtly altered function, and later, to a highly abnormal micro-circulation and to atherosclerotic large vessels. It has not yet been resolved whether platelets are significant contributors to the genesis of micro- and macrovascular disease, or largely innocent carriers of evidence of a damaged circulation.

7.7.2   vWF IN DIABETES MELLITUS

vWF is a circulating glycoprotein that has two main functions; to act as a carrier protein for factor VIII and as a platelet/collagen ligand. In the latter role, vWF acts as an adhesion molecule to promote platelet adhesion by binding to the platelet GpIb/IX receptor and to exposed subendothelial collagen. Elevated concentrations of vWF have been described in both IDDM [122] and NIDDM [71, 123] sub-jects. Although there is substantial evidence that vWF relates to macrovascular disease in non-diabetic subjects, there are interesting associations described with microvascular disease in both NIDDM and IDDM subjects. Levels of vWF are reported as elevated in the presence of microalbuminuria [53, 124–126] and there are indications that levels are lower prior to the development of microalbumin-uria [124] and may predict its development [125]. Similarly, vWF has been reported to predict deterioration of neuropathy in a mixed group of predominantly IDDM sub-jects [127] and levels of vWF are elevated in NIDDM subjects with retinopathy [128].

These results have to be viewed with a degree of caution as there are complex clinical relationships between micro- and macrovas-cular disease that may be confusing the issue. However, vWF consistently appears as a risk marker for arterial disease and it is likely that the elevated levels seen in both NIDDM and IDDM indicate endothelial cell involvement and vascular damage. Very little work has been carried out on the genetics of vWF in relation to disorders other than von Wille-brand's disease, although we have been unable to find a relationship between a com-mon polymorphism in exon 12 and levels of vWF in NIDDM subjects [123]. Recent work from our group has identified common poly-morphisms in the vWF promoter that are related to extent of atheroma in non-diabetic subjects (D Heywood, unpublished) and these polymorphisms may be useful markers for the study of vascular disease in diabetic subjects in the future.

7.8 CONCLUSIONS

The development of atherothrombotic disease in diabetic subjects is the result of complex interactions promoting increased smooth muscle proliferation, atheroma formation, plaque rupture and thrombus formation. The high incidence of cardiovascular disease in both IDDM and NIDDM makes it likely that common factors such as hyperglycaemia and protein glycosylation are intimately involved in the pathological processes leading to myocardial infarction. However, the mechanisms involved in converting poor metabolic control to myocardial infarction are unclear and probably involve multiple interrelated systems.

Abnormalities of haemostasis are strong candidates for a role in the development of vascular disease in both diabetic and non-diabetic subjects. Fibrin deposition forms an important part of the atheromatous plaque and the development of a thrombus is part of the final insult that leads to vascular obstruction and ischaemic tissue injury and death. Both IDDM and NIDDM are characterized by a bewildering array of haemostatic abnormalities that superficially can be interpreted as indicating the presence of a hypercoagulable state. The clinical evidence to support this view is weak as neither IDDM nor NIDDM is associated with increased venous thrombotic disorders.

Clinically, premature myocardial infarction occurs in subjects with multiple risk such as family history, diabetes, smoking, dyslipidaemia and lack of exercise, and there is an inexorable momentum developed towards vascular disease. A more plausible view of the multiple changes in haemostasis is that they occur in response to the effects of other risk factors and then interact with them to further increase vascular risk. A similar example would be the dyslipidaemia characteristic of NIDDM that occurs in relation to the development of insulin resistance and then contributes to vascular risk.

There are likely to be a number of processes involved in the haemostatic changes observed in diabetes, some of which could account for some of the subtle differences between NIDDM and IDDM. Hyperglycaemia, glycosylation and dyslipdaemia may lead to endothelial cell damage leading to increased vWF, PAI-1 and tPA, while hepatic effects increase fibrinogen and perhaps factor VII. These changes would be common to both NIDDM and IDDM. The development of insulin resistance in NIDDM would lead to further increases in PAI-1, factor VII and to a lesser extent, fibrinogen.

An interesting question arises as to whether it is possible to develop a global view of the role of haemostasis in vascular disease that applies to both diabetic and non-diabetic subjects. It is worth noting that the consistent risk markers in all populations are fibrinogen and vWF. Both have important roles as ligands for platelet glycoproteins and have a major role in platelet adhesion, aggregation and activation. Endothelial cell damage leads to vWF binding to exposed collagen and to GpIb/IX which enhances expression of GpIIb/IIIa which binds fibrinogen. Factor XIIIa is important in platelet/fibrinogen binding and itself leads to local cross-linking of fibrin which enmeshes the developing platelet aggregate. The inhibition of fibrinolysis due to increased PAI-1 would further cement these processes.

The metabolic abnormalities associated with diabetes mellitus would create an environment in which these processes could flourish, by initially enhancing endothelial cell damage and atheroma formation and subsequently enhancing platelet aggregation and clot formation. If this is correct, the development of new therapeutic strategies such as GpIIb/IIIa inhibitors, fibrinogen-lowering agents and lipid-modulating agents are likely to be of particular benefit in the management of the cardiovascular complications of diabetes.

REFERENCES

1. Ratnoff, O.D. and Forbes, C.D. *Disorders of Hemostasis*, 3rd edn, 1996, W.B. Saunders, Philadelphia,
2. Gaffney, P.J. and Longstaff, C. An overview of fibrinolysis. In *Haemostasis and Thrombosis*, 3rd edn, Vol. 2, (eds A.L. Bloom, C.D. Forbes, D.P. Thomas and E.G.D. Tuddenham), Churchill Livingstone, Edinburgh, 1994, pp. 549–74.
3. Bachmann, F. Fibrinolysis. In *Thrombosis and Haemostasis*, (eds M. Verstraete, J. Vermylen, R. Lijnen and J. Arnout), Leuven University Press, 1987, pp. 227–65.
4. Booth, N.A. and Bennett, B. Fibrinolysis and thrombosis, *Baillieres Clin. Haematol.*, 1994, **7**, 559–72.
5. Lane, D.A., Mannucci, P.M., Bauer, K.A., et al. Inherited thrombophilia: part 2. *Thromb. Haemost.*, 1996, **76**, 824–34.
6. Franks, P.J., Wright, D.D., Moffatt, C.J., Stirling, J., Fletcher, A.E., Bulpitt, C.J. and McCollum, C.N. Prevalence of venous disease: a community study in west London. *Eur. J. Surg.*, 1992, **158**, 143–7.
7. Veth, G., Meuwissen, O.J., van Houwelingen, H.C. and Sixma, J.J. Prevention of postoperative deep vein thrombosis by a combination of subcutaneous heparin with subcutaneous dihydroergotamine or oral sulphinpyrazone. *Thromb. Haemost.*, 1985, **54**, 570–73.
8. Bergqvist, D., Bergentz, S.E., Bornmyr, S., Husberg, B., Konrad, P. and Ljungner, H. Deep vein thrombosis after renal transplantation: a prospective analysis of frequency and risk factors. *Eur. Surg. Res.*, 1985, **17**, 69–74.
9. Saarinen, J., Sisto, T., Laurikka, J., Salenius, J.P. and Tarkka, M. The incidence of postoperative deep vein thrombosis in vascular procedures, FINNVASC Study Group. *Vasa*, 1995, **24**, 126–9.
10. Lynch, A.F., Bourne, R.B., Rorabeck, C.H., Rankin, R.N. and Donald, A. Deep vein thrombosis and continuous passive motion after total knee arthroplasty. *J. Bone Joint Surg.*, 1988, **70**, 11–14.
11. Goldhaber, S.Z., Grodstein, F., Stampfer, M.J., Manson, J.E., Colditz, G.A., Speizer, F.E., Willett, W.C. and Hennekens, C.H. A prospective study of risk function for pulmonary embolism in women. *J. Am. Med. Assoc.*, 1997, **277**, 642–5.
12. Conlan, M.G., Folsom, A.R., Finch, A., Davis, C.E., Sorlie, P., Marcucci, G. and Wu, K.K. Associations of factor VIII and von Willebrand factor with age, race, sex, and risk factors for atherosclerosis. The Atherosclerosis Risk in Communities (ARIC) Study. *Thromb. Haemost.*, 1993, **70**, 380–5.
13. Fuller, J.H., Keen, H., Jarrett, R.J., Omer, T., Meade, T.W., Chakrabarti, R., North. W.R. and Stirling, Y. Haemostatic variables associated with diabetes and its complications. *Br. Med. J.*, 1979, **2**, 964–6.
14. Ostermann, H. and van de Loo, J. Factors of the hemostatic system in diabetic patients: a survey of controlled studies. *Haemostasis*, 1986, **16**, 386–416.
15. el Khawand, C., Jamart, J., Donckier, J., Chatelain, B., Lavenne, E., Moriau, M. and Buusschaert, M. Hemostasis variables in type 1 diabetic patients without demonstrable vascular complications. *Diabetes Care*, 1993, **16**, 1137–45.
16. Juhan-Vague, I., Alessi, M.C. and Vague, P. Thrombogenic and fibrinolytic factors and cardiovascular risk in non-insulin-dependent diabetes mellitus. *Ann. Med.*, 1996, **28**, 371–80.
17. Kwaan, H.C. Changes in blood coagulation, platelet function, and plasminogen-plasmin system in diabetes. *Diabetes*, 1992, **31**, 32–5.
18. Colwell, J.A., Lyons, T.J., Klein, R.L. and Lopes-Virella, M.F. New concepts about the pathogenesis of atherosclerosis and thrombosis in diabetes mellitus. In *The Diabetic Foot*, 5th edn, (ed. M.J. Levin), Mosby, St Louis, MO, 1993, pp. 79–114.
19. Schneider, D.J., Nordt, T.K. and Sobel, B.E. Attenuated fibrinolysis and accelerated atherogenesis in type II diabetic patients. *Diabetes*, 1993, **42**, 1–7.
20. Juhan-Vague, I., Alessi, M.C. and Vague, P. Increased plasma plasminogen activator inhibitor 1 levels: a possible link between insulin resistance and atherothrombosis. *Diabetologia*, 1991, **34**, 457–62.
21. Bruno, G., Cavallo-Perin, P., Bargero, G., Borra, M., D'Errico, N. and Pagano, G. Association of fibrinogen with glycemic control and albumin excretion rate in patients with

non-insulin-dependent diabetes mellitus. *Ann. Intern. Med.*, 1996, **125**, 653–7.

22. Gruden, G., Cavallo-Perin, P., Bazzan, M., Stella, S., Vuolo, A. and Pagano, G. PAI-1 and factor VII activity are higher in IDDM patients with microalbuminuria. *Diabetes*, 1994, **43**, 426–9.

23. Ibbotson, S.H., Walmsley, D., Davies, J.A. and Grant, P.J. Generation of thrombin activity in relation to factor VIII:C concentrations and vascular complications in type 1 (insulin-dependent) diabetes mellitus. *Diabetologia*, 1992, **35**, 863–7.

24. Ceriello, A., Quatraro, A., Marchi, E., Barbanti, M. and Giugliano, D. Impaired fibrinolytic response to increased thrombin activation in type 1 diabetes mellitus: effects of the glycosaminoglycan sulodexide. *Diabet. Metab.*, 1993, **19**, 225–9.

25. Ceriello, A., Taboga, C., Giacomello, R. *et al.* Fibrinogen plasma levels as a marker of thrombin activation in diabetes. *Diabetes*, 1994, **43**, 430–2.

26. Grant, P.J., Stickland, M.H., Wiles, P.G., Gaffney, P.J., Davies, J.A. and Prentice, C.R.M. Acute changes in blood glucose concentration do not promote thrombin generation or fibrin breakdown in type 1 diabetes. *Diabet. Med.*, 1988, **5**, 867–70.

27. Jones, R.L. Fibrinopeptide-A in diabetes mellitus. Relation to levels of blood glucose, fibrinogen disappearance, and hemodynamic changes. *Diabetes*, 1985, **34**, 836–43.

28. Eriksson, J., Taimela, S. and Koivisto, V.A. Exercise and the metabolic syndrome. *Diabetologia*, 1997, **40**, 125–35.

29. Donahue, R.P., Abbott, R.D., Reed, D.M. and Yano, K. Post challenge glucose concentration and coronary heart disease in men of Japanese ancestry: Honolulu Heart Program. *Diabetes*, 1987, **36**, 689–92.

30. Jarrett, R.J., McCartney, P. and Keen, H.. The Bedford Survey: ten year mortality rates in newly diagnosed diabetics, borderline diabetics and normoglycaemic controls and risk indices for coronary heart disease in borderline diabetics. *Diabetologia*, 1982, **22**, 79–84.

31. Garcia, M.J., McNamara, P.M., Gordon, T. and Kannel, W.B. Morbidity and mortality in diabetics in the Framingham population. Sixteen year follow-up study. *Diabetes*, 1974, **23**, 105–11.

32. Fuller, J.H., Shipley, M.J., Rose, G., Jarrett, R.J. and Keen, H. Mortality from coronary heart disease and stroke. Relation to degree of glycaemia: The Whitehall Study. *Br. Med. J.*, 1983, **287**, 867–70.

33. Lee, P., Jenkins, A., Bourke, C. *et al.* Prothrombotic and antithrombotic factors are elevated in patients with type 1 diabetes complicated by microalbuminuria. *Diabet. Med.*, 1993, **10**, 122–8.

34. Carmassi, F., Morale, M., Puccetti, R. *et al.* Coagulation and fibrinolytic system impairment in insulin dependent diabetes mellitus. *Thromb. Res.*, 1992, **67**, 643–54.

35. Dubrey, S.W., Reaveley, D.R., Seed, M., Lane, D.A., Ireland, H., O'Donnell, M., O'Connor, B., Noble, M.I. and Lesie, R.D. Risk factors for cardiovascular disease in IDDM. A study of identical twins. *Diabetes*, 1994, **43**, 831–5.

36. Morishita, E., Asakura, H., Jokaji, H. *et al.* Hypercoagulability and high lipoprotein(a) levels in patients with type II diabetes mellitus. *Atherosclerosis*, 1996, **120**, 7–14.

37. Avellone, G., Di Garbo, V., Cordova, R. *et al.* Blood coagulation and fibrinolysis in obese NIDDM patients. *Diabet. Res.*, 1994, **25**, 85–92.

38. Vanninen, E., Laitinen, J. and Uusitupa, M. Physical activity and fibrinogen concentration in newly diagnosed NIDDM. *Diabetes Care*, 1994, **17**, 1031–8.

39. Acang, N. and Jalil, F.D. Hypercoagulation in diabetes mellitus. *Southeast Asian J. Trop. Med. Public Health*, 1993, **24** (suppl 1), 263–6.

40. Lee, A.J., Lowe, G.D., Woodward, M. and Tunstall-Pedoe, H. Fibrinogen in relation to personal history of prevalent hypertension, diabetes, stroke, intermittent claudication, coronary heart disease, and family history: the Scottish Heart Health Study. *Br. Heart. J.*, 1993, **69**, 338–42.

41. Ganda, O.P. and Arkin, C.F. Hyperfibrinogenemia. An important risk factor for vascular complications in diabetes. *Diabetes Care*, 1992, **15**, 1245–50.

42. Missov, R.M., Stolk, R.P., van der Bom, J.G., Hofman, A., Bots, M.L., Pols, H.A. and Grobbee, D.E. Plasma fibrinogen in NIDDM: the Rotterdam study. *Diabetes Care*, 1996, **19**, 157–9.

43. Rodriguez, B.L., Curb, J.D., Burchfield, C.M., Huang, B., Sharp, D.S., Lu, G.Y., Fujimoto, W. and Yano, K. Impaired glucose tolerance, diabetes, and cardiovascular disease risk factor

profiles in the elderly. The Honolulu Heart Programme. *Diabetes Care,* 1996, **19,** 587–90.

44. Memeh, C.U. Differences between plasma viscosity and proteins of type 1 and 2 diabetic Africans in early phase of diabetes. *Horm. Metab. Res.,* 1993, **25,** 21–3.

45. Ho, C.H., Wang, S.P. and Jap, T.S. Hemostatic risk factors of coronary artery disease in the Chinese. *Int. J. Cardiol.,* 1995, **51,** 79–84.

46. Robbins, D.C., Knowler, W.C., Lee, E.T., Yeh, J., Go, O.T., Welty, T., Fabsitz, R. and Howard, B.V. Regional differences in albuminuria among American Indians: an epidemic of renal disease. *Kidney Int.,* 1996, **49,** 557–63.

47. Knight, T., Smith, Z., Lockton, J.A., Sahota, P., Bedford, A., Toop, M., Kernohan, E. and Baker, M.R. Ethnic differences in risk markers for heart disease in Bradford and implications for preventive strategies. *J. Epidemiol. Community Health,* 1993, **47,** 89–95.

48. Burchfiel, C.M., Curb, J.D., Sharp, D.S., Rodriguez, B.L., Arakaki, R., Chyou, P.H. and Yano, K. Distribution and correlates of insulin in elderly men. The Honolulu Heart Program. *Arterio. Thromb. Vasc. Biol.,* 1995, **15,** 2213–21.

49. Mansfield, M.W., Heywood, D.M. and Grant, P.J. Circulating levels of factor VII, fibrinogen and von Willebrand factor and features of insulin resistance in first degree relatives of patients with NIDDM. *Circulation,* 1996, **94,** 2171–6.

50. Meade, T.W., Chakrabarti, R., Haines, A.P., North, W.R. and Stirling, Y. Characteristics affecting fibrinolytic activity and plasma fibrinogen concentrations. *Br. Med. J.,* 1979, **1,** 153–6.

51. Montgomery, H.E., Clarkson, P., Nwose, O.M., Mikailidis, D.P., Japgroop, I.A., Dollery, C., Moult, J., Benhizia, F., Deanfield, J., Jubb, M., World, M., McEwan, J.R., Winder, A. and Humphries, S. The acute rise in plasma fibrinogen concentration with exercise is influenced by the G453A polymorphism of the b fibrinogen gene. *Arterio. Thromb. Vasc. Biol.,* 1996, **16,** 386–91.

52. Jones, S.L., Close, C.F., Mattock, M.B., Jarrett, R.J., Keen, H. and Viberti, G.C. Plasma lipid and coagulation factor concentrations in insulin dependent diabetics with microalbuminuria. *Br. Med. J.,* 1989, **298,** 487–90.

53. Knobl, P., Schernthaner, G., Schnack, C. *et al.* Thrombogenic factors are related to urinary albumin excretion rate in type 1 (insulin-dependent) and type 2 (non-insulin-dependent) diabetic patients. *Diabetologia,* 1993, **36,** 1045–50.

54. Schleiffer, T., Hellstern, P., Freitag, M. and Brass, H. Plasminogen activator inhibitor 1 activity and lipoprotein(a) in nephropathic patients with non-insulin-dependent diabetes mellitus versus patients with nondiabetic nephropathy. *Haemostasis,* 1994, **24,** 49–54.

55. Ernst, E., Resch, K.L. Fibrinogen as a cardiovascular risk factor: a meta-analysis and review of the literature. *Ann. Intern. Med.,* 1993, **118,** 956–63.

56. Yudkin, J.S., Forrest, R.D., Jackson, C.A. Microalbuminuria as predictor of vascular disease in non-diabetic subjects. Islington Diabetes Survey. *Lancet,* 1988, **ii,** 530–3.

57. Agewal, S., Fagerberg, B., Attvall, S., Ljungman, S., Urbanavicius, V., Tengborn, L. and Wikstrand, J. Microalbuminuria, insulin sensitivity and haemostatic factors in non-diabetic treated hypertensive men. Factor Intervention Study Group. *J. Intern. Med.,* 1995, **237,** 195–203.

58. Meade, T.W., Chakrabarti, R., Haines, A.P. *et al.* Haemostatic function and cardiovascular death: early results of a prospective study. *Lancet,* 1980, **i,** 1050–3.

59. Violi, F., Criqui, M., Longoni, A. and Castiglioni, C. Relation between risk factors and cardiovascular complications in patients with peripheral vascular disease. Results from the A.D.E.P. study. *Atherosclerosis,* 1996, **120,** 25–35.

60. Kannel, W.B., D'Agostino, R.B. and Belanger, A.J. Update on fibrinogen as a cardiovascular risk factor. *Ann. Epidemiol.,* 1992, **2,** 457–66.

61. Hamsten, A., Iselius, L., De Faire, U. and Blomback, M. Genetic and cultural inheritance of plasma fibrinogen concentration. *Lancet,* 1987, **ii,** 988–90.

62. Friedlander, Y., Elkana, Y., Sinnreich, R. and Kark, J.D. Genetic and environmental sources of fibrinogen variability in Israeli families: the Kibbutzim Family Study. *Am. J. Hum. Genet.,* 1995, **56,** 1194–206.

63. Humphries, S.E., Ye, S., Talmud, P.J., Bara, L., Wilhelmsen, L. and Tiret, L. European Atherosclerosis Research Study: Genotype at the fibrinogen locus (G455A b-gene) is association with differences in plasma fibrinogen

levels in young men and women from different regions in Europe. *Arterio. Thromb. Vasc. Biol.*, 1995, **5**, 96–104.

64. de Maat, M.P.M., de Knijff, P., Green, F.R., Thomas, A.E., Jespersen, J. and Kluft, C. Gender related association between b-fibrinogen genotype and plasma fibrinogen levels and linkage disequilibrium at the fibrinogen locus in Greenland Inuit. *Arterio. Thromb. Vasc. Biol.*, 1995, **5**, 856–60.

65. Carter, A., Catto, A.J., Bamford, J.M. and Grant, P.J. Gender specific associations of the fibrinogen B· 448 polymorphism, fibrinogen levels and acute cerebrovascular disease. *Arterio. Thromb. Vasc. Biol.*, 1997, **17**, 589–94.

66. Snowden, C., Houlston, R., Laker, M.F., Kesteven, P., Alberti, K.G. and Humphries, S.E. Plasma fibrinogen levels and fibrinogen genotype in non-insulin-dependent diabetics. *Disease Markers*, 1992, **10**, 159–67.

67. Fowkes, F.G., Common, J.M., Smith, F.B., Wood, J., Donnan, P.T. and Lowe, G.D.O. Fibrinogen genotype and risk of peripheral atherosclerosis. *Lancet*, 1992, **339**, 693–6.

68. Behague, I., Poirier, O., Nicaud, V. *et al.* β fibrinogen gene polymorphisms are associated with plasma fibrinogen and coronary artery disease in patients with myocardial infarction. The ECTIM study. *Circulation*, 1996, **93**, 440–9.

69. Carter, A.M., Mansfield, M.W., Stickland, M.H. and Grant, P.J. Fibrinogen β gene -455 G/A polymorphism and fibrinogen levels: risk factors for coronary artery disease in subjects with non-insulin-dependent diabetes mellitus. *Diabetes Care*, 1996, **19**, 1265–8.

70. Kario, K., Matsuo, T., Kobayashi, H., Matsuo, M., Sakata, T. and Miyata, T. Activation of tissue factor-induced coagulation and endothelial cell dysfunction in non-insulin-dependent diabetic patients with microalbuminuria. *Arterio. Thromb. Vasc. Biol.*, 1995, **15**, 1114–20.

71. Knobl, P., Schernthaner, G., Schnack, C. *et al.* Haemostatic abnormalities persist despite glycaemic improvement by insulin therapy in lean type 2 diabetic patients. *Thromb. Haemost.*, 1994, **71**, 692–7.

72. Donders, S.H., Lustermans, F.A. and van Wersch, J.W. Glycometabolic control, lipids, and coagulation parameters in patients with non-insulin-dependent diabetes mellitus. *Int. J. Clin. Lab. Res.*, 1993, **23**, 155–9.

73. Christe, M., Fritschi, J., Lammle, B., Tran, T.H., Marbet, G.A., Berger, W. and Duckert, F. Fifteen coagulation and fibrinolysis parameters in diabetes mellitus and in patients with vasculopathy. *Thromb. Haemost.*, 1984, **52**, 138–43.

74. van Wersch, J.W. A chromogenic assay for coagulation factor VII: analytical performance characteristics and application in several diseases. *Int. J. Clin. Lab. Res.*, 1993; **23**, 221–4.

75. Mansfield, M.W., Heywood, D.M. and Grant, P.J. Sex differences in coagulation and fibrinolysis in white subjects with non-insulin-dependent diabetes mellitus. *Arterio Thromb. Vasc. Biol.*, 1996, **16**, 160–4.

76. Miller, G.J., Walter, S.J., Stirling, Y., Thompson, S.G., Esnouf, M.P. and Meade, T.W. Assay of factor VII activity by two techniques: evidence of increased conversion of VII to aVII in hyperlipidaemia, with possible implications for ischaemic heart disease. *Br. J. Haematol.*, 1985, **59**, 249.

77. Simpson, H.C.R., Meade, T.W., Stirling, Y., Mann, J.I., Chakrabarti, R. and Woolf, L. Hypertriglyceridaemia and hypercoagulability. *Lancet*, 1983, **i**, 78–90.

78. Miller, G.J., Martin, J.C., Mitropoulos, K.A., Reeves, B.E.A., Thompson, R.L., Meade, T.W., Cooper, J.A. and Cruikshank, J.K. Plasma FVII is activated by postprandial triglyceridaemia irrespective of dietary fat composition. *Atherosclerosis*, 1991, **86**, 163–71.

79. Van der Bom, J.G., Bots, M.L., Van Vilet, H.H.D.M., Hofman, A. and Grobbee, D.E. Factor VII coagulant activity is related to blood lipids in the elderly. The Rotterdam Study. *Fibrinolysis*, 1994, **8**, 132–14.

80. Heywood, D., Mansfield, M.W. and Grant, P.J. Factor VII gene polymorphisms, factor VII:C levels and features of insulin resistance in non-insulin-dependent diabetes mellitus: A link with vascular risk. *Thromb. Haemostas.*, 1996, **75**, 401–7.

81. Heinrich, J., Balleisen, L., Schulte, H., Assmann, G. and van de Loo, J. Fibrinogen and factor VII in the prediction of coronary risk. Results from the PROCAM study in healthy men. *Arterio. Thromb.*, 1994, **14**, 54–9.

82. Cortellaro, M., Baldassarre, D., Cofrancesco, E., Tremoli, E., Colombo, A., Boschetti, C. and Paoletti, R. Relation between hemostatic variables and increase of common carotid intima-

media thickness in patients with peripheral arterial disease. *Stroke,* 1996, **27,** 450–4.

83. Humphries, S.E., Green, F.R., Temple, A., Dawson, S., Henney, A., Kelleher, C.H., Wilkes, H., Meade, T.W., Wiman, B. and Hamsten, A. Genetic factors determining thrombosis and fibrinolysis. *Ann. Epidemiol.,* 1992, **2,** 371–85.

84. Heywood, D.M., Ossei-Gerning, N. and Grant, P.J. Association of factor VII:C levels with environmental and genetic factors in patients with ischaemic heart disease and coronary atheroma characterised by angiography. *Thromb. Haemost.,* 1996, **76,** 161–5.

85. Lane, D.A., Green, F., Scarabin, P.Y., Nicaud, V., Bara, L., Humphries, S., Evans, A., Luc, G., Cambou, J.P., Arveiler, D. and Cambien, F. Factor VII Arg/Gln353 polymorphism determines factor VII coagulation activity in patients with myocardial infarction (MI) and control subjects in Belfast and in France but is not a strong indicator of MI risk in the ECTIM study. *Atherosclerosis,* 1996, **119,** 119–27.

86. Mansfield, M.W. and Grant, P.J. Fibrinolysis and diabetes mellitus. In *Fibrinolysis in Disease. Molecular and Hemovascular Aspects of Fibrinolysis,* (ed. P. Glas-Greenwalt), CRC Press, Boca Raton, 1996, pp. 172–83.

87. Gough, S.C.L. and Grant, P.J. The fibrinolytic system in diabetes mellitus. *Diabet. Med.,* 1991, **8,** 898–905.

88. Walmsley, D., Hampton, K.K. and Grant, P.J. Contrasting fibrinolytic responses in Type 1 (insulin-dependent) and Type 2 (non-insulin-dependent) diabetes. *Diabet. Med.,* 1991, **8,** 954–9.

89. Fisher, B.M., Quinn, J.D., Rumley, A., Lennie, S.E., Small, M., MacCuish, A.C. and Lowe, G.D.O. Effects of acute insulin-induced hypoglycaemia on haemostasis, fibrinolysis and haemorheology in insulin-dependent diabetic patients and control subjects. *Clin. Sci.,* 1991, **80,** 525–31.

90. Mahmoud, R., Raccah, D., Alessi, M.C., Aillaud, M.F., Juhan-Vague, I. and Vague, P. Fibrinolysis in insulin dependent diabetic patients with or without nephropathy. *Fibrinolysis,* 1992, **6,** 105–9.

91. Grant, P.J. Polymorphisms of coagulation/fibrinolysis genes: gene-environment interactions and vascular risk. *Prostaglandins Leukot. Essent. Fatty Acids,* 1997, **57,** 473–7.

92. Grant, P.J., Ruegg, M. and Medcalf, R.L. Basal expression and insulin mediated induction of PAI-1 mRNA in Hep G2 cells. *Fibrinolysis,* 1991, **5,** 81–6.

93. Kooistra, T., Bosma, P.J., Tons, H.A.M., van den Berg, A.P., Meyer, P. and Princen, H.M.G. Plasminogen activator inhibitor 1: biosynthesis and mRNA level are increased by insulin in cultured human hepatocytes. *Thromb. Haemost.,* 1989, **91,** 2185–93.

94. Grant, P.J., Kruithof, E.K.O., Felley, C.P., Felber, J.P. and Bachmann, F. Short term infusions of insulin, triacylglycerol and glucose do not cause acute increases in plasminogen activator inhibitor-1 concentrations in man. *Clin. Sci.,* 1990, **79,** 513–16.

95. Potter van Loon, B.J., deBart, A.C.W., Radder, J.K., Frolich, M., Kluft, C. and Meinders, A.E. Acute exogenous hyperinsulinaemia does not result in elevation of plasma plasminogen activator inhibitor-1 (PAI-1) in humans. *Fibrinolysis,* 1990, **4,** 93–4.

96. Maiello, M., Boeri, D., Podesta, F. *et al.* Increased expression of tissue plasminogen activator and its inhibitor and reduced fibrinolytic potential of human endothelial cells cultured in elevated glucose. *Diabetes,* 1992, **41,** 1009–15.

97. Sironi, L., Mussoni, L., Prati, L., Baldassarre, D., Camera, M., Banfi, C. and Tremoli, E. Plasminogen activator inhibitor type 1 synthesis and mRNA expression in HepG2 cells are regulated by VLDL. *Arterio. Thromb. Vasc. Biol.,* 1996, **16,** 89–96.

98. Hamsten, A., De Faire, U., Walldius, G. *et al.* Plasminogen activator inhibitor in plasma: risk factor for recurrent myocardial infarction. *Lancet,* 1987, **ii,** 3–9.

99. Ridker, P.M., Hennekens, C.H., Stampfer, M.J., Manson, J.E. and Vaughan, D.E. Prospective study of endogenous tissue plasminogen activator and risk of stroke. *Lancet,* 1994, **343,** 940–3.

100. Erikkson, P., Kallin, B., van't Hooft, F.M., Båvenholm, P. and Hamsten, A. Allele-specific increase in basal transcription of the plasminogen-activator inhibitor 1 gene is associated with myocardial infarction. *Proc. Natl Acad. Sci. USA,* 1995, **92,** 1851–5.

101. Dawson, S.J., Wiman, B., Hamsten, A., Green, F., Humphries, S.E. and Henney, A.M. The two allele sequences of a common polymorphism in the promoter of the plasminogen

activator inhibitor-1 (PAI-1) gene respond differently to interleukin-1 in HepG2 cells. *J. Biol. Chem.*, 1993, **268**, 10739–45.

102. Panahloo, A., Mohamed-Ali, V., Lane, A., Green, F., Humphries, S.E. and Yudkin, J.S. Determinants of the plasminogen activator inhibitor-1 activity in treated NIDDM and its relation to a polymorphism in the plasminogen activator inhibitor 1 gene. *Diabetes*, 1995, **44**, 37–42.

103. Mansfield, M.W., Stickland, M.H. and Grant, P.J. Environmental and genetic factors in relation to elevated circulating levels of plasminogen activator inhibitor-1 in Caucasian patients with non-insulin dependent diabetes mellitus. *Thromb. Haemost.*, 1995, **74**, 842–7.

104. Ossei-Gerning, N., Mansfield, M.W., Stickland, M.H., Wilson, I.J. and Grant, P.J. Plasminogen activator inhibitor-1(PAI-1) promoter 4G/5G genotype and levels in relation to a history of myocardial infarction in patients characterised by coronary angiography. *Arterio. Thromb. Vasc. Biol.*, 1997, **17**, 33–7.

105. Mansfield, M.W., Stickland, M.H. and Grant, P.J. Plasminogen activator inhibitor-1 (PAI-1) promoter polymorphism and coronary artery disease in non-insulin-dependent diabetes. *Thromb. Haemost.*, 1995, **74**, 1032–4.

106. The 4G/5G genetic polymorphism in the promoter of the plasminogen activator inhibitor-1 (PAI-1) gene is associated with differences in plasma PAI-1 activity but not with risk of myocardial infarction in the ECTIM Study. *Thromb. Haemost.*, 1995, **74**, 837–41.

107. Ridker, P.M., Hennekens, C.H., Lindpaintner, K., Stampfer, M.J. and Miletich, J.P. Arterial and venous thrombosis is not associated with the 4G/5G polymorphism in the promoter of the plasminogen activator inhibitor gene in a large cohort of US men. *Circulation*, 1997, **95**, 59–62.

108. Winocour, P.D. Platelet abnormalities in diabetes mellitus. *Diabetes*, 1992, **41**, 26–31.

109. Colwell, J.A. and Halushka, P.V. Platelet function in diabetes mellitus. *Br. J. Haematol.*, 1980, **40**, 521–6.

110. Jackson, C.A., Greaves, M., Boulton, A.J.M., Ward, J.D. and Preston, F.E. Near-normal glycaemic control does not correct abnormal platelet reactivity in diabetes mellitus. *Clin. Sci.*, 1984, **67**, 551–5.

111. Daví, G., Catalano, I., Averna, M., Notarbartolo, A., Strano, A., Ciabattoni, G. and Patrono, C. Thromboxane biosynthesis and platelet function in type II diabetes mellitus. *N. Engl. J. Med.*, 1990, **322**, 1769–74.

112. García Frade, L.J., de la Calle, H., Alava, I., Navarro, J.L., Creighton, L.J. and Gaffney, P.J. Diabetes mellitus as a hypercoagulable state: its relationship with fibrin fragments and vascular damage. *Thromb. Res.*, 1987, **47**, 533–540.

113. Fritschi, J., Christe, M., Lämmle, B., Marbet, G.A., Berger, W. and Duckert, F. Platelet aggregation, β-thromboglobulin and platelet factor 4 in diabetes mellitus and in patients with vasculopathy. *Thromb. Haemost.*, 1984, **52**, 236–9.

114. Cho, N.H., Becker, D., Dorman, J.S. *et al.* Spontaneous whole blood platelet aggregation in insulin-dependent diabetes mellitus: an evaluation in an epidemiologic study. *Thromb. Haemost.*, 1989, **61**, 127–30.

115. Tschoepe, D., Roesen, P., Kaufmann, L., Schauseil, S., Kehrel, B., Ostermann, H. and Gries, F.A. Evidence for abnormal platelet glycoprotein expression in diabetes mellitus. *Eur. J. Clin. Invest.*, 1990, **20**, 166–70.

116. Lee, M., Paton, R.C., Passa, P. and Caen, J.P. Fibrinogen binding and ADP- induced aggregation in platelets from diabetic subjects. *Thromb. Res.*, 1981, **24**, 143–50.

117. Burrows, A.W., Chavin, S.I. and Hockaday, T.D.R. Plasma-thromboglobulin concentrations in diabetes mellitus. *Lancet*, 1978, **i**, 235–7.

118. Zahavi, J. and Zahavi, M. Platelet function in type 1 diabetes mellitus (letter). *N. Engl. J. Med.*, 1988, **319**, 1665–6.

119. van Oost, B.A., Veldhuyzen, B., Timmermans, A.P.M. and Sixma, J.J. Increased urinary β-thromboglobulin excretion in diabetes assayed with a modified RIA kit-technique. *Thromb. Haemost.*, 1983, **49**, 18–20.

120. Mustard, J.F. and Packham, M.A. Platelets and diabetes mellitus. *N. Engl. J. Med.*, 1984, **311**, 665–7.

121. Alessandrini, P., McRae, J., Feman, S. and FitzGerald, G.A. Thromboxane biosynthesis and platelet function in type 1 diabetes mellitus. *N. Engl. J. Med.*, 1988, **319**, 208–12.

122. Moriau, M. and Buysschaert, M. Hemostasis variables in type 1 diabetic patients without demonstrable vascular complications. *Diabetes Care*, 1993, **16**, 1137–45.

123. Heywood, D.M., Mansfield, M.W. and Grant, P.J. Levels of von Willebrand factor with features of the metabolic syndrome and a common vWF gene polymorphism in type 2 diabetes mellitus. *Diabet. Med.,* 1996, **13,** 720–5.

124. Stehouwer, C.D., Fischer, H.R., van Kuijk, A.W., Polak, B.C. and Donker, A.J. Endothelial dysfunction precedes development of microalbuminuria in IDDM. *Diabetes,* 1995, **44,** 561–4.

125. Myrup, B., Mathiesen, E.R., Ronn, B. and Deckert, T. Endothelial function and serum lipids in the course of developing microalbuminuria in insulin-dependent diabetes mellitus. *Diabetes Res.,* 1994, **26,** 33–9.

126. Yaqoob, M., Patrick, A.W., McCelland, P., Stevenson, A., Mason, H., White, M.C. and Bell, G.M. Relationship between markers of endothelial dysfunction, oxidant injury and tubular damage in patients with insulin-dependent diabetes mellitus. *Clin. Sci.,* 1993, **85,** 557–62.

127. Dent, M.T., Preston, F.E. and Ward, J.D. Elevated von Willebrand factor antigen predicts deterioration in diabetic peripheral nerve function. *Diabetologia,* 1996, **39,** 336–43.

128. Morise, T., Takeuchi, Y., Kawano, M., Koni, I. and Takeda, R. Increased plasma levels of immunoreactive endothelin and von Willebrand factor in NIDDM Patients. *Diabetes Care,* 1995, **18,** 87–9.

INSULIN RESISTANCE AND ARTERIAL DISEASE IN DIABETES: A UNIFYING HYPOTHESIS

John S. Yudkin

8.1 INTRODUCTION

This chapter outlines some new observations on the associations of diabetes, insulin resistance and vascular disease. While insulin resistance in itself would be of interest to a limited band of metabolic physiologists and biochemists, its importance, and that of the metabolic syndrome, is of wider relevance because of the association of many of its component parts with cardiovascular disease. Throughout the whole chapter, the cardiovascular system and its health will be the spectre at the feast, even where the processes under discussion seem far removed from the blood vessel wall.

The chapter includes a definition of insulin resistance, and describes how it is measured and what are the consequences to carbohydrate metabolism when insulin sensitivity is reduced. The diverse but overlapping definitions of the metabolic syndrome thought to be caused by insulin resistance are outlined, with more detail on a few new members of the cluster. Some of these appear readily comprehensible under the dominant paradigm but others need a deep belief in the primacy of insulin resistance to accept them as a consequence of such a mechanism. The views expressed include that demonstration of correlation is not proof of causation, that the ability of a measure to predict the development of future pathology does not impute

aetiology and that only the demonstration that the removal of the putative cause results in prevention of the putative consequence can truly be taken as proof [1].

There is some creative speculation, suggesting that there may be a much better explanation for the associations described, by attributing them to a common antecedent. Several such antecedents have been proposed and there are many people deeply enamoured with their pet hypotheses. Some data are presented relating to the possible role of both intrauterine growth retardation and impaired endothelial function in the aetiology of both insulin resistance and its associated phenotypic features.

An alternative proposal is presented for a common antecedent: the pro-inflammatory cytokines interleukin-6 (IL-6) and tumour necrosis factor-α (TNF-α), secreted in the main from adipocytes. Thereby, the role of adipose tissue in the cluster of variables comprising the metabolic syndrome, which has had its advocates and its detractors, is brought back to the centre of the debate. This common antecedent hypothesis is able to explain not only the clustering of the disparate parts of the metabolic syndrome with insulin resistance and obesity, but also the association of all of these with endothelial dysfunction and cardiovascular disease. Suggestions are put forward as to how this might be tested.

8.2　THE INSULIN RESISTANCE SYNDROME: WHAT IS IT AND WHO BELONGS?

8.2.1　WHAT IS INSULIN RESISTANCE?

The metabolic effects of insulin include actions on the metabolism of fat, carbohydrate and protein, on ion transport mechanisms and on cell growth, and the modulation of cell differentiation and programmed cell death. Nevertheless, the regulation of insulin secretion by the pancreatic islets is largely mediated through the ambient concentration of plasma glucose. This implies that sensitivity to, or resistance to, insulin action is generally understood to refer to the enhanced, or impaired, ability of insulin to lower plasma glucose concentration. It does this both by stimulating glucose uptake by insulin-sensitive tissues (predominantly skeletal muscle) and by inhibiting liver glucose production from glycogen or from gluconeogenic precursors.

The gold standard for measuring insulin sensitivity is the euglycaemic hyperinsulinaemic clamp. At the usual concentrations of insulin employed for such clamps, it is peripheral glucose uptake which is the limiting pathway [2]. Under normal circumstances, there is substantial spare capacity for islet cell production of insulin, such that removal of as much as half of the pancreas generally has little impact on glucose tolerance [3]. Similarly, the pancreas can tolerate substantial increases in insulin resistance, either by liver or by skeletal muscle, without the development of fasting hyperglycaemia, because additional insulin can be secreted to maintain normoglycaemia [4]. For this reason, fasting hyperinsulinaemia is often used in population studies as a surrogate for insulin resistance; studies show strong enough correlations between fasting insulin concentrations [5] or those adjusted for levels of glucose [6], with direct measures of insulin sensitivity to make this assumption a reasonable one. When insulin resistance is associated with normal fasting glucose levels, intolerance to a carbohydrate load may be manifest, if the pancreas is working close to its maximum capacity, but it is only with deterioration of pancreatic function that frank diabetes, with fasting hyperglycaemia, occurs [4]. The existence of a large population of insulin-resistant, but glucose-tolerant, subjects has been recognized for some 20 or more years [7], and studies too numerous to mention have documented that these individuals are at substantially increased risk of future development of non-insulin dependent diabetes (NIDDM) [8].

8.2.2　INSULIN RESISTANCE AND THE METABOLIC SYNDROME

As if being a harbinger of NIDDM were not enough, the evil reputation of insulin resistance as a risk factor for heart disease grew by leaps and bounds when its name started being linked with a wide variety of other usual suspects [9]. Thus Modan described associations of hyperinsulinaemia with hypertension, obesity and abnormalities of membrane sodium transport [10]. Ferrannini showed an association between essential hypertension and insulin resistance [11] and mechanisms were proposed whereby insulin itself might mediate an elevation in blood pressure: Landsberg related hyperinsulinaemia to excessive activation of the sympathetic nervous system [12] and de Fronzo related it to renal sodium retention [13]. While other candidates continue to claim primacy for the description of clusters of risk factors with insulin resistance, it was Reaven, in his Lilly Lecture in 1988, who described the cluster under the title syndrome X [14], unfortunately ignorant of the fact that cardiologists had already patented this term for the syndrome of ischaemic chest pain with normal coronary arteries.

The syndrome described by Reaven comprised insulin resistance, in combination with hypertension and dyslipidaemia, i.e. elevated concentrations of very low density lipoprotein (VLDL) triglyceride and reduced concentrations of high density lipoprotein (HDL) cholesterol. In addition, the predisposition to glucose intolerance and NIDDM was an important factor, but the other risk factors are clearly abnormal in insulin-resistant subjects before the onset of glucose intolerance.

8.2.3   THE RELEVANCE OF OBESITY AND PHYSICAL ACTIVITY

The importance of obesity as a contributor to insulin resistance cannot be overstated. In the general population, both global adipose tissue mass (as indicated by body mass index, or as measured by impedance methods or by underwater weighing) and central obesity (as indicated by waist circumference or its ratios, or as measured using computerized tomographic or magnetic resonance imaging scans) are associated strongly both with insulin resistance and with the dyslipidaemia, hypertension and glucose intolerance with which it clusters [15–17]. However, Reaven disputes that obesity is a component of the metabolic syndrome, arguing that insulin resistance in lean subjects is associated with all the same phenotypic abnormalities outlined above [14] and, in some of these studies, subjects have also been matched for waist–hip ratio [18, 19]. Nevertheless, in studies in which accurate documentation of total and intra-abdominal fat has been performed, the strength of the association between insulin resistance and either hypertension or dyslipidaemia is substantially weakened [20].

An additional confounding variable which must be taken into account in studies on insulin resistance is that of physical activity. Physical fitness increases insulin sensitivity [21], perhaps in proportion to increases in muscle blood flow, and concomitantly reduces blood pressure, elevates HDL-cholesterol and lowers triglyceride levels, even without weight reduction. This is relevant in studies in healthy subjects, but potentially more important as a confounding factor when insulin resistance is documented in cross-sectional studies of patient populations, such as those with coronary heart disease (CHD) [22].

8.2.4   CAN INSULIN RESISTANCE EXPLAIN DYSLIPIDAEMIA AND HYPERTENSION?

The mechanism of the dyslipidaemia found in association with insulin resistance is not fully clear, but at least in part relates to overproduction of VLDL by the liver. This is probably a consequence of oversupply of substrate rather than a direct influence of insulin resistance on hepatic triglyceride synthesis. Insulin in low concentrations suppresses lipolysis by adipose tissue, and the dose–response curve for this effect is shifted to the right in insulin resistant subjects [14]. As a consequence, the supply of non-esterified fatty acids (NEFA) available for hepatic lipogenesis is increased. Furthermore, because intraperitoneal adipose tissue is less sensitive to insulin than is subcutaneous fat [23], this over-release of NEFA is particularly the case in subjects with visceral obesity, when the fatty acids from intraperitoneal fat drain directly into the liver through the portal vein.

Insulin stimulates the action of lipoprotein lipase (LPL) [24], the enzyme responsible for clearance of both dietary and hepatically secreted triglyceride-rich lipoproteins, so that in insulin-resistant states, impaired clearance of these particles would be an expected consequence. There is a well documented, but again poorly understood, link between hypertriglyceridaemia and low concentrations of HDL-cholesterol. It is suggested to be a consequence of the impaired exchange of apolipoproteins and cholesterol, mediated by cholesteryl ester transfer protein, between VLDL and HDL lipoproteins [25].

The link between insulin resistance and hypertension is more problematic. Blood pressure is curious, in that the human body has such a vested interest in keeping it normal that any trend which is likely to affect the status quo will be strongly opposed by a series of reflexes to restore normality. The two main mechanisms which have been invoked to explain the link between insulin resistance and hypertension – sympathetic nervous system activation and sodium retention – have been alluded to above. Both hypotheses rely on the influence of hyperinsulinaemia in elevating blood pressure, rather than on insulin resistance being responsible. This means that the influence of insulin on the kidney and on the sympathetic nervous system must remain fully competent even in the presence of insulin resistance in skeletal muscle and adipose tissue. While there is some evidence that this may be the case for both organs [26, 27], the observation that the hyperinsulinaemia of patients with insulinoma is not associated with hypertension [28] does raise questions as to whether insulin itself can raise blood pressure.

8.2.5 INSULIN RESISTANCE AND CHD

Besides a link between insulin resistance and several of the classic risk factors for vascular disease, there is a long-running debate as to whether insulin resistance, or more probably the consequent hyperinsulinaemia, is an independent risk factor for atherothrombotic vascular disease. For over 20 years, much energy has been expended by both proponents and opponents of this view [29, 30]. There are data, largely from animal studies [31] and well summarized by Stout [29], that insulin may be pro-atherogenic. However, the main arguments are based on the interpretation of three prospective population studies which showed weak and inconsistent relationships between elevated insulin concentrations, either fasting or post-glucose load, and incident coronary heart disease (CHD) in men [32–34].

Among the additional problems of these studies were the absence of positive results in women [34] and lack of data on important

confounding variables, such as HDL-cholesterol and central obesity [30]. This debate has major practical relevance to the management of diabetes, and it is a relief that the results of the UK Prospective Diabetes Study, in which over 5000 patients with newly diagnosed NIDDM have been randomized between five different therapies, should finally answer the question as to which therapy for NIDDM is able to reduce (CHD) risk [35].

Another area in which the relevance of insulin resistance to cardiovascular disease is contentious is the therapy of hypertension. It has been argued that deleterious effects of thiazides and beta-blockers on insulin resistance negated any cardiovascular benefits consequent upon blood pressure lowering [36]. Whereas concerns about the metabolic effects of hypotensive agents are legitimate, it is unrealistic to expect that the elevated risk of CHD in hypertensive people could be fully reversed within two or three years; meta-analysis of the available trial data provides a more informative picture [37]. Even though angiotensin-converting enzyme inhibitors and alpha-blockers are generally neutral or even positive in their effects on insulin resistance [38], data are still awaited showing that stroke risk can be reduced by 38% or CHD risk by 16% with these agents [39].

Two recent studies which have addressed the issue of hyperinsulinaemia and CHD must be mentioned. A Canadian study has shown powerful predictive ability of hyperinsulinaemia for CHD in 196 subjects over five years follow-up, even when controlling for obesity and concentrations of HDL-cholesterol [40], a defect of earlier studies. Furthermore, a recent paper from the British Regional Heart Study, also controlling for HDL-cholesterol, has supported an independent predictive role for hyperinsulinaemia, although only men were studied [41]. While these studies confront some of the problems of earlier ones, two issues remain. First, a number of new risk factors have been found to cluster with insulin resistance and the question of the true independence of hyper-insulinaemia as a risk factor will continue until other new prospective studies also incorporate these potential confounders. Second, is the nature of evidence itself. Epidemiologists love to get involved in heated, almost theological, debates on risk factors: confounders, under- and over-correction, colinearity etc. But no observational study can answer the question of aetiology, whatever is measured and however carefully. The proof of causation requires evidence that when a risk factor is removed, so is the risk [1]. While this is now the case with cholesterol [42] and blood pressure [36], such proof of causation does not exist for insulin or insulin resistance.

8.3   THE INSULIN RESISTANCE SYNDROME CLUB: NEW APPLICANTS FOR MEMBERSHIP

The universally agreed components of the metabolic syndrome are dyslipidaemia, hypertension and glucose intolerance, along with hyperinsulinaemia or insulin resistance [14]. The various authors who have written on this topic have sometimes appended additional candidates, including obesity (central or global) [10, 43] or hyperuricaemia [44]. However, a number of other risk factors for CHD have emerged during the last 10 years, each of which is also associated with insulin resistance (Figure 8.1). And it is, curiously, the increasing tortuosity of the arguments as to how these new risk factors can be explained on the basis of insulin resistance which has led to the paradigm shift: a search for a common antecedent.

8.3.1   PLASMINOGEN ACTIVATOR INHIBITOR-1

The fibrinolytic system plays an important role in maintaining patency of blood vessels. Plasminogen activation to plasmin is under physiological regulation by tissue plasminogen activator (tPA), and the major inhibitor of this serine protease is plasminogen activator

inhibitor-1 (PAI-1) [45]. This molecule is expressed by hepatocytes, endothelial cells and platelets [46] and liver production of PAI-1 is powerfully influenced by both insulin resistance [47] and by insulin itself [48]. Additionally, VLDL is able to induce expression of PAI-1 by endothelial cells [49]. In consequence, there are strong correlations between concentrations of PAI-1 and measures of both insulin and insulin resistance in both non-diabetic and diabetic populations [50–52]. Of all the new candidates for membership, PAI-1 has the strongest claim. Furthermore, the studies with isolated hepatocytes and with liver cell lines provide strong evidence for a cause and effect relationship both with insulin resistance and with insulin.

8.3.2   PRO-INSULIN-LIKE MOLECULES

The advent of highly specific two-site monoclonal antibody assays for insulin and for its precursor molecules, pro-insulin and des-31,32-pro-insulin [53], led to a major, but short-lived period of doubt regarding the accuracy of all previous studies on the role of insulin deficiency in the aetiology of NIDDM [54]. While it is the case that most of the previous polyclonal insulin assays cross-reacted fully with these precursor molecules, in non-diabetic subjects this led to only around 10% over-estimation of concentrations of 'true' insulin [55]. In NIDDM subjects, however, the contribution of the precursor molecules is much larger [53] and, in this situation, subjects are substantially more insulin-deficient than appears the case when non-specific insulin assays are used [54].

Rather more curious than the contribution of the pro-insulin-like molecules to apparent insulin status is their role in cardiovascular risk. Absolute concentrations of pro-insulin correlate with measures of insulin resistance rather than with β-cell dysfunction [56]. Furthermore, both in diabetic [57] and non-diabetic subjects [55, 58], concentrations of these molecules appear to correlate as

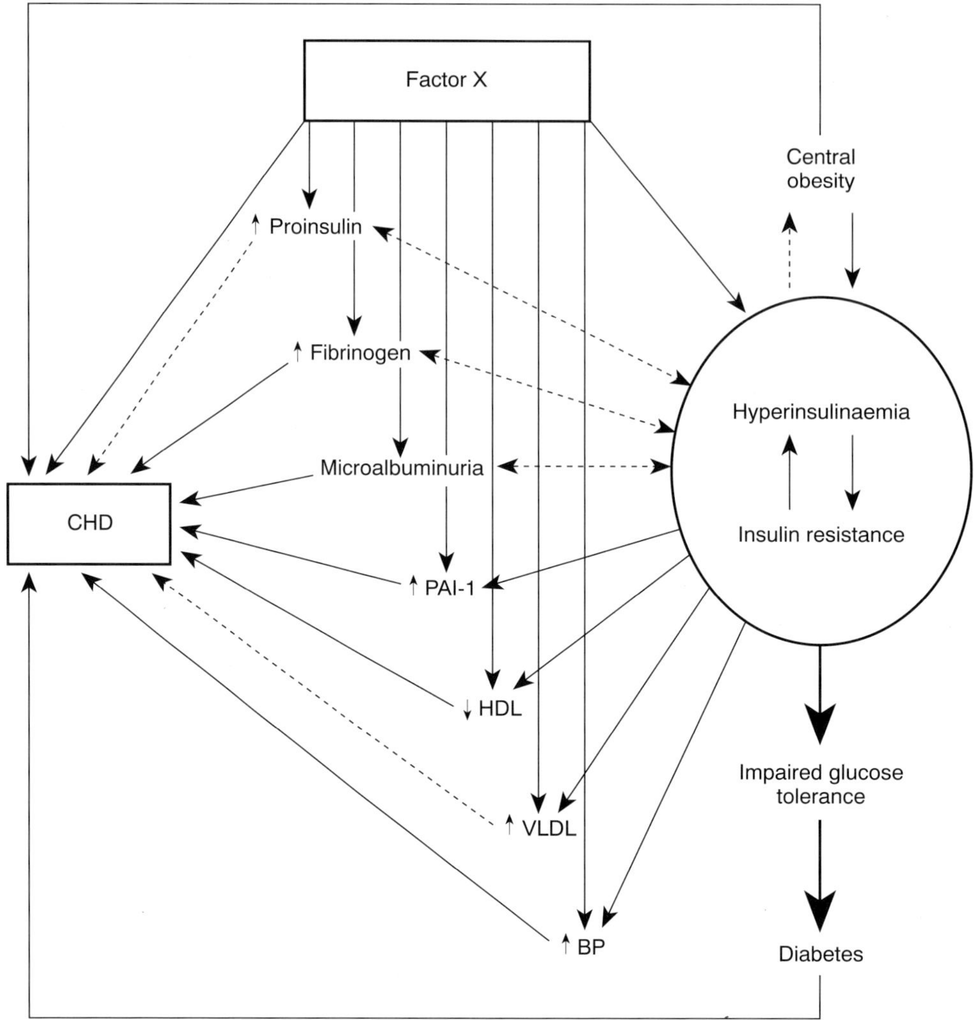

Figure 8.1 The expanded insulin resistance syndrome. CHD, cardiac heart disease; PAI-1, plasminogen activator inhibitor-1; HDL, high density lipoprotein; VLDL, very low density lipoprotein; BP, blood pressure.

strongly as, or more strongly than, do those of insulin with several components of the metabolic cluster, and with CHD itself [59]. This observation in itself makes it improbable that these molecules are driving the metabolic syndrome, bearing in mind that both their concentrations and their activity on the insulin receptor are substantially less than those of insulin [53]. Furthermore, in two studies of NIDDM subjects, in which concentrations of pro-insulin-like molecules, but not those of insulin, were altered by therapy with either sulphonylureas or insulin, we found no changes of levels of lipids or blood pressure when those of pro-insulin were altered by as much as 40% [60, 61]. Nevertheless, in both studies, levels of PAI-1 altered in parallel with those of pro-insulin [60, 61]. The conclusion must be that pro-insulin-like molecules cluster with other features of the metabolic syndrome, and may play a role in regulation of PAI-1 but not of other parts of the syndrome. However, the strength of the relationships of the features of the cluster with concentrations of the precursor molecules does question the interpretation, based on weaker correlations, that insulin resistance is driving the metabolic syndrome.

8.3.3   MICROALBUMINURIA

The excretion of increased amounts of albumin in the urine in diabetic patients predicts not only renal failure but also an increased risk of cardiovascular disease [62]. Furthermore, microalbuminuria may be present in non-diabetic subjects, where it is also accompanied by substantially increased CHD risk [63]. The degree of excess risk is probably substantially greater than can be explained by the abnormalities in blood pressure, lipids and coagulation which accompany microalbuminuria. As a possible explanation both for the risk factors clustering with microalbuminuria and for the excess incidence of CHD, in both diabetic and non-diabetic subjects, microalbuminuria is accompanied by insulin resistance [64–66].

While such an observation may explain one part of a paradox, it merely shifts the puzzle. If there is a correlation between increased albumin excretion rate and reduced insulin action, which way does the arrow go in the cause-and-effect diagram? It has been postulated that hyperinsulinaemia may increase endothelial permeability [67], but physiological hyperinsulinaemia does not induce microalbuminuria in normal glucose tolerant subjects [68]. Far more likely is the possibility

that something else is driving both, the consequences of a common antecedent.

8.3.4   FIBRINOGEN

Another association which is difficult to explain on the basis of current concepts of the mechanisms of insulin action is that between hyperinsulinaemia and elevated concentrations of fibrinogen [55]. In subjects with CHD, fibrinogen levels may be raised as a consequence of an acute phase response [69], with parallel activation of stress hormones producing insulin resistance [70]. It is more difficult, however, to understand the strength of the correlations between fibrinogen and insulin levels in a healthy population [55, 71]. While a common antecedent is probable, the mechanism remains puzzling.

8.4   INSULIN RESISTANCE AND ITS ASSOCIATES: CONSEQUENCES OF A COMMON ANTECEDENT?

There are, then, several more phenotypes which cluster with insulin resistance than was the case when the earlier descriptions of the cluster were outlined. Some of these new members, such as fibrinogen and microalbuminuria, are powerful predictors of CHD, both in diabetic and non-diabetic populations [72, 73], whereas others, such as pro-insulin and PAI-1, have been linked with CHD only in cross-sectional studies [59, 74, 75]. What is their relationship with insulin resistance? With PAI-1, microalbuminuria and fibrinogen associated, the possibility that insulin resistance is the central mechanism becomes ever more improbable. It is more likely that these phenomena are all the consequence of a different mechanism, further upstream from the cluster (Figure 8.1). The first candidate for antecedence is the small baby syndrome.

8.5   THE SMALL BABY SYNDROME

Barker and Hales and their groups have studied several populations in which records of birth weight or early growth were linked to cardiovascular disease or its risk factors up to 60 or 70 years later [76–78]. Early reports showed that low birth weight was able to predict glucose intolerance [76, 78] and CHD [79] later in life, while other studies found links between low birth weight and hypertension [77]. More detailed birth records were able to provide a derived ponderal index, a measure of fatness, or thinness, at birth. The thin neonate, especially if it became a fat adult, was found later to develop glucose intolerance, hypertension, hypertriglyceridaemia and raised fibrinogen levels. It also had raised concentrations of pro-insulin-like molecules and PAI-1 [77, 80]. Additional investigation showed that these thin babies did indeed show insulin resistance in adulthood [81]. There are also data to suggest that IDDM patients with nephropathy were more likely to have been growth retarded *in utero* than those without renal involvement [82]. Our observation that non-diabetic subjects with microalbuminuria are shorter in adult stature than normoalbuminuric individuals [83] may be related to this. It is possible, then, that the small or thin baby develops the full panoply of risk factors of the metabolic cluster, including those which are difficult to explain on the basis of insulin resistance.

Although these observations provide a tentative common explanation for the cluster, such an explanation begs several questions. First, is the small baby link to adult disease a consequence of maternal nutrition during pregnancy? A number of observations in animals have suggested that protein deprivation during pregnancy can lead to reduced pancreatic function [84], raised blood pressure [85] and altered liver zonation with increased synthesis of gluconeogenic enzymes [86]. However, despite some soft data in humans on maternal diet and neonatal anthropometry [87] or maternal protein intake and offspring's blood pressure [88], the likelihood is that, at least in western society, the major

determinant of fetal growth is placental function and not maternal diet. Also, we have found no evidence from subjects exposed *in utero* to the siege of Leningrad that acute protein calorie malnutrition produces either diabetes or elevated levels of any other cardiovascular risk factor in the offspring [89]. It nevertheless remains possible that nutritional influences earlier in the mother's life may be responsible for the high risk of diabetes in the small babies born to undernourished women in many parts of the developing world [90].

The second question which the observations of the small baby syndrome do not resolve is that of mechanism. One relevant observation is that fetuses which manifest growth retardation in the third trimester of pregnancy show poor renal development, with lower nephron numbers than appropriate size for dates fetuses, without any catch-up in nephron number postnatally [91]. While these findings may or may not be relevant to the later development of microalbuminuria or hypertension, they may point to a common theme between growth retardation and cardiovascular risk. In fetuses showing poor growth in late pregnancy, the cardiac output of the left side of the fetal heart exceeds that of the right side, maintaining blood supply to the brain at the expense of that to the abdominal viscera and legs [9]. If poor capillarization were to limit the vascularization of glomerular tufts, pancreatic islets, liver and skeletal muscle, the consequence might be oligonephropathy, poor islet function, altered zonation of the liver and poor delivery of insulin and substrate to the main sites of insulin-sensitive glucose disposal [93, 94]. The fact that low skeletal muscle capillary density may play an important role in limiting insulin action has been suggested by studies of muscle biopsies in 41 Pima Indian and 23 Caucasian non-diabetic subjects [95]. Furthermore, recent observations from Stehouwer's group have shown powerful relationships between low birth weight, impaired capillary recruitment, poor

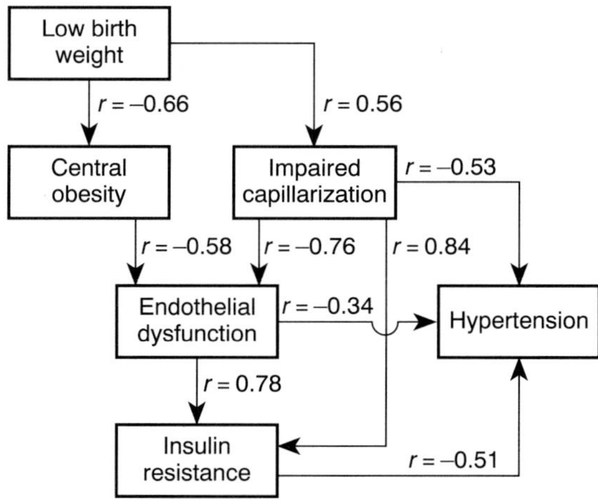

Figure 8.2 The relationships between birth weight, central obesity, capillary recruitment, endothelial dysfunction and insulin sensitivity in 18 healthy subjects. Redrawn from [96].

endothelial dependent vasodilatation and insulin resistance in a detailed study in 18 healthy subjects with a wide range of insulin sensitivity [96] (Figure 8.2). This offers a possible unifying vascular mechanism for the consequences of growth retardation.

Indeed, the health of blood vessels may be vital to the maintenance of metabolic and haemostatic balance, as well as of major relevance to the prevention of cardiovascular disease. And the integrity, or disease, of the endothelium, whether a consequence of shear stress resulting from growth retardation and undercapillarization or from damage acquired later in life, may underlie several of the features of the metabolic cluster [94].

8.6 ENDOTHELIAL DYSFUNCTION AS A COMMON ANTECEDENT OF INSULIN RESISTANCE AND THE METABOLIC CLUSTER

Could the endothelium be responsible for the metabolic cluster attributed to insulin resistance? And what about insulin action itself? The endothelium is more than a passive lining of blood vessels. The list of products of the endothelial cell has been growing ever longer, with consequent important roles in vascular tone (nitric oxide, endothelin), platelet aggregation (prostacyclin) and fibrinolysis (tPA, PAI-1). Moreover, the endothelium binds to its luminal surface enzymes which contribute importantly to the health of the vascular tree, including angiotensin-converting enzyme and LPL. It could, then, be speculated that endothelial damage is potentially at the root of several components of the metabolic cluster, including hypertension, impaired clearance of triglyceride-rich lipoproteins and increased expression of PAI-1 [94], as well as of atherothrombotic disease itself [97]. But what about insulin resistance *per se*?

During a prolonged period of hyperinsulinaemia, vasodilatation of resistance vessels occurs, with a consequent increase in blood flow to limb skeletal muscle [98]. This action of insulin is mediated by nitric oxide and blocked by inhibitors of nitric oxide synthase, implying that it is endothelially mediated [99]. Baron's group has estimated that as much of 40% of insulin action on peripheral glucose uptake could be mediated by the enhanced delivery of hormone and substrate to insulin-sensitive tissues as a consequence of this endothelial action [98], but there is substantial debate about whether the increased blood flow is physiologically relevant and whether it is the cause or consequence of insulin's stimulation of muscle glucose utilization [100].

There is additional evidence that the endothelium makes an important contribution to insulin action, but whether this is relevant to endothelial dysfunction is more speculative. Insulin receptors on skeletal muscle are accessible to insulin in the interstitial space, but not to intraluminal insulin. Direct measurement of insulin concentrations in interstitial fluid is possible by microdialysis, although certain assumptions are necessary to correct for the extremely low recovery of molecules of this size across the dialysis membrane. Using this approach, Jansson and colleagues have found a two- to threefold gradient of insulin across the vascular wall, both basally and during a hyperinsulinaemic clamp [101]. Similar conclusions are reached by Bergman *et al.* from studies in humans using measures of lymph insulin or mathematical modelling of glucose kinetics during the intravenous glucose tolerance test and in experimental animals during hyperinsulinaemic clamps [102–104]. Furthermore, Bergman has presented data showing that the access of insulin to the interstitial fluid compartment is rate-limiting, not only for its action on glucose disposal, but also for its suppression of hepatic glucose output [102, 105]. This single gateway hypothesis depends on a systemic signal modulated by interstitial insulin, which may well be adipose tissue-generated non-esterified fatty acids (Figure 8.3). As to whether insulins transport into the interstitium is active or passive, receptor-mediated or concentration-dependent, the findings are unclear [106, 107], as is the effect of capillary endothelial dysfunction, inflammation, membrane structure or levels of circulating metabolites on this transport.

When cardiologists or clinical pharmacologists use the term endothelial dysfunction, they are usually referring to some abnormality of resistance vessel response, for example to acetylcholine or to shear stress. If, however, active functioning of the endothelium is necessary for the ability of insulin to reach its receptor, it is the health of capillary endothelium which is relevant [94]. To assess endothelial well-being at this order of vessel, such measures as transcapillary escape rate of albumin or release of endothelial proteins may be more appropriate. There are some limited studies linking insulin resistance to endothelial dysfunction in population or clinical investigative studies. Thus Petrie *et al.* found correlations between limb blood flow response to monomethyl arginine, an inhibitor of endothelial nitric-oxide-dependent vasodilatation, and whole body glucose uptake in healthy subjects [108]. The European Concerted Action on Thrombosis (ECAT) study has found correlations of fasting insulin concentrations with those of von Willebrand factor, a marker of (capillary) endothelial damage, in 1484 subjects with angina [71]. We have shown relationships of a more direct measurement of insulin resistance, using the insulin suppression test, with von Willebrand factor concentrations in 33 subjects with NIDDM [94]. However, in an attempt to look more closely at relationships between endothelial dysfunction and insulin action, we have serendipitously come up with a series of novel observations which provide an alternative, and more radical, hypothesis to relate features of the metabolic cluster, including the new members.

8.7 PRO-INFLAMMATORY CYTOKINES, THE ACUTE PHASE RESPONSE AND INSULIN RESISTANCE

In order to investigate further the possible role of endothelial dysfunction as an explanation for the metabolic cluster, we explored the relationships between four markers of endothelial dysfunction (Table 8.1a) and the cluster of insulin resistance variables (Table 8.1b) in 107 non-diabetic subjects [109]. Furthermore, because of the relationships we had found between insulin concentrations and those of

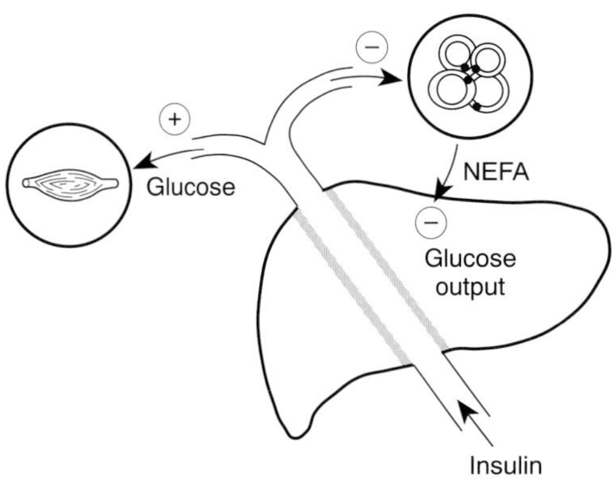

Figure 8.3 The single gateway hypothesis. NEFA, Non-esterified fatty acids. Redrawn from [102].

fibrinogen [55], we created an acute phase cluster (Table 8.1c), comprising fibrinogen and C-reactive protein (CRP), two classic acute phase proteins, with circulating levels of two pro-inflammatory cytokines: IL-6, the major determinant of hepatic synthesis of CRP [110], and TNF-α. The method used was to derive a Z score for each variable, so as to create a unit-free value, and then to calculate a mean Z score for each cluster. This approach was taken to reduce the influences of biological variability on each measure used alone. It also circumvents the problem of co-linearity among the individual components of each score, which would make the usual multivariate approach less suitable. There was, indeed, a relationship between the sum score of insulin resistance and that of endothelial dysfunction ($r = 0.32$, $p = 0.0008$) (Figure 8.4a), but the strength of this relationship was dwarfed by that between the metabolic cluster and the acute phase score ($r = 0.59$, $p < 0.00005$) (Figure 8.4b). The third of these correlations, between endothelial and acute

Table 8.1 Groupings for Z scores

---

a The endothelial dysfunction Z score
Thrombomodulin
Cellular fibronectin
von Willebrand factor
Albumin excretion rate

b The insulin resistance Z score
Systolic blood pressure
Diastolic blood pressure
Triglyceride
High density lipoprotein cholesterol (inverse)
Insulin sensitivity (inverse)
Body mass index
Waist-to-hip ratio
Subscapular-to-triceps ratio

c The acute phase Z score
Fibrinogen
C-reactive protein
Interleukin-6
Tumour necrosis factor-α

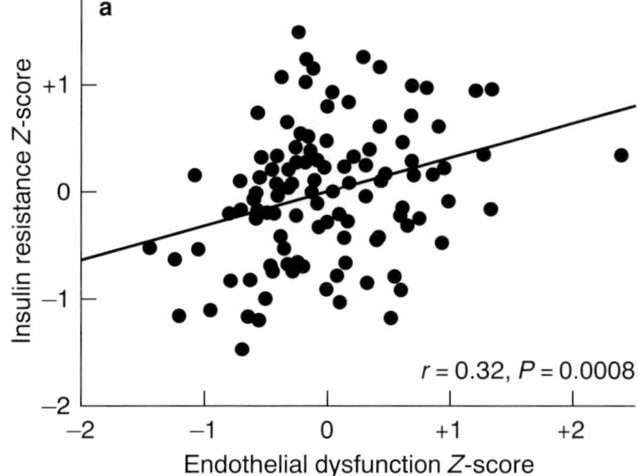

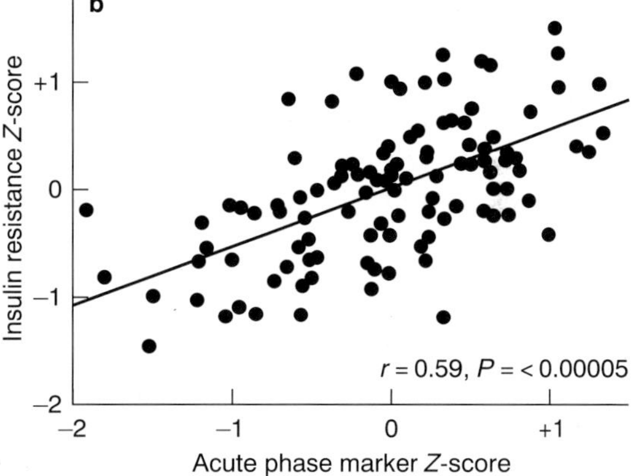

Figure 8.4 Relationship between (a) endothelial dysfunction Z score and insulin resistance Z score and (b) acute phase marker Z score and insulin resistance Z score.

phase scores, was also significant ($r = 0.43$, $p < 0.00005$).

How much of the link between the insulin resistance and acute phase cluster is because of confounding? Removing the three measures of obesity from the insulin resistance cluster score weakened the relationship with the acute phase score only slightly ($r = 0.53$, $p < 0.00005$), suggesting that this link was largely independent of adiposity. Moreover, in multiple regression models, the relationship between acute phase markers and the insulin resistance cluster remained significant when age, gender, smoking and prevalent CHD were included in the model (partial $r = 0.60$, $p<0.00005$). However, the relationship between the endothelial and insulin resistance scores was substantially weakened in such a model (partial $r = 0.18$, $p = 0.061$). Furthermore, if the acute phase and endothelial scores were included in the same model, the former remained significantly associated with insulin resistance score (partial $r = 0.61$, $p<0.00005$) but not the latter (partial $r = -0.02$, $p = 0.82$).

Concentrations of TNF-α were related to all insulin resistance variables, including proinsulin-like molecules, tPA and PAI-1, as well as to markers of endothelial damage (Table 8.2). Concentrations of IL-6 were also related to several of the insulin resistance cluster and endothelial markers, including albumin excretion rate. In general, the relationships for C-reactive protein were stronger than those for IL-6.

These observations suggest that, even in healthy subjects, insulin resistance and the cluster of variables with which it is associated may be consequences of circulating levels of pro-inflammatory cytokines. Alternatively, these levels may reflect tissue concentrations of the factor(s) responsible for the components of the insulin resistance cluster. Moreover, these same compounds may also be responsible for the endothelial damage with which insulin resistance is associated, including raised levels of von Willebrand factor and of albumin excretion. Is there any biological plausibility in this hypothesis? It is clear that TNF-α has a number of such actions, including inhibiting the tyrosine phosphorylation of insulin receptor substrate-1 induced by insulin binding [111, 112], suppressing the action of LPL [113], stimulating lipolysis [114] and impairing endothelial function [115]. Several of these actions are shared by IL-6 [116–118] and recent evidence suggests that, in states of inflammation, the increase in circulating concentrations of soluble IL-6 receptor may increase the effect of IL-6 on secretion of soluble adhesion molecules by endothelial cells [119]. In such a fashion, it might be possible that the production of these cytokines, and their overspill into insulin-sensitive tissues such as skeletal muscle and

Table 8.2 Relationships of acute phase markers and concentrations of pro-inflammatory cytokines with metabolic syndrome variables and with markers of endothelial dysfunction in 107 subjects

	Tumour necrosis factor-α[†]	*Interleukin-6[†]*	*C-reactive protein[†]*
Insulin sensitivity[†]	−0.35***	−0.09	−0.22*
Triglyceride[†]	0.37***	0.03	0.27**
High density lipoprotein cholesterol	0.27**	−0.26**	−0.21*
Systolic blood pressure	0.33***	0.31**	0.34***
Intact proinsulin[†]	0.33**	0.16	0.16
Des 31,32 proinsulin[†]	0.28**	0.11	0.08
PAI-1 antigen	0.35***	0.18	0.19*
Tissue plasminogen activator antigen	0.40***	0.32**	0.40***
von Willebrand factor	0.38***	0.11	0.31***
Thrombomodulin[†]	0.32**	−0.05	0.13
Cellular fibronectin[†]	0.36***	0.13	0.28**
Mean albumin excretion rate[†]	0.25*	0.20*	0.07

[†] Data logarithmically transformed.
* $p<0.05$.
** $p<0.01$.
*** $p<0.001$.

adipose tissue, could produce the cluster previously ascribed to a primary defect in insulin action, as well as endothelial damage. But where do these cytokines come from in apparently healthy middle-aged people on the practice register of a London general practitioner?

8.8 THE ROLE OF INFECTIONS AND ADIPOSE TISSUE?

The most likely source of such pro-inflammatory cytokines might seem to be macrophages activated by some occult infection. For this reason we explored relationships with titres of immunoglobulin G antibodies to three organisms which may have a role in atherogenesis [120–122]. Both the acute phase score and concentrations of C-reactive protein correlated weakly with titres of *Helicobacter pylori*, *Chlamydia pneumoniae* and cytomegalovirus antibodies (Table 8.3). However, the only significant correlation seen between titres of such antibodies and concentrations of cytokines was that of IL-6 with *Helicobacter pylori* [109].

Both TNF-α and IL-6 are expressed in adipose tissue [123, 124]. Using the technique of inferior epigastric vein cannulation, we have recently described the release of IL-6, but not of TNF-α, from a subcutaneous adipose tissue bed *in vivo*, this release increasing significantly up to five hours after a high carbohydrate meal [125]. We have estimated, rather surprisingly, that in these healthy people, up to 40% of total body production of IL-6 comes from adipose tissue. In the 107 healthy subjects in whom we had analysed clustering, we found that both the acute phase score as a whole, and the concentrations of IL-6, TNF-α and C-reactive protein, were strongly related to measures of total, and particularly central, obesity (Table 8.3) [109].

These observations suggest that adipose tissue synthesizes and produces substances which, via autocrine, paracrine or endocrine mechanisms, influence insulin signalling, lipoprotein metabolism and endothelial and hepatic expression of procoagulant molecules, as well as other properties of the endothelium. It might also be the case that signalling of insulin action to the liver is mediated from the periphery via modulation of adipose tissue NEFA release by such cytokines [102]. The influence of adipose tissue-generated TNF-α on insulin signalling has been suggested by studies of its expression by adipocytes [123] and of its effect on the phosphorylation of tyrosine and serine residues of insulin receptor substrate-1 [111, 112]. Effects of this cytokine on lipid metabolism and on endothelium are also recognized [113, 115].

The relationship of concentrations of circulating levels of this cytokine both to the components of the metabolic cluster and to markers of endothelial dysfunction might imply an endocrine role for this cytokine, and the relationship with measures of obesity would imply an adipose tissue origin. However, the failure to find an arteriovenous difference of this cytokine across a single adipose tissue bed [125] would make this source of TNF-α less likely unless there are major regional differences in its production. It may suggest that circulating concentrations represent a complex of the cytokine with one of its soluble receptors, which themselves are expressed in [126], and may be secreted by, adipose tissue. The role of IL-6 as the main regulator of hepatic synthesis of CRP [110] implies an endocrine role for this cytokine, and our finding that it is secreted by adipose tissue [125] provides an explanation of the relationship between the acute phase response and obesity. The influence of IL-6 on lipid metabolism [116] and endothelial function [118, 119] are known, albeit less well documented than those of TNF-α. The relationships of levels of CRP with a number of features of the insulin resistance cluster and of endothelial dysfunction implies that the cytokine may have a greater role in these

Table 8.3 Relationships of acute phase markers and concentrations of pro-inflammatory cytokines with antibody titres to *Helicobacter pylori*, *Chlamydia pneumoniae* and cytomegalovirus, and to measures of obesity in 107 subjects

	Insulin resistance cluster score	Endothelial marker score	Acute phase marker score	Tumour necrosis factor-α[†]	Interleukin-6[†]	C-reactive protein[†]
Helicobacter phylori titre ($n = 80$)	0.12	−0.08	0.27*	0.18	0.28*	0.24*
Chlamydia pneumoniae titre ($n = 70$)	0.25*	−0.12	0.28*	0.21	0.15	0.25*
Cytomegalovirus titre ($n = 80$)	0.09	0.11	0.30**	0.21	0.17	0.23*
Body mass index	‡	0.26***	0.45***	0.33***	0.19*	0.41***
Waist-to-hip ratio	‡	0.29***	0.49***	0.51***	0.41***	0.32**
Subscapular-to-triceps ratio	‡	0.22**	0.33**	0.37***	0.26**	0.21*

[†] Data logarithmically transformed.
[‡] Included in calculation of variable.
* $p<0.05$.
** $p<0.01$.
*** $p<0.001$.

disturbances than is implied by the correlations in Table 8.3. IL-6 is the main regulator of hepatic expression of CRP, but unlike the acute phase protein [127] has a short circulating half life [128].

8.9   A NEW PARADIGM FOR INSULIN RESISTANCE, OBESITY, ENDOTHELIAL DYSFUNCTION AND CARDIOVASCULAR DISEASE

There has recently been much interest in evidence suggesting that atherosclerosis is an inflammatory disease, with levels of CRP both representing disease activity [69] and acting as a prognostic marker [69, 129, 130]. What is now being proposed is that inflammation may underlie the atherosclerotic process, not as a result of chronic infection with *Helicobacter*, *Chlamydia* or cytomegalovirus, but because of adipocyte-generated cytokines.

What is being suggested is a new explanation: that the relationship of the cluster of variables previously ascribed to insulin resistance is because they are all produced by actions of proinflammatory cytokines. The hypothesis is that this mechanism may exist in healthy individuals, particularly in obese subjects, in whom adipose tissue may be the source of these cytokines. The hypothesis further proposes an explanation for the association of the metabolic cluster and of obesity with endothelial dysfunction, and may underlie the link between adiposity, particularly that which is centrally distributed, and CHD [131]. There are some studies relating early growth retardation to increased visceral adiposity [96, 132], even allowing for the possibility of the small baby hypothesis operating through cytokine-type mechanisms (Figure 8.2). Although there are no data, it is possible that in disease states, increased release of these cytokines could help explain the insulin resistance of stress and that seen in people with CHD. Yet it must be recognized that, based as they are on a series of cross-sectional correlations, these conjectures are castles built on sand. Could it be, for example, that adipose tissue releases some other signal, such as NEFA, which modulates insulin action and produces the associated changes, and that levels of other adipose tissue products are merely reflecting those of the true culprit? Furthermore, despite the strength of some of these correlations shown in Figures 8.2 and 8.4, it is improbable that insulin resistance, any more than arterial disease, has a single cause. Apportioning the population variance of insulin resistance to cytokines, NEFA, early growth retardation, capillarization, endothelial damage or other factors remains a task for the future.

The imputation of causation to the relationship between two variables requires studies of the effects of interventions. What are the effects of administering the cytokines, or of neutralizing their actions? Administration of TNF-α produces alterations of lipid metabolism [133] and of endothelial protein expression [115], although effects on insulin signalling *in vivo* have not been investigated. For IL-6, data are more limited. Yet for neither cytokine has the effect of very small elevations of concentrations, similar to those in obese but healthy individuals, been documented. There are conflicting data in mice and in humans on the effects of neutralizing TNF-α with monoclonal antibodies or soluble receptors [134, 135], although it would be improbable that an autocrine or paracrine effect of the cytokine would be affected. If the cytokines in peripheral blood represent overspill from adipose tissue, the concentrations which act locally on the adipocyte may be much higher [134, 136] and it may be possible to study these directly by microdialysis. What is also unclear is whether the levels of TNF-α and IL-6 measured in the circulation represent free or bound cytokine and whether the concentrations of these molecules approximate to those which influence cell signalling. Finally, the cytokines studied represent only two of a large family of molecules expressed by adipose tissue, including the classic example of an adipose tissue signal: leptin [137]. It is possible that other members of this family may share effects of TNF-α on metabolic signalling and endothelial cell function. Indeed, it could be proposed that the actions of TNF-α and IL-6 on insulin action, and on LPL and lipolysis, could play a part in the adipostatic mechanism [138], whereby increases in fat cell size result in metabolic changes which limit further increases in adipose tissue mass in the face of continuing positive energy balance.

8.10   CONCLUSIONS

Insulin is a hormone which stops us getting diabetes. For the last 20 or more years, it has been getting a bad press by being associated, in population studies, with several cardiovascular risk factors and also with heart disease itself. Yet it is guilt by association, and has led to major anxieties about, for example, the wisdom of using highly effective treatments for hypertension and even of treating diabetic patients, suboptimally controlled on tablets, with the one treatment which is physiologically relevant. The possibility is that insulin resistance is not the prime mover and that it is reflecting the action of the grim reaper which the overstretched adipocyte churns out in the face of positive energy balance.

REFERENCES

1. Bradford Hill, A. The environment and disease: association or causation? *Proc. R. Soc. Med.*, 1965, **58**, 295–300.
2. DeFronzo, R.A., Tobin, J.D. and Andres, R. Glucose clamp technique: a method for quantifying insulin secretion and resistance. *Am. J. Physiol.*, 1979, **237**, E214–23.
3. Kendall, D.M., Sutherland, D.E.R., Najarian, J.S., Goetz, F.C. and Robertson, R.P. Effects of hemipancreatectomy on insulin secretion and glucose tolerance in healthy humans. *N. Engl. J. Med.*, 1990, **322**, 898–903.
4. Rudenski, A.S., Matthews, D.R., Levy, J.C. and Turner, R.C. Understanding 'insulin resistance': both glucose resistance and insulin resistance are required to model human diabetes. *Metabolism*, 1991, **40**, 908–17.
5. Laakso, M. How good a marker is insulin level for insulin resistance? *Am. J. Epidemiol.*, 1993, **137**, 959–65.
6. Matthews, D.R., Hosker, J.P., Rudenski, A.S., Naylor, B.A., Treacher, D.F. and Turner, R.C. Homeostasis model assessment; insulin resistance and β-cell function from fasting plasma glucose and insulin concentrations in man. *Diabetologia*, 1985, **28**, 412–19.
7. Shen, S.-W., Reaven, G.M. and Farquhar, J.W. Comparison of impedance to insulin-mediated glucose uptake in normal subjects and in subjects with latent diabetes. *J. Clin. Invest.*, 1970, **49**, 2151–60.
8. Yki–Järvinen, H. Role of insulin resistance in the pathogenesis of NIDDM. *Diabetologia*, 1995, **38**, 1378–88.
9. Rains, C. (as Captain Louis Renault) in *Casablanca*. Screenplay by J.J. Epstein, P.G. Epstein and H. Koch. Director M. Curtiz, Hollywood, CA, 1942.
10. Modan, M., Halkin, H., Almog, S., Lusky, A., Eshkol, A., Sheki, M., Shitrit, A. and Fuchs, Z. Hyperinsulinemia: a link between hypertension, obesity and glucose intolerance. *J. Clin. Invest.*, 1985, **75**, 809–17.
11. Ferrannini, E., Buzzigoli, G., Bonadonna, R., Giorico, M.A., Oleggini, M., Graziadei, L., Pedrinelli, R., Brandi, L. and Bevilacqua, S. Insulin resistance in essential hypertension. *N. Engl. J. Med.*, 1987, **317**, 350–7.
12. Landsberg, L. Diet, obesity and hypertension; an hypothesis involving insulin, the sympathetic nervous system, and adaptive thermogenesis. *Q. J. Med.*, 1986, **236**, 1081–90.
13. DeFronzo, R.A. The effect of insulin on renal sodium metabolism. A review with clinical implications. *Diabetologia*, 1981, **21**, 165–71.
14. Reaven, G.M. Role of insulin resistance in human disease. *Diabetes*, 1988, **37**, 1595–607.
15. Hollenbeck, C. and Reaven, G.M. Variations in insulin-stimulated glucose uptake in healthy individuals with normal glucose tolerance. *J. Clin. Endocrinol. Metab.*, 1987, **64**, 1169–73.
16. Golay, A., Chen, Y-DI, and Reaven, G.M. Effect of differences in glucose tolerance on insulin's ability to regulate carbohydrate and free fatty acid metabolism in obese individuals. *J. Clin. Endocrinol. Metab.*, 1986, **62**, 1081–8.

17. Peiris, A.N., Stagner, J.I., Vogel, R.L., Nakagawa, A. and Samols, E. Body fat distribution and peripheral insulin sensitivity in healthy men: role of insulin pulsatility. *J. Clin. Endocrinol. Metab.*, 1992, **75,** 290–3.

18. Facchini, F., Chen, Y.D., Clinkingbeard, C., Jeppesen, J. and Reaven, G.M. Insulin resistance, hyperinsulinemia, and dyslipidemia in nonobese individuals with a family history of hypertension. *Am. J. Hypertens.*, 1992, **5,** 694–9.

19. Yip, J.W., Facchini, F., Chen, I. and Reaven, G.M. Insulin resistance in patients with essential hypertension can occur in the absence of microalbuminuria. *Am. J. Hypertens.*, 1996, **9,** 959–63.

20. Boyko, E.J., Leonetti, D.L., Bergstrom, R.W., Newell–Morris, L. and Fujimoto, W.Y. Visceral adiposity, fasting plasma insulin, and blood pressure in Japanese Americans. *Diabetes Care*, 1995, **18,** 174–81.

21. Ebeling, P., Bourey, R., Koranyi, L., Tuominen, J.A., Groop, L.C., Henriksson, J. and Mueckler, M. Mechanism of enhanced insulin sensitivity in athletes. Increased blood flow, muscle glucose transport protein (GLUT–4) concentration, and glycogen synthase activity. *J. Clin. Invest.*, 1993, **92,** 1623–31.

22. Bressler, P., Bailey, S.R., Matsuda, M. and DeFronzo, R.A. Insulin resistance and coronary artery disease. *Diabetologia*, 1996, **39,** 1345–50.

23. Björntorp, P. 'Portal' adipose tissue as a generator of risk factors for cardiovascular disease and diabetes. *Arteriosclerosis*, 1990, **10,** 493–6.

24. Frayn, K.N. and Coppack, S.W. Insulin resistance, adipose tissue and coronary heart disease. *Clin. Sci.*, 1992, **82,** 1–8.

25. Tall, A.R. Plasma cholesteryl ester transfer protein and high-density lipoproteins: new insights from molecular genetic studies. *J. Intern. Med.*, 1995, **237,** 5–12.

26. Skøtt, P., Vaag, A., Bruun, N.E., Hother-Nielsen, O., Gall, M.A., Beck-Nielsen, H. and Parving, H.H. Effect of insulin on renal sodium handling in hyperinsulinaemic type 2 (non-insulin-dependent) diabetic patients with peripheral insulin resistance. *Diabetologia*, 1991, **34,** 275–81.

27. O'Hare, J.A., Minaker, K.L., Meneilly, G.S., Rowe, J.W., Pallotta, J.A. and Young, J.B. Effect of insulin on plasma norepinephrine and 3, 4-dihydroxyphenylalanine in obese men. *Metabolism*, 1989, **38,** 322–9.

28. Sawicki, P.T., Heinemann, L., Starke, A. and Berger, M. Hyperinsulinaemia is not linked with blood pressure elevation in patients with insulinoma. *Diabetologia*, 1992, **35,** 649–52.

29. Stout, R.W. Insulin and atheroma. 20 year perspective. *Diabetes Care*, 1990, **13,** 631–55.

30. Jarrett, R.J. Is insulin atherogenic? *Diabetologia*, 1988, **31,** 71–5.

31. Pyörälä, K. Relationship of glucose tolerance and plasma insulin to the incidence of coronary heart disease: results from two population studies in Finland. *Diabetes Care*, 1979, **2,** 131–41.

32. Ducimetière, P., Eschwège, E., Papoz, L., Richard, J.-L., Claude, C.R. and Rosselin, G. Relationship of plasma insulin levels to the incidence of myocardial infarction and coronary heart disease mortality in a middle-aged population. *Diabetologia*, 1980, **19,** 205–10.

33. Welborn, T.A. and Wearne, K. Coronary heart disease incidence and cardiovascular mortality in Busselton with reference to glucose and insulin concentrations. *Diabetes Care*, 1979, **2,** 154–60.

34. Stout, R.W. Development of vascular lesions in insulin-treated animals fed on a normal diet. *BMJ*, 1970, **3,** 685–7.

35. UK Prospective Diabetes Study (UKPDS) 17. A 9–year update of a randomized, controlled trial on the effect of improved metabolic control on complications in non-insulin-dependent diabetes mellitus. *Ann. Intern. Med.*, 1996, **124,** 136–45.

36. Black, H.R. The coronary artery disease paradox: the role of hyperinsulinemia and insulin resistance and implications for therapy. *J. Cardiovasc. Pharmacol.*, 1990, **15** (suppl, 5), S26–S38.

37. Collins, R., Peto, R., MacMahon, S., Hebert, P., Fiebach, N.H., Eberlein, K.A., Godwin, J., Qizilbash, N., Taylor, J.O. and Hennekens, C.H. Blood pressure, stroke, and coronary heart disease. Part 2, short-term reductions in blood pressure: Overview of randomised drug trials in their epidemiological context. *Lancet*, 1990, **335,** 827–38.

38. Berne, C., Pollare, T. and Lithell, H. Effects of antihypertensive treatment on insulin sensitivity with special reference to ACE inhibitors. *Diabetes Care*, 1991, **14** (suppl. 4) 39–47.

39. Hebert, P.R., Moser, M., Mayer, J., Glynn, R.J. and Hennekens, C.H. Recent evidence on drug therapy of mild to moderate hypertension and decreased risk of coronary heart disease. *Arch. Intern. Med.*, 1993, **153**, 578–81.

40. Després J.P., Lamarche, B., Mauriège, P., Cantin, B., Dagenais, G.R., Moorjani, S. and Lupien, P.-J. Hyperinsulinemia as an independent risk factor for ischemic heart disease. *N. Engl. J. Med.*, 1996, **334**, 952–7.

41. Perry, I.J., Wannamethee, G., Whincup, P.H., Shaper, A.G., Walker, M.K. and Alberti, K.G.M.M. Serum insulin and incident coronary heart disease in middle-aged British men. *Am. J. Epidemiol.*, 1996, **144**, 224–34.

42. Scandinavian Simvastatin Survival Study Group. Randomized trial of cholesterol lowering in 4444 patients with coronary heart disease: the Scandinavian Simvastatin Survival Study (4S). *Lancet*, 1994, **344**, 1383–9.

43. Kaplan, N.M. The deadly quartet: upper-body obesity, glucose intolerance, hypertriglyceridemia, and hypertension. *Arch. Intern. Med.*, 1989, **149**, 1514–20.

44. Vuorinen-Markkola, H. and Yki-Järvinen, H. Hyperuricemia and insulin resistance. *J. Clin. Endocrinol. Metab.*, 1994, **78**, 25–9.

45. Chmielewska, J., Ranby, M. and Wiman, B. Evidence for a rapid inhibitor to tPA in plasma. *Thromb. Res.*, 1983, **31**, 427–63.

46. Panahloo, A. and Yudkin, J.S. Diminished fibrinolysis in diabetes mellitus and its implication for diabetic vascular disease. *Coronary Artery Dis.*, 1996, **7**, 723–31.

47. Anfosso, F., Chomiki, N., Alessi, M.C., Vague, P. and Juhan-Vague, I. Plasminogen activator inhibitor-1 synthesis in the human hepatoma cell line Hep G2: metformin inhibits the stimulating effect of insulin. *J. Clin. Invest.*, 1993, **91**, 2185–93.

48. Kooistra, T., Bosma, P.J., Töns, H.A.M., van den Berg, A.P., Meyer, P. and Princen, H.M.G. Plasminogen activator inhibitor 1: biosynthesis and mRNA level are increased by insulin in cultured human hepatocytes. *Thromb. Haemost.*, 1989, **62**, 723–8.

49. Stiko-Rahm, A., Wiman, B., Hamsten, A. and Nilsson, J. Secretion of plasminogen activator inhibitor-1 from cultured human umbilical vein cells is induced by very low density lipoprotein. *Arteriosclerosis*, 1990, **10**, 1067–73.

50. Juhan Vague, I., Roul, C., Alessi, M.C., Ardissone, J.P., Heim, M. and Vague, P. Increased plasminogen activator inhibitor activity in non insulin dependent diabetic subjects: relationship with plasma insulin. *Thromb. Haemostat.*, 1989, **61**, 370–3.

51. Nagi, D.K., Mohamed-Ali, V., Jain, S.K., Walji, S. and Yudkin, J.S. Plasminogen activator inhibitor (PAI-1) activity is elevated in Asian and caucasian subjects with non-insulin-dependent (Type 2) diabetes but not in those with impaired glucose tolerance (IGT) or non-diabetic Asians. *Diabet. Med.*, 1996, **13**, 59–64.

52. Potter van Loon, B.J., Kluft, C., Radder, J.K., Blankenstein, M.A. and Meinders, A.E. The cardiovascular risk factor plasminogen activator inhibitor type 1 is related to insulin resistance. *Metabolism*, 1993, **42**, 945–9.

53. Yudkin, J.S. Circulating proinsulin-like molecules. *J. Diabet. Complications*, 1993, **7**, 113–23.

54. Temple, R.C., Carrington, C.A., Luzio, S.D., Owens, D.R., Schneider, A.E., Sobey, W.J. and Hales, C.N. Insulin deficiency in non-insulin-dependent diabetes. *Lancet*, 1989, **i**, 293–5.

55. Mohamed–Ali, V., Gould, M.M., Gillies, S., Goubet, S., Yudkin, J.S. and Haines, A.P. Association of proinsulin-like molecules with lipids and fibrinogen in non-diabetic subjects – evidence against a modulating role for insulin. *Diabetologia*, 1995, **38**, 1110–16.

56. Phillips, D.I., Clark, P.M., Hales, C.N. and Osmond, C. Understanding oral glucose tolerance: comparison of glucose or insulin measurements during the oral glucose tolerance test with specific measurements of insulin resistance and insulin secretion. *Diabet. Med.*, 1994, **11**, 286–92.

57. Nagi, D.K., Hendra, T.J., Ryle, A.J., Cooper, T.M., Temple, R.C., Clark, P.M.S., Schneider, A.E., Hales, C.N. and Yudkin, J.S. The relationship of concentrations of insulin, intact proinsulin and 32–33 split proinsulin with cardiovascular risk factors in type 2 (non-insulin dependent) diabetic subjects. *Diabetologia*, 1990, **33**, 532–7.

58. Haffner, S.M., Mykkanen, L., Stern, M.P., Valdez, R.A., Heisserman, J.A. and Bowsher, R.R. Relationship of proinsulin and insulin to cardiovascular risk factors in non diabetic subjects. *Diabetes*, 1993, **42**, 1297–302.

59. Yudkin, J.S., Denver, A.E., Mohamed-Ali, V., Ramaiya, K.L., Nagi, D.K., Goubet, S., McLarty, D.G. and Swai, A. The relationships of concentrations of insulin and of proinsulin-like molecules with coronary heart disease

prevalence and incidence. A study of two ethnic groups. *Diabetes Care,* 1997, **20,** 1093–100.

60. Jain, S.K., Nagi, D.K., Slavin, B.M., Lumb, P.J. and Yudkin, J.S. Insulin therapy in type 2 diabetic subjects suppresses plasminogen activator inhibitor (PAI-1) activity and proinsulin-like molecules independently of glycaemic control. *Diabet. Med.,* 1993, **10,** 27–32.

61. Panahloo, A., Mohamed-Ali, V., Andrés, C., Denver, A.E. and Yudkin, J.S. Effect of insulin versus sulphonylurea therapy on cardiovascular risk factors and fibrinolysis in type II diabetes. *Metabolism,* 1998, **47,** 637–43.

62. Mogensen, C.E. Microalbuminuria predicts clinical proteinuria and early mortality in maturity-onset diabetes. *N. Engl. J. Med.,* 1984, **310,** 356–60.

63. Yudkin, J.S. Microalbuminuria in non-diabetic individuals – a prognostic index of cardiovascular disease. *Int. Yearbook Nephrol. Dialysis Transpl.,* 1994, **9,** 59–74.

64. Nosadini, R., Cipollina, M.R., Solini, A., Sambataro, M., Morocutti, A., Doria, A., Fioretto, P., Brocco, E., Muollo, B. and Frigato, F. Close relationship between microalbuminuria and insulin resistance in essential hypertension and non-insulin dependent diabetes mellitus. *J. Am. Soc. Nephrol.,* 1992, **3,** S56–S63.

65. Yip, J., Mattock, M.B., Morocutti, A., Sethi, M., Trevisan, R. and Viberti, G. Insulin resistance in insulin-dependent diabetic patients with microalbuminuria. *Lancet,* 1993, **342,** 883–7.

66. Foyle, W.-J., Carstensen, E., Fernández, M. and Yudkin, J.S. A longitudinal study of associations of microalbuminuria with the insulin resistance syndrome and sodium–lithium countertransport in non-diabetic subjects. *Arterioscler. Thromb. Vasc. Biol.,* 1995, **15,** 1330–7.

67. Nestler, J.E., Barlascini, C.O., Tetrault, G.A., Fratkin, M.J., Clore, J.N. and Blackard, W.G. Increased transcapillary escape rate of albumin in nondiabetic men in response to hyperinsulinemia. *Diabetes,* 1990, **39,** 1212–17.

68. Catalano, C., Muscelli, E., Galvan, A.Q., Baldi, S., Masoni, A., Gibb, I., Torffvit, O., Seghieri, G. and Ferrannini, E. Effect of insulin on systemic and renal handling of albumin in nondiabetic and NIDDM subjects. *Diabetes,* 1997, **46,** 868–75.

69. Haverkate, F., Thompson, S.G., Pyke, S.D.M., Gallimore, J.R. and Pepys, M.B. Production of C-reactive protein and risk of coronary events in stable and unstable angina. *Lancet,* 1997, **349,** 462–6.

70. Oswald, G.A., Smith, C.C., Betteridge, D.J. and Yudkin, J.S. Determinants and importance of stress hyperglycaemia in non-diabetic patients with myocardial infarction. *BMJ,* 1986, **293,** 917–22.

71. Juhan Vague, I., Thompson, S.G. and Jespersen, J. on behalf of the ECAT Angina Pectoris Study Group. Involvement of the hemostatic system in the insulin resistance syndrome. A study of 1500 patients with angina pectoris. *Arterioscler. Thromb.,* 1993, **13,** 1865–73.

72. Meade, T.W., Mellows, S., Brozovic, M., Miller, G.J., Chakrabarti, R.R., North, W.R., Haines, A.P., Stirling, Y., Imeson, J.D. and Thompson, S.G. Haemostatic function and ischaemic heart disease: principal results of the Northwick Park Heart Study. *Lancet,* 1986, **ii,** 533–7.

73. Yudkin, J.S., Forrest, R.D. and Jackson, C.A. Microalbuminuria as predictor of vascular disease in non-diabetic subjects: Islington Diabetes Survey. *Lancet,* 1988, **ii,** 530–3.

74. Gray, R.P., Yudkin, J.S. and Patterson, D.L. Enzymatic evidence of impaired reperfusion in diabetic patients after thrombolytic therapy for acute myocardial infarction: a role for plasminogen activator inhibitor? *Br. Heart. J.,* 1993, **70,** 530–6.

75. Hamsten, A., de Faire, U., Walldius, G., Dahlen, G., Szamosi, A., Landou, C., Blomback, M. and Wiman, B. Plasminogen activator inhibitor in plasma: a risk factor for recurrent myocardial infarction. *Lancet,* 1987, **ii,** 3–9.

76. Hales, C.N., Barker, D.J.P., Clark, P.M.S., Cox, L.J., Fall, C., Osmond, C. and Winter, P.D. Fetal and infant growth and impaired glucose tolerance at age 64. *BMJ,* 1991, **303,** 1019–22.

77. Barker, D.J.P., Hales, C.N., Fall, C.H.D., Osmond, C., Phipps, K. and Clark, P.M.S. Type 2 (non–insulin–dependent) diabetes mellitus, hypertension and hyperlipidaemia (syndrome X): relation to reduced fetal growth. *Diabetologia,* 1993, **36,** 62–7.

78. Hales, C.N., Barker, D.J.P. and Martyn, C.N. Type 2 (non-insulin-dependent) diabetes mellitus: the thrifty phenotype hypothesis. *Diabetologia,* 1992, **46,** 595–601.

79. Barker, D.J.P., Winter, P.D., Osmond, C., Margetts, B. and Simmonds, S.J. Weight in infancy

and death from ischaemic heart disease. *Lancet*, 1989, **ii**, 577–80.

80. Barker, D.J.P., Meade, T.W., Fall, C.H.D., Lee, A., Osmond, C., Phipps, K. and Stirling, Y. Relation of fetal and infant growth to plasma fibrinogen and factor VII concentrations in adult life. *BMJ*, 1992, **304**, 148–52.

81. Phillips, D.I.W., Barker, D.J.P., Hales, C.N., Hirst, S. and Osmond, C. Thinness at birth and insulin resistance in adult life. *Diabetologia*, 1994, **37**, 150–4.

82. Rossing, P., Tarnow, L., Nielsen, F.S., Hansen, B.V., Brenner, B.M. and Parving, H.H. Low birth weight. A risk factor for development of diabetic nephropathy? *Diabetes*, 1995, **44**, 1405–7.

83. Gould, M.M., Mohamed-Ali, V., Goubet, S.A., Yudkin, J.S. and Haines, A.P. Microalbuminuria: associations with height and sex in non-diabetic subjects. *BMJ*, 1993, **306**, 240–2.

84. Snoeck, A., Remacle, C., Reusens, B. and Hoet, J. Effect of a low protein diet during pregnancy on the fetal rat endocrine pancreas. *Biol. Neonate*, 1990, **5**, 107–18.

85. Langley, S.C. and Jackson, A.A. Increased systolic blood pressure in adult rats induced by fetal exposure to maternal low protein diets. *Clin. Sci.*, 1994, **86**, 217–22.

86. Desai, M., Crowther, N.J., Ozanne, S.E., Lucas, A. and Hales, C.N. Adult glucose and lipid metabolism may be programmed during fetal life. *Biochem. Soc. Trans.*, 1995, **23**, 331–5.

87. Godfrey, K., Robinson, S., Barker, D.J.P., Osmond, C. and Cox ,V. Maternal nutrition in early and late pregnancy in relation to placental and fetal growth. *BMJ*, 1996, **312**, 410–14.

88. Campbell, D.M., Hall, M.H., Barker, D.J.P., Cross, J., Shiell, A.W. and Godfrey, K.M. Diet in pregnancy and the offspring's blood pressure 40 years later. *Br. J. Obstet. Gynaecol.*, 1996, **103**, 273–80.

89. Stanner, S.A., Bulmer, K., Andrés, C., Lantseva, O., Borodina, V., Poteen, V.V. and Yudkin, J.S. Malnutrition in utero as a determinant of diabetes and coronary heart disease in adult life: The Leningrad Siege Study. *BMJ*, 1997, **315**, 1342–9.

90. Stein, C.E., Fall, C.H.D., Kumaran, K., Osmond, C., Cox, V. and Barker, D.J.P. Fetal growth and coronary heart disease in South India. *Lancet*, 1996, **348**, 1269–73.

91. Hinchliffe, S.A., Lynch, M.R., Sargent, P.H., Howard, C.V. and Van Velzen, D. The effect of intrauterine growth retardation on the development of renal nephrons. *Br. J. Obstet Gynaecol.*, 1992, **99**, 296–301.

92. Rizzo, G. and Arduini, D. Fetal cardiac function in intrauterine growth retardation. *Am. J. Obstet. Gynecol.*, 1991, **165**, 876–82.

93. Yudkin, J.S. Hyperinsulinaemia, insulin resistance, microalbuminuria and the risk of coronary heart disease. *Ann. Med.*, 1996, **28**, 433–8.

94. Pinkney, J., Stehouwer, C.D.A., Coppack, S.W. and Yudkin, J.S. Endothelial dysfunction: cause of the insulin resistance syndrome? *Diabetes*, 1997, **46** (suppl. 2), S9–S13.

95. Lillioja, S., Young, A.A., Culter, C., Ivy, J.L., Abbott, W.G.H., Zawadzki, J.K., Yki-Järvinen, H., Christin, L., Secomb, T.W. and Bogardus, C. Skeletal muscle capillary density and fiber type are possible determinants of *in vivo* insulin resistance in man. *J. Clin. Invest.*, 1987, **80**, 415–24.

96. Serné, E.H., Stehouwer, C.D.A., Ter Maaten, J.C., Donker, A.J.M. and Gans, R.O.B. Insulin resistance and hypertension: role for microcirculation? *Diabetologia*, 1997, **40** (suppl. 1), A256.

97. Ross, R. The pathogenesis of atherosclerosis: an update. *N. Engl. J. Med.*, 1986, **314**, 488–500.

98. Baron, A.D. Cardiovascular actions of insulin in humans. Implications for insulin sensitivity and vascular tone. *Ballières Clin. Endocrinol. Metab.*, 1993, **7**, 961–85.

99. Zeng, G. and Quon, M.J. Insulin-stimulated production of nitric oxide is inhibited by wortmannin. Direct measurement in vascular endothelial cells. *J. Clin. Invest.*, 1996, **98**, 894–8.

100. Raitakari, M., Nuutila, P., Ruotsalainen, U., Laine, H., Teräs, M., Iida, H., Mäkimattila, S., Utriainen, T., Oikonen, V., Sipilä, H., Haaparanta, M., Solin, O., Wegelius, U., Knuuti, J. and Yki-Järvinen, H. Evidence for dissociation of insulin stimulation of blood flow and glucose uptake in human skeletal muscle. Studies using $[^{15}O]H_2O$, $[^{18}F]$fluoro-2-deoxy-D-glucose, and positron emission tomography. *Diabetes*, 1996, **45**, 1471–7.

101. Jansson, P.A., Fowelin, J.P., von Schenck, H.P., Smith, U.P. and Lönnroth, P.N. Measurement by microdialysis of the insulin concentration

in subcutaneous interstitial fluid. *Diabetes,* 1993, **42,** 1469–73.

102. Bergman, R.N. New concepts in extracellular signalling for insulin action: the single gateway hypothesis. *Recent Progr. Horm. Res.,* 1997, **52** 359–85.

103. Castillo, C., Bogardus, C., Bergman, R., Thuillez, P. and Lillioja, S. Interstitial insulin concentrations determine glucose uptake rates but not insulin resistance in lean and obese men. *J. Clin. Invest.,* 1994, **93,** 10–16.

104. Yang, Y.J., Hope, I.D., Ader, M. and Bergman, R.N. Insulin transport across capillaries is rate limiting for insulin action in dogs. *J. Clin. Invest.,* 1989, **84,** 1620–8.

105. Bradley, D.C., Poulin, R.A. and Bergman, R.N. Dynamics of hepatic and peripheral insulin effects suggest common rate-limiting step *in vivo. Diabetes,* 1993, **42,** 296–306.

106. King, G.L. and Johnson, S.M. Receptor-mediated transport of insulin across endothelial cells. *Science,* 1985, **227,** 1583–6.

107. Stiel, G.M., Ader, M., Moore, D.M., Rebrin, K. and Bergman, R.N. Transendothelial insulin transport is not saturable *in vivo.* No evidence for a receptor-mediated process. *J. Clin. Invest.,* 1996, **97,** 1497–503.

108. Petrie, J.R., Ueda, S., Webb, D.J., Elliott, H.I. and Connell, J.M.C. Endothelial nitric oxide production and insulin sensitivity. A physiological link with implications for pathogenesis of cardiovascular disease. *Circulation,* 1996, **93,** 1331–3.

109. Yudkin, J.S., Stehouwer, C.D.A., Emeis, J.J. and Coppack, S.W. Insulin resistance syndrome and endothelial damage – role of adipose tissue-derived proinflammatory cytokines. *Diabetologia,* 1997, **40** (suppl. 1), A305.

110. Heinrich, P.C., Castell, J.V. and Andus, T. Interleukin-6 and the acute phase response. *Biochem. J.,* 1990, **265,** 621–36.

111. Hotamisligil, G.S., Budavari, A., Murray, D.L. and Spiegelman, B.M. Reduced tyrosine kinase activity of the insulin receptor in obesity-diabetes: central role of tumor necrosis factor-α. *J. Clin. Invest.,* 1994, **94,** 1543–9.

112. Hotamisligil, G.S., Peraldi, P., Budavari, A., Ellis, R., White, M.F. and Spiegelman, B.M. IRS-1-mediated inhibition of insulin receptor tyrosine kinase activity in TNF-α- and obesity-induced insulin resistance. *Science,* 1996, **271,** 665–8.

113. Kawakami, M., Pekala, P.H., Lane, M.D. and Cerami, A. Lipoprotein lipase suppression in 3T3-L1 cells by an endotoxin-induced mediator from exudate cells. *Proc. Natl Acad. Sci. USA,* 1982, **82,** 912–16.

114. Hardardóttir, I., Grünfeld, C. and Feingold, K.R. Effects of endotoxin and cytokines on lipid metabolism. *Curr. Opin. Lipidol.,* 1994, **5,** 207–15.

115. van der Poll, T., van Deventer, S.J.H., Pasterkamp, G., van Mourik, J.A., Büller, H.R. and ten Cate, J.W. Tumour necrosis factor induces von Willebrand factor release in healthy humans. *Thromb. Haemostas.,* 1992, **67,** 623–6.

116. Greenberg, A.S., Nordan, R.P., McIntosh, J., Calvo, J.C., Scow, R.O. and Jablons, D. Interleukin 6 reduces lipoprotein lipase activity in adipose tissue of mice *in vivo* and in 3T3-L1 adipocytes: a possible role for interleukin 6 in cancer cachexia. *Cancer Res.,* 1992, **52,** 4113–16.

117. Van Snick, J. Interleukin-6: an overview. *Annu. Rev. Immunol.,* 1990, **8,** 253–78.

118. Watson, C., Whittaker, S., Smith, N., Vora, A.J., Dumonde, D.C. and Brown, KA. IL-6 acts on endothelial cells to preferentially increase their adherence for lymphocytes. *Clin. Exp. Immunol.,* 1996, **105,** 112–19.

119. Romano, M., Sironi, M., Toniatti, C., Polentarutti, N., Fruscalla, P., Ghezzi, P., Faggioni, R., Luini, W., van Hinsbergh, V., Sozzani, S., Bussolino, F., Poli, V., Cillberto, G. and Mantovani, A. Role of IL-6 and its soluble receptor in induction of chemokines and leukocyte recruitment. *Immunity,* 1997, **6,** 1–20.

120. Patel, P., Mendall, M.A., Carrington, D., Strachan, D.P., Leatham, E., Molineaux, N., Levy, J., Blakeston, C., Seymour, C.A., Camm, A.J. and Northfield, T.C. Association of *Helicobacter pylori* and *Chlamydia pneumoniae* infections with coronary heart disease and cardiovascular risk factors. *BMJ,* 1995, **311,** 711–14.

121. Miettinen, H., Lehto, S., Saikku, P., Haffner, S.M., Rönnemaa, T., Pyörälä, K. and Laakso, M. Association of *Chlamydia pneumoniae* and acute coronary heart disease events in non-insulin dependent diabetic and non-diabetic subjects in Finland. *Eur. Heart J.,* 1996, **17,** 682–8.

122. Javier Nieto, F., Adam, E., Sorlie, P., Farzadegan, H., Melnick, J.L., Comstock, G.W. and

Szklo, M. Cohort study of cytomegalovirus infection as a risk factor for carotid intimal-medial thickening, a measure of subclinical atherosclerosis. *Circulation,* 1996, **94,** 922–7.

123. Hotamisligil, G.S., Arner, P., Caro, J.F., Atkinson, R.L. and Spiegelman, B.M. Increased adipose tissue expression of tumour necrosis factor-α in human obesity and insulin resistance. *J. Clin. Invest.,* 1995, **95,** 2409–15.

124. Purohit, A., Ghilchik, M.W., Duncan, L., Wang, D.Y., Singh, A., Walker, M.M. and Reed, M.J. Aromatase activity and interleukin-6 production by normal and malignant breast tissue. *J. Clin. Endocrinol. Metabol.,* 1995, **80,** 3052–8.

125. Mohamed-Ali, V., Goodrick, S., Rawesh, A., Miles, J.M., Katz, D.R., Yudkin, J.S. and Coppack, S.W. Subcutaneous adipose tissue secretes interleukin-6 but not tumour necrosis factor-α *in vivo. J. Clin. Endocrinol. Metab.,* 1997, **82,** 4196–200.

126. Hotamisligil, G., Arner, P., Atkinson, R.L. and Spiegelman, B.M. Differential regulation of the p80 tumor necrosis factor receptor in human obesity and insulin resistance. *Diabetes,* 1997, **46,** 451–5.

127. Vigushin, D.M., Pepys, M.B. and Hawkins, P.N. Metabolic and scintigraphic studies of radioiodinated human C-reactive protein in health and disease. *J. Clin. Invest.,* 1993, **90,** 1351–7.

128. Castell, J.V., Geiger, T., Gross, V., Andus, T., Walter, E., Hirano, T., Kishimoto, T. and Heinrich, P.C. Plasma clearance, organ distribution and target cells of interleukin-6/hepatocyte-stimulating factor in the rat. *Eur. J. Biochem.,* 1988, **177,** 357–61.

129. Liuzzo, G., Biasucci, L.M., Gallimore, J.R., Grillo, R.L., Rebuzzi, A.G., Pepys, M.B. and Maseri, A. The prognostic value of C-reactive protein and serum amyloid A protein in severe unstable angina. *N. Engl. J. Med.,* 1994, **331,** 417–24.

130. Maseri, A., Biasucci, L.M. and Liuzzo, G. Inflammation in ischaemic heart disease. *BMJ,* 1996, **312,** 1049–50.

131. Fontbonne, A., Thibult, M., Eschwège, E. and Ducimetière, P. Body fat distribution and coronary heart disease mortality in subjects with impaired glucose tolerance and diabetes mellitus: the Paris Prospective Study, a 15 year follow-up. *Diabetologia,* 1992, **35,** 464–8.

132. Law, C.M., Barker, D.J., Osmond, C., Fall, C.H. and Simmonds, S.J. Early growth and abdominal fatness in adult life. *J. Epidemiol. Community Health,* 1992, **46,** 184–6.

133. Hotamisligil, G.S., Budavari, A., Murray, D. and Spiegelman, B.M. Reduced tyrosine kinase activity of the insulin receptor in obesity-diabetes. *J. Clin. Invest.,* 1994, **94,** 1543–9.

134. Hotamisligil, G.S., Shargill, N.S. and Spiegelman, B.M. Adipose expression of tumor necrosis factor-alpha: direct role in obesity-linked insulin resistance. *Science,* 1993, **259,** 87–91.

135. Ofei, F., Hurel, S., Newkirk, J., Sopwith, M. and Taylor, R. Effects of an engineered human anti-TNF-alpha antibody (CDP571) on insulin sensitivity and glycemic control in patients with NIDDM. *Diabetes,* 1996, **45,** 881–5.

136. Hotamisligil, G.S. and Spiegelman, B.M. Tumor necrosis factor α: a key component of the obesity-diabetes link. *Diabetes,* 1994, **43,** 1271–8.

137. Zhang, Y., Proenca, R., Maffei, M., Barone, M., Leopold, L. and Friedman, J.M. Positional cloning of the mouse obese gene and its human homologue. *Nature,* 1994, **372,** 425–32.

138. Weigle, D.S. Appetite and the regulation of body composition. *Fed. Am. Soc. Exp. Biol. J.,* 1994, **8,** 302–10.

PART THREE

THE PATHOGENESIS OF DIABETIC MICROANGIOPATHY

THE ROLE OF GLYCAEMIA IN THE PATHOGENESIS OF MICROANGIOPATHY

Kenneth M. MacLeod

9.1 INTRODUCTION

The diagnosis of diabetes rests on the demonstration of hyperglycaemia which if it was persistent would be sufficient to be associated with unique long-term complications. The triumvirate of diabetes-specific microangiopathic complications – retinopathy, nephropathy and neuropathy – have as their final common denominator exposure to chronic hyperglycaemia. The weight of evidence from animal studies, epidemiological studies, cross-sectional and small-scale interventional human studies has long since implicated hyperglycaemia in the causation of microangiopathy. Koch's postulates for causality were finally established for hyperglycaemia in the aetiology of microangiopathy in human diabetes in 1993 when the North American Diabetes Control and Complications Trial (DCCT) demonstrated the power of intensive glycaemic control to prevent the development and retard the progression of the microvascular complications of diabetes [1].

In this chapter, the glucose hypothesis is reviewed, the epidemiological evidence which incriminates glucose in the pathogenesis of the microvascular complications of diabetes is considered and the evidence from observational and interventional studies which allow assessment of the clinical impact of glycaemic control on microangiopathic outcomes is reviewed. The phenomenon of 'glucose re-entry' is discussed, the circumstantial evidence implicating hypoglycaemia in the pathogenesis of microangiopathy is considered and, finally, the question of what else, other than glucose, determines microangiopathy is briefly considered.

9.2 THE GLUCOSE HYPOTHESIS

The 'glucose hypothesis' roots the initiation and progression of the microangiopathic complications of diabetes (retinopathy, nephropathy and neuropathy) in exposure to chronic hyperglycaemia. At its most simple, it proposes that hyperglycaemia causes these complications and that achieving and sustaining normoglycaemia will prevent them. Indeed, so closely intertwined are current concepts of microangiopathy and hyperglycaemia, that the accepted glycaemic thresholds for the diagnosis of diabetes are based on the epidemiological association with retinopathy [2]. Patients with moderate glucose intolerance, not associated with retinopathy, were classified as having impaired glucose tolerance; those with more extreme hyperglycaemic decompensation (fasting plasma glucose >7.8 mmol/l), which is associated in long-term studies with retinopathy were categorized as having diabetes [3].

The common characteristics of the microangiopathic complications of diabetes include: their association with increased disease duration [4]; their predilection for tissues in which glucose and its metabolites accumulate by mass action in proportion to the prevailing plasma glucose concentration and independent of insulin; the common early morphological abnormalities of microvascular structure, particularly basement membrane thickening [5–7]; the occurrence of the same spectrum of complications in different clinical forms of diabetes in which the metabolic profiles, other than hyperglycaemia, are not concurrent; and the absence of microvascular complications in disorders other than diabetes. All these shared characteristics suggest a common pathogenic mechanism and a central role for glucose [3]. The pathogenic mechanisms of glucotoxicity are considered in detail in Chapter 10.

9.3 INDIRECT EVIDENCE INCRIMINATING GLUCOSE IN THE PATHOGENESIS OF MICROANGIOPATHY

9.3.1 STUDIES OF INDIVIDUALS WITH IMPAIRED GLUCOSE TOLERANCE AND THOSE WITH NEWLY DIAGNOSED DIABETES

The prevalence of retinopathy in US and UK community studies of subjects with impaired glucose tolerance, has been variously estimated at 1.3% in Bedford, UK [8], 1% in the Pima Indians [9] and 1.5% in the Rancho Barnardo Californian study [10, 11]. These consistently low prevalence rates were not significantly different from those seen in individuals with normal glucose tolerance at least in the Californian studies. This minimal level of non-significant, non-specific retinopathy (no proliferative disease was detected in any study and only non-specific blot haemorrhages or microaneurysms were reported) suggest that an elevated blood glucose concentration is the key initiator of the microangiopathic retinal process and that

hyperglycaemia is certainly an essential prerequisite for the development of significant, diabetes-specific, sight-threatening retinopathy. The UK Prospective Diabetes Study (UKPDS), using the sophisticated technique of four-field fundal photography, documented the prevalence of diabetic retinopathy as 21% at diagnosis but this may simply reflect the long duration between onset of hyperglycaemia and diagnosis of diabetes in this group [12]. The common concurrence of multiple other vascular risk factors, particularly hypertension and dyslipidaemia, in these patients may also increase the potential of a given glycaemic burden to initiate and progress diabetic retinal microangiopathy.

In contrast to type 1 diabetes, the prevalence of hypertension, macro- and microalbuminuria is higher at the onset of type 2 diabetes [13–16]. Again, although this could represent a long period of silent hyperglycaemia preceding the diagnosis of diabetes, an alternative hypothesis is that renal microvascular changes are related to some antecedent of type 2 diabetes. This contention is supported by the fact that Mykkanen *et al.* have shown the microalbuminuria predicts the development of type 2 diabetes [16]. Microalbuminuria then may be a central facet of the insulin-resistant syndrome rather than a renal response to sustained hyperglycaemia. Consistent with this hypothesis, the prevalence of microalbuminuria in patients with impaired glucose tolerance has been shown to lie somewhere between that of normal and patients with type 2 diabetes [15, 17–20].

Franklyn *et al.* have made similar observations with respect to neuropathy [22]. In the San Luis Valley Colorado study they found that subjects with impaired glucose tolerance (IGT) had a prevalence of peripheral sensorimotor neuropathy (10.6%) intermediate between that of those with normal glucose tolerance and those with type 2 diabetes (3.9 % and 25.8%, respectively) [21].

These observations raise the possibility that the conventional glycaemic thresholds for microangiopathy are too high and that, with the application of more sensitive screening techniques, a higher prevalence of micro-angiopathy at lower levels of glycaemia may emerge. The data are however consistent with the hypothesis that sustained hyperglycaemia predictably promotes microangiopathy.

9.3.2   PATIENTS WITH MATURITY ONSET DIABETES OF THE YOUNG

Maturity onset diabetes of the young (MODY) represents unusual and well-defined genetic causes of diabetes, characterized by an early onset of dominantly inherited non-insulin-dependent diabetes. Several different subtypes of MODY are recognized. Gluco-kinase, which catalyses the phosphorylation of glucose to glucose-6-phosphate, and repre-sents the first rate-limiting step in glucose metabolism, acts as the pancreatic β cell glu-cose sensor [22]. Patients with glucokinase mutations have an altered pancreatic 'glucose set-point' and a consistent biochemical phe-notype, with mild fasting hyperglycaemia (6–9 mmol/l), present from early childhood and associated with minimal deterioration in glucose tolerance with age [23, 24]. Treatment of glucokinase MODY with diet is usually adequate and microvascular complications are rare [23, 25, 26]. MODY 1 and MODY 3, recently ascribed to mutations in the tran-scription factors hepatocyte nuclear factor 4α (HNF-4α) and hepatocyte nuclear factor 1α (HNF-1α) respectively [27, 28], are also dis-eases associated with defective islet cell insu-lin production. In contrast to glucokinase MODY, however, MODY 1 (HNF-4α) and MODY 3 (HNF-3α) are associated with pro-gressive deficiency of insulin secretion, pro-gressive and more significant hyperglycaemia and a much higher prevalence of microangio-pathic complications [29]. This is further evi-dence that, irrespective of the aetiology of

diabetes and the duration of disease, the degree of hyperglycaemia is the major factor determining the prevalence of microangio-pathy.

9.3.3   RELATIONSHIP OF MICROVASCULAR COMPLICATIONS TO DURATION OF DISEASE AND DEGREE OF HYPERGLYCAEMIA

Retrospective observational and non-random-ized prospective studies have confirmed the strength of the relationship between degree and duration of hyperglycaemia and the prevalence and severity of microangiopathy and paved the way for the definitive pro-spective randomized controlled trials [4, 10, 30, 31].

In 1960 Johnsson published the results of an observational study comparing the preva-lence of retinopathy and nephropathy in two groups of insulin-treated diabetic subjects who had achieved different degrees of glycae-mia. After 25 years of follow-up, patients who had consistently achieved urine free from glu-cose had significantly less retinopathy and nephropathy (9 versus 61%) than the control group who had simply avoided symptomatic polyuria [32]. The glycosuria-free patients ('intensively controlled') did however have a significantly increased experience of hypogly-caemia, with 25% of them (compared with 5% of controls) having had more than 20 episodes of hypoglycaemia coma in the 25 years of follow-up. Johnsson, pointing to the fact that no patients with more than 20 comas had overt proteinuria and 50% had normal fundi, concluded that the evidence favoured tight glycaemic control. Reviewing the study and initiating the debate on the risk/benefit ratio for tight control which has continued ever since, Lawrence confirmed that frequent hypoglycaemic coma as evidence of tight con-trol minimized the risk of complications but

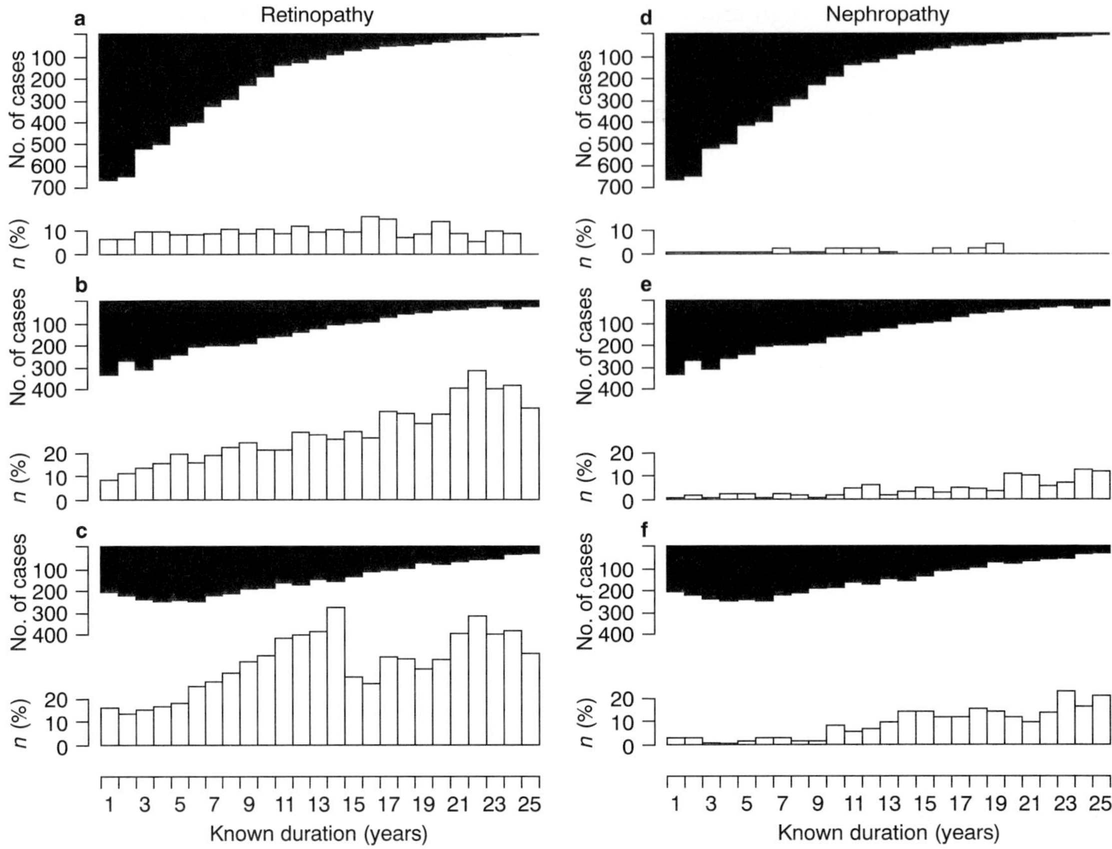

Figure 9.1 Prevalence of diabetic complications related to duration of diabetes and quality of glycaemic control. (a–c) Retinopathy; (d–f) nephropathy; similar effects are seen for neuropathy. a,d, Good glycaemic control; b,e, intermediate glycaemic control; c, f, poor glycaemic control; *n*, disease as a percentage of control. Modified with permission from [4].

suggested that 20 hypoglycaemia comas was excessive [33].

In 1978, Pirart reported the prevalence of microangiopathy in approximately 4400 patients followed from 1947 for up to 25 years. On the basis of clinical and biochemical data collected annually, he classified them retrospectively into three groups: those with 'good', 'fair' and 'poor' glycaemic control. He clearly demonstrated that the prevalence of retinopathy, neuropathy and nephropathy were increased with increasing disease duration and with poor glycaemic control [4]. The

results from his elegant data set are summarized in Figure 9.1.

9.3.4 OBSERVATIONAL STUDIES: DIABETIC RETINOPATHY IN FOCUS

Retinopathy is the most frequent complication of type 1 diabetes and after a lag phase of around four years, the frequency of background retinopathy increases rapidly with duration of diabetes [34, 35], affecting 1 of 100 patients in the fifth year and 11 of 100 in the fourteenth year. The development of background retinopathy is necessary but not sufficient for the development of proliferative retinopathy, which is the leading cause of blindness in type 1 diabetes [36]. In contrast, the incidence rate of proliferative retinopathy increases rapidly between 10 and 15 years of diabetes but subsequently develops at the constant rate of 3 per 100 previously unaffected patients annually, irrespective of whether they have had diabetes for 20 or 40 years [37].

The incidence of proliferative retinopathy relates directly to the glycaemic burden during the years immediately preceding the onset of this complication [37, 38]. Janka *et al.* found that when long-duration patients with type 1 diabetes and background retinopathy were followed for four years, individuals in the highest quartile of glycosylated haemoglobin were found to develop preproliferative or proliferative retinopathy 20 times more than that those in the lowest quartile [39]. Similarly, in the Wisconsin Epidemiologic Study of Diabetic Retinopathy the glycosylated haemoglobin was a significant predictor of progression to neovascularization. The group in the highest quartile of glycosylated haemoglobin had 22 times greater risk than the lower group and the predictive power of glycated haemoglobin persisted even after adjusting for age, sex, duration of diabetes and severity of retinopathy at baseline [40]. Further supportive evidence was provided by Chase *et al.*, who compared the prevalence of retinopathy in 230 patients with type 1 diabetes of more than five years' duration. No subjects with good control (glucated haemoglobin HbA1c <9%) had retinopathy while 37% of those with poor control (HbA1c >12.3%) had this complication [30].

The progression of diabetic retinopathy appears to be a complex multi-stage process with progression and regression determined by the interplay of haemodynamic and metabolic factors. Two stages are defined, background retinopathy followed by neovascularization and the evidence suggests that although hyperglycaemia is critical in the evolution of the retinopathic process, differing glycaemic thresholds and several other metabolic, haemodynamic and autocrine factors may influence the emergence of background retinopathy and the progression to proliferative disease.

9.3.5 OBSERVATIONAL STUDIES: DIABETIC NEPHROPATHY IN FOCUS

The clinical syndrome of diabetic nephropathy is characterized by persistent proteinuria and rising arterial blood pressure culminating in renal failure or premature death due to macroangiopathy, particularly coronary artery disease. The incidence rate of diabetic nephropathy has been shown in many studies to increase with duration of diabetes during the first 15 years and then to decline [41, 42]. In the older epidemiological studies after a five-year lag period the incidence rises to its peak of 2.5 per 100 annually during the second decade of diabetes and then declines to an annual rate of about 1 per 100 among the previously unaffected individuals. This pattern of declining incidence after the second decade suggests that only a subset of patients are susceptible to renal damage in the presence of diabetes.

The early observational studies documented that poor glycaemic control was an important determinant of nephropathy. In patients with type 1 diabetes and poor glycaemic control during the first decade of diabetes there was a 4.5-fold higher risk for individuals in the highest compared to the lowest quartile of glycaemic index [41, 43]. Glycaemic index represents a derived surrogate of average glycaemic control which in these pre-glycosylated haemoglobin days was calculated by determining the proportion of clinic visits in which severe hyperglycaemia was present. Interestingly clinic non-attenders had the highest risk of persistent proteinuria [41, 43].

The accumulating strength of the epidemiological data pointing to an association between hyperglycaemia and microangiopathy heralded the clinical intervention trials of the last 20 years. These trials were made more feasible by technical developments permitting more physiological insulin delivery as well as better means of assessing glycaemic control.

9.4   INTERVENTIONAL STUDIES

9.4.1   ANIMAL STUDIES

In animal models of diabetes, studies of the progression of microangiopathy equivalents have demonstrated the impact of improved glycaemic control to arrest the progression of retinopathy and glomerulopathy in spontaneously diabetic rats [44] and alloxan-induced diabetic dogs [45, 46]. Complete regression of the early histological hallmarks of diabetic nephropathy and restoration of normal anatomy was observed within two months of transplanation of kidneys from diabetic rats into normal rats [47]. Similarly the pathognomonic feature of diabetic glomerulopathy appeared after two months in the kidneys taken from non-diabetic animals and transplanted into diabetic animals [47]. Successful islet cell transplantation with the achievement of normoglycaemia also results in reduction in glomerular volume and mesangial expansion in diabetic rats [48].

9.4.2   HUMAN STUDIES

The ultimate test of the glucose hypothesis would be the prevention of the microangiopathic complications of diabetes in patients intensively treated to achieve and maintain normoglycaemia. Given the limitations of even present-day insulin regimens (delivery of insulin to the peripheral rather than portal circulation, subcutaneous rather than intravenous administration, intermittent rather than continuous therapy, loss of feed-back control etc.) the goal of sustained normoglycaemia is unrealistic for the vast majority of patients. The alternative approach which has been implemented successfully is a comparison of the prevalence and progression of microangiopathy in patients with differing degrees of glycaemic control.

9.4.3   THE EVIDENCE IN INSULIN-DEPENDENT DIABETES MELLITUS

Pre-DCCT

The earliest randomized clinical trials of the ability of tight glycaemic control to retard the progression of microangiopathy were of insufficient size and duration to definitively answer the question. They did, however, successfully demonstrate that intensive and conventional treatment regimens could achieve significant separation between groups in terms of quality of glycaemic control, illustrating the viability and underlining the need for well-conducted studies to test the hypothesis robustly. These studies included the Kroc study involving North American and UK centres [49, 50], the Danish Steno study [51, 52] and the Norwegian Oslo study [53–56]. They suggested that tight glycaemic control reduced the rate of development and progression of microalbuminuria and, after an initial deterioration, tended to limit progression of diabetic retinopathy. However, the results were not entirely convincing. In the Kroc study, after eight months follow-up 13 of the 32 patients randomized to continuous subcutaneous insulin infusion (CSII) showed progression of their retinopathy by at least one level, compared with only nine of 33 patients in the conventional treatment group. However, this result was only of borderline statistical significance. When the results were re-examined after 24 months follow-up, the conclusions were reversed with a marginal advantage in favour of intensive control (four of 29 progressed compared with seven of 31 in the conventional treated groups [49, 50]. Similarly in the Steno study, at 12 months there was a tend towards accelerated retinopathy in the CSII group (10 of 15 patients progressed compared with five of 15 in the conventional group) but again at 24 months the trend had reversed in favour of intensive control [51, 52]. In the Oslo study, after two years fewer retinal microaneurysms and haemorrhages had developed in patients treated with CSII or multiple insulin injections compared with those given conventional treatment, in whom the number had increased significantly ($p < 0.01$). Motor nerve conduction velocity deteriorated in conventionally treated patients but was unchanged after one year and improved after two years in those randomized to CSII. No change occurred in the urinary albumin excretion rates [54].

Two further studies of similar design but with five-year follow-up data contributed to the evidence. Verrillo *et al.* randomized patients with type 1 diabetes of between 15 and 30 years' duration to intensive or conventional therapy [57]. The treatment regimens successfully separated the two groups in terms of glycaemic control. The intensively treated patients achieved a glycated haemoglobin some 2% lower than the conventionally treated patients and maintained this for the five years of the study. Despite this, retinopathy progressed at a similar rate in both groups. In a larger study of similar design, the Stockholm Diabetes Intervention Study, 102 patients with type 1 diabetes were randomized to intensive or conventional control. In this study, the glycated haemoglobin was 1.5% lower in the intensively treated group and this difference was sustained over the first five years of the study. Over a further four years of follow-up, there was a steady improvement in glycaemic control in the conventionally treated group. At five years, 10 of the 44 patients in the intensively treated group had progressed to proliferative retinopathy compared with 15 of the 52 patients in the control group. At nine years, 12 of the 44 patients in the intensively treated group and 27 of the 52 in the control group had progressed, a statistically significant difference in favour of tight glycaemic control [58, 59].

A meta-analysis of 16 randomized trials of the impact of intensive therapy to reduce the progression of retinopathy and nephropathy was published just preceding the DCCT in 1993 [60]. In the intensive therapy group, the risk of retinopathy progression was insignificantly higher after 6–12 months of intensive glycaemic control (odds ratio 2.11). After more than two years of intensive therapy, the risk of retinopathy was lower (odds ratio 0.49; 95% confidence interval 0.28–0.95; $p = 0.011$). The risk of nephropathy progression was also decreased significantly (odds ratio 0.34; 95% confidence interval 0.29–0.58; $p > 0.001$) by intensive control. The incidence of severe hypoglycaemia increased by 9.1 episodes per 100 person-years in the intensively treated group and, only in patients managed with continuous subcutaneous insulin infusion, the incidence of diabetic ketoacidosis increased by 12.6 episodes per 100 person-years [60]. The effects of long-term intensive glycaemic control on the progression of retinopathy and nephropathy are summarized in Figures 9.2 and 9.3.

Taken together and summarized by the results of the meta-analysis, these observational studies demonstrated that the weight of evidence supported the contention that sustained intensive glycaemic control provided effective secondary prevention, significantly reducing the risk of progression of microangiopathy. Individually though, the studies were criticized for methodological reasons including: retrospective analysis; insufficient power; short duration; lack of an integrated measure of long-term glycaemic control (pre-HbA1c); failure to address the question of primary prevention and failure to separate patients with type 1 and type 2 diabetes. Given these criticisms, there was no

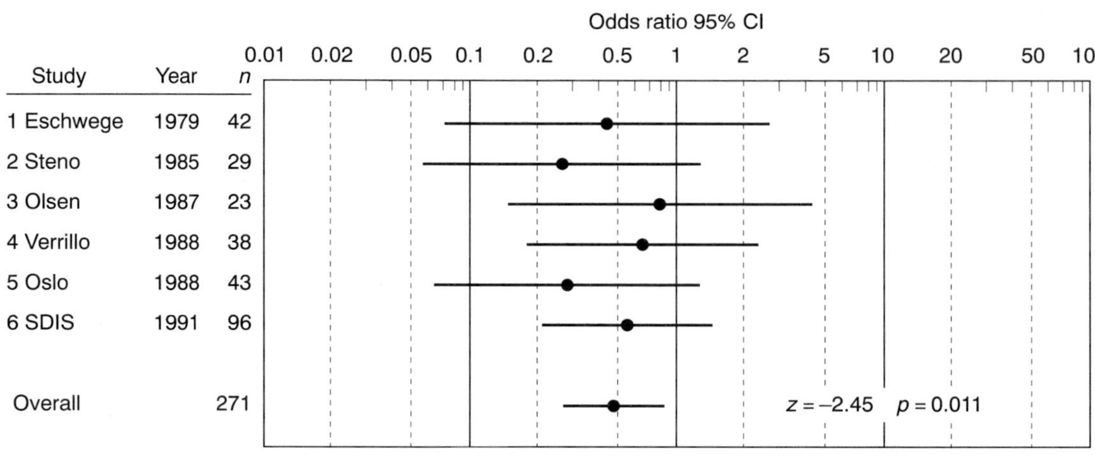

Figure 9.2 Meta-analysis of effects of intensive glycaemic control on diabetic retinopathy. Data analysed by Der Simonian and Laird method and presented as odds ratio (95% CI) on log scale. *n*, number of patients. Modified from [60].

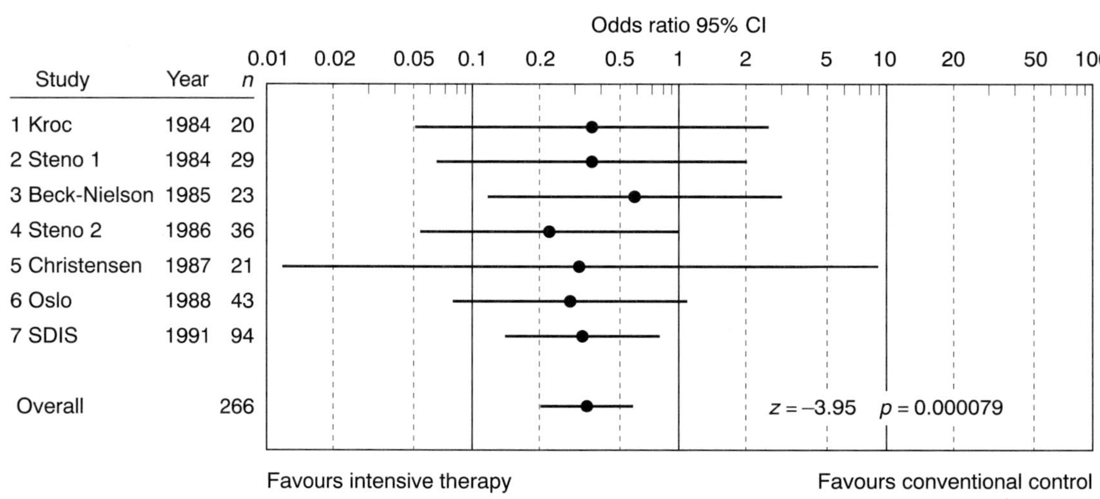

Figure 9.3 Meta-analysis of effects of intensive glycaemic control on diabetic nephropathy. *n*, number of patients. Modified from [60].

international consensus amongst clinical diabetologists that intensive glycaemia control should be a priority of diabetes management; further evidence was needed.

DCCT

The landmark multi-centre North American DCCT Research Group settled the argument when they published the results of their large prospective randomized controlled trial assessing the impact of intensive versus conventional glycaemic control on the development and progression of the micro-angiopathic complications of diabetes [1]. A total of 1441 patients with insulin-dependent diabetes mellitus (IDDM) were randomly assigned to intensive or conventional therapy. Of the 1441, 726 had no retinopathy at base-line (the primary prevention group) and 715 had mild retinopathy (the secondary inter-vention group). Those randomized to inten-sive therapy used either an external insulin infusion pump or multiple daily subcuta-neous insulin injections adjusted according to frequent capillary blood glucose measure-ments with the aim of achieving pre-prandial blood glucose concentrations in the 3.9–6.7 mmol/l range and post-prandial concentra-tions of less than 10 mmol/l. Those random-ized to conventional therapy continued with one or two daily insulin injections. The patients were followed for a mean of 6.5 years, and the appearance and progression of retinopathy and other complications were assessed regularly.

In the primary prevention cohort, intensive therapy reduced the adjusted mean risk for development of retinopathy by 76% (95% confidence intervals 62–85%) compared with conventional therapy. In the secondary-inter-vention group, intensive therapy slowed the progression of retinopathy by 54% (95% con-fidence interval, 39–66%) and reduced the development of proliferative or severe retin-opathy by 47% (95% confidence interval 14–67%). In the two cohorts combined, inten-sive therapy reduced the occurrence of micro-albuminuria (urinary albumin excretion $\geq$40 mg per 24 hours) by 39% (95% confidence interval, 21–52%), that of albuminuria (uri-nary albumin excretion $\geq$300 mg per 24 hours) by 54% (95% confidence interval, 19–74%) and that of clinical neuropathy by 60% (95% confidence interval 38–74%). The

data pertaining to retinopathy and nephro-pathy are shown in Figures 9.4 and 9.5 repro-duced from DCCT, 1993.

The chief adverse event associated with intensive therapy was a two- to threefold increase in severe hypoglycaemia. This important clinical study then clearly demon-strated the power of intensive insulin therapy to delay the onset and retard the progression of diabetic microangiopathy (retinopathy, nephropathy and neuropathy) in IDDM, a message which is being enthusiastically adopted and applied by diabetologists world-wide. Importantly, the study revealed that good glycaemic control incurred benefit for those patients who already had clinical evi-dence of early micorangiopathy. This con-trasts with data from studies in patients with advanced microangiopathy in whom inten-sive glycaemic control (even by pancreatic transplantation) did not retard progression of the late stages of diabetic retinopathy or nephropathy [61, 62]. The extent to which the microangiopathic processes may be reversed with improvements in glycaemic control may depend on the extent of the microangiopathy when these manoeuvres are initiated. Improved glycaemic control for example is relatively ineffective in delaying the progres-sion of established diabetic nephropathy.

Post-DCCT

The Stockholm Diabetes Intervention Study has recently reported 10-year follow-up data [63]. HbA1c (normal range 3.9–5.7%) was reduced from 9.5 $\pm$ 1.4% (mean $\pm$ SD) in the intensified therapy group and 9.4 $\pm$ 1.4% (mean $\pm$ SD) in the standard therapy group to a mean (during 10 years of follow-up) of 7.2 $\pm$ 0.6% and 8.3 $\pm$ 1.0% respectively ($p <$ 0.001). Serious retinopathy (63 versus 33%, p = 0.003), nephropathy (26 versus 7%, p = 0.012) and symptoms of neuropathy (32 ver-sus 14%, p = 0.041) were more common in the standard therapy group after 10 years. HbA1c and age emerged as the only independent

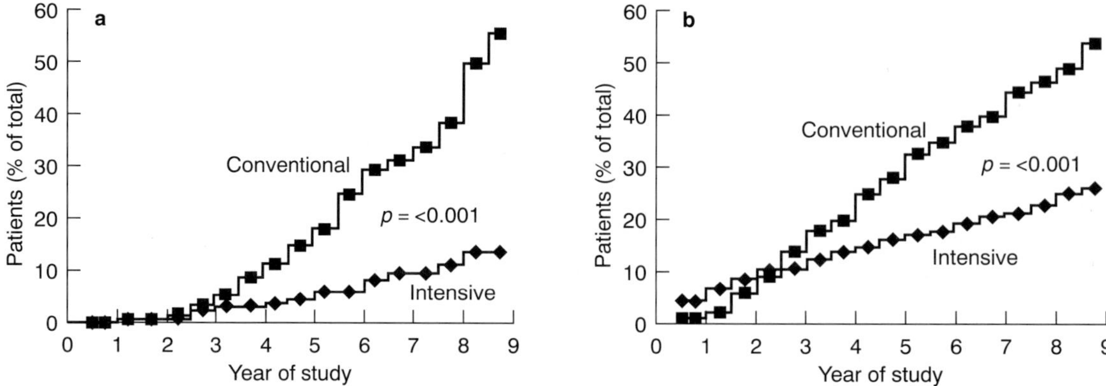

Figure 9.4 The effect of intensive treatment of diabetes on the development and progression of retinopathy in insulin-dependent diabetes mellitus. (a) Primary prevention cohort; (b) secondary prevention cohort. Modified from [60].

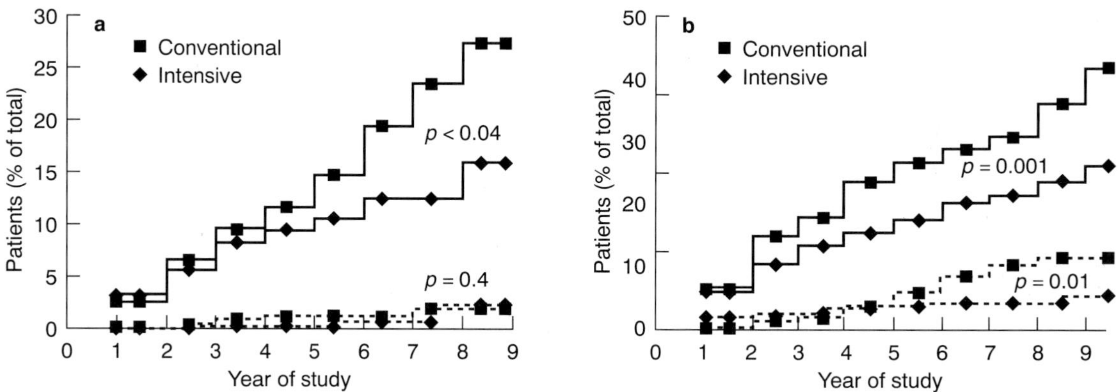

Figure 9.5 The effect of intensive treatment of diabetes on the development and progression of nephropathy in insulin-dependent diabetes mellitus expressed as the cumulative incidence of urinary albumin excretion $\geq$300 mg per 24 h (---) and $\geq$40 mg/l (——). (a) Primary prevention cohort; (b) secondary prevention cohort. Modified from [1].

risk factors for the development of complications. Self-reported well-being increased to a greater degree and severe hypoglycaemia was 2.25 times more common in the intensified therapy group, but cognitive function was similar in both groups and there was no relationship between cognitive function and severe hypoglycaemia. These longer-term results increase confidence that the reduction in the long-term microvascular complications as a consequence of intensive glycaemic control is sustained and associated with increased well-being and an acceptable side effect profile [63].

9.5 TIGHT CONTROL IN TYPE 2 DIABETES: THE EVIDENCE

The incidence and progression of microangiopathy in type 2 diabetes is difficult to determine precisely because of the insidious onset of the disease, the delay in diagnosis and the potential for numerous other facets of the insulin-resistance syndrome to influence the evolution of the microangiopathy. Despite these difficulties, abundant evidence incriminates hyperglycaemia in the pathogenesis of diabetic retinopathy, the prototype microangiopathic complication [40, 64]. Although the benefit of intensive therapy in type 2 diabetes is less certain, the Wisconsin study suggests that hyperglycaemia is also the principal orchestrator of the microangiopathic complications in this group of patients [64, 65]. The levels of HbA1c appear to predict progression of retinopathy [66, 67].

A study, smaller in scale but broadly similar in design to the DCCT, has examined the impact of intensive glycaemic control on the frequency and severity of microvascular complications in patients with type 2 diabetes [68]. In this Japanese study, 110 recently diagnosed non-obese patients with type 2 were randomly assigned to conventional insulin therapy (CIT) or to multiple insulin injection therapy (MIT). A total of 55 patients with no retinopathy and urinary albumin excretion rates <30 mg/24 h at baseline were evaluated in the primary-prevention cohort and 55 patients with background retinopathy and urinary albumin excretion rates >30 but <300 mg/24 h were evaluated in the secondary intervention cohort.

The cumulative percentages for the development and progression of retinopathy after six years were 7.7% for the MIT group and 32% for the CIT group in the primary-prevention cohort ($p = 0.039$), and 19.2% for the MIT group and 44% for the CIT group in the secondary-intervention cohort ($p = 0.049$). The cumulative percentages of the development and progression in retinopathy after six years were 7.7% for the MIT group and 28% for the CIT group in the primary prevention cohort ($p = 0.032$), and 11.5% and 32.0%, respectively, for the MIT and CIT groups in the secondary prevention cohort ($p = 0.044$). In neurological tests after six years, the MIT group showed significant improvement in nerve conduction velocities, while the CIT group showed significant deterioration in the

median nerve conduction velocities and vibration threshold. Although both postural hypotension and the coefficient of variation of R–R interval tended to improve in the MIT group, they deteriorated in the CIT group.

Thus at least in this Japanese population, intensive glycaemic control achieved by multiple insulin injection therapy, prevented the onset and retarded the progression of microangiopathy and proved to be as powerful an intervention to minimize microangiopathy as in type 1 patients. These data are reproduced in Figures 9.6 and 9.7 and summarized in Table 9.1.

There is no definitive evidence against intensive glycaemic control in patients with type 2 diabetes. Some have suggested that the weight gain and hyperinsulinaemia, which can be associated with intensive insulin therapy, may attenuate and even negate the overall benefit of intensive therapy, perhaps by accelerating the large vessel complications which are the major causes of morbidity and premature death in type 2 diabetes [66]. However clinically unlikely this seems, it remains true that there is no definitive evidence proving that intensive control prevents or retards macroangiopathy. In the DCCT study for example, the macrovascular complication rates were too low to determine an effect of intensive insulin therapy [1] and this was also true in the Japanese study of intensive control in type 2 diabetes [68]. In the absence of definite benefit caution is required, particularly since the controversial University Group Diabetes Program (UGDP) study failed to confirm an advantage for intensive therapy either in terms of micro- or macroangiopathy and indeed raised a suspicion of excess cardiovascular mortality in the sulphonylurea (tolbutamide) treated group [69]. Although there has been much critical debate over the validity of the UGDP result [70] it seems premature to discard the study without conclusive evidence to the contrary from larger and better conducted trials.

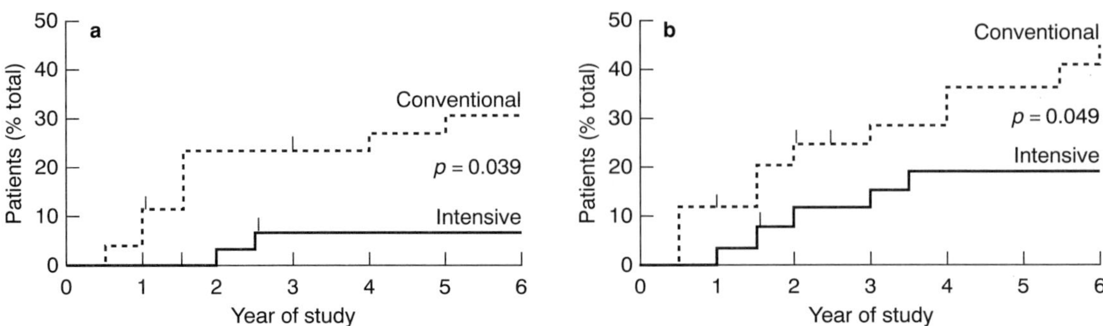

Figure 9.6 Intensive insulin therapy and the progression of retinopathy in Japanese patients with non-insulin dependent diabetes. (a) Primary prevention cohort; (b) secondary prevention cohort. Modified with permission from [68].

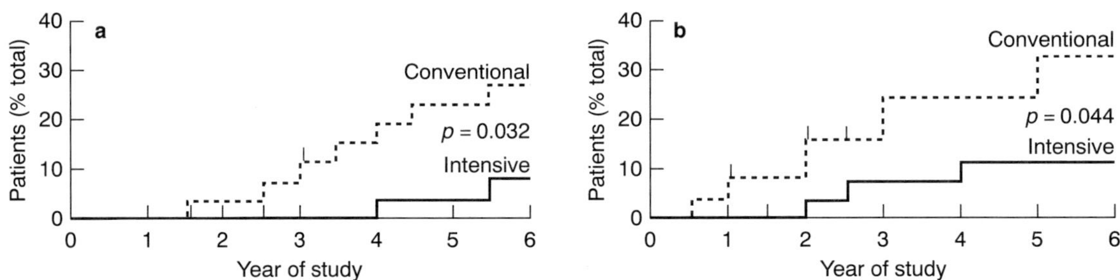

Figure 9.7 Intensive insulin therapy and the progression of nephropathy in Japanese patients with non-insulin dependent diabetes. (a) Primary prevention cohort; (b) secondary prevention cohort. Modified from [68].

The UKPDS will provide information to assist the selection of the most effective therapeutic strategy (insulin/sulphonylureas/metformin) to minimize micro- and macro-angiopathic complications in newly diagnosed type 2 diabetes. However, the early indications are that it may not have the power to determine specifically whether intensive insulin therapy can modify the macrovascular morbidity in patients with newly-diagnosed type 2 diabetes [71–74]. The UKPDS will give us valuable information on the natural history of type 2 diabetes and the relative efficacy of the varied possible therapeutic approaches from diagnosis, but it will not determine the role of intensification of glycaemic control in long-standing patients with poor glycaemic control.

A feasibility study has been performed to determine whether individuals in the late stages of type 2 diabetes could be safely and successfully randomized to receive standard insulin therapy (1–2 doses/day) or intensive insulin therapy (with or without a sulphonyl-urea) with the goal of achieving a nearly normal HbA1c level in the latter group [73–75]. The prospective study included 153 men of 60 ± 6 years who had a known duration of diabetes of 7.8 ± 4 years. They were randomly assigned to a standard insulin treatment group (one morning injection per day) or to an intensive therapy group designed to attain near normoglycaemia and a clinically significant separation of glycated haemoglobin values. A four-step plan for progressive intensification of insulin therapy was

Table 9.1 Comparative efficacy of intensive glycaemic control to prevent the onset and delay the progression of microangiopathy in type 1 and type 2 diabetes. Taken from [68]

Complications	Primary-prevention cohort			Secondary-intervention cohort			Combined cohort
	CT event rate	IT event rate	RR (%)	CT event rate	IT event rate	RR (%)	RR (%)
Kumamoto study in patients with NIDDM							
≥ 2-Step sustained retinopathy (scale of 19 stages)	5.3	1.3	76*	7.3	3.2	56*	65* (69)**
Severe non-proliferative or proliferative retinopathy	–	–	–	2.0	1.2	40*	40*
Photocoagulation	–	–	–	2.0	1.2	40*	40*
Urinary albumin excretion (mg/24 h)							
≥ 30	3.3	1.3	62*	4.0	1.9	52*	57* } (70)**
> 300	1.3	0	100*	1.3	0	100*	100* }
DCCT in patients with IDDM							
≥ 3-Step sustained retinopathy (scale of 25 stages)	4.7	1.2	76**	7.8	3.7	54**	63**
Severe non-proliferative or proliferative retinopathy	–	–	–	2.4	1.1	47**	47**
Photocoagulation	–	–	–	2.3	0.9	56**	51**
Urinary albumin excretion (mg/24 h)							
≥ 40	3.4	2.2	34**	5.7	3.6	43**	39**
≥ 300	0.3	0.2	44**	1.4	0.6	56**	54**

CT, conventional therapy; IT, intensive therapy, RR, risk reduction. Event rate is the rate of development and progression of complications per 100 patient-years. RR represents the comparison of intensive with conventional insulin injection therapy.
* Expressed as a percentage and calculated using crude relative risk analysis in the Kumamoto study.
** Expressed as a percentage and calculated using proportional-hazards analysis in the Kumamoto study and DCCT.

used in the group, aiming for tight glycaemic control. The mean follow-up was 27 months.

After six months, the mean HbA1c was at or below 7.3% and remained 2% lower than the standard group for the duration of the trial (mean HbA1c 7.1 versus 9.2%, $p < 0.001$). The reduction in mean HbA1c in the intensive group was achieved by a single injection of evening intermediate insulin, alone or in addition to glipizide. Retinopathy was assessed at baseline, 12 and 24 months by seven-field stereo fundus photography performed at each of the five participating centres and read centrally. In this relatively short period of follow-up, near normalization of glycaemic control did not cause transient deterioration of retinal morphology, neither did it prevent the onset or retard the progression of the retinopathy [76]. There was, however, a very high macrovascular event rate (cardiovascular death, myocardial infarction, stroke, congestive heart failure, coronary angioplasty etc.): 61 events were seen in 40 patients with 10 deaths, i.e. a large vessel event rate of approximately 12% per year [75] which is 4–6-fold higher than that seen in trials of recently diagnosed patients [68, 69, 71, 72]. Severe hypoglycaemia was uncommon in this group (two events per 100 patients per year) and not significantly different between groups, neither were there any between group differences in weight, blood pressure or plasma lipids. The evidence from this study suggests that stepped insulin therapy in type 2 diabetes patients who have failed glycaemic control on pharmacological therapy is effective in maintaining near normoglycaemia for more than 2 years without excessive hypoglycaemia, weight gain, hypertension, dyslipidaemia or acceleration of retinopathy [75, 76].

It is clear that patients with type 2 diabetes who remain poorly controlled despite attempts at lifestyle modification (diet and exercise) and pharmacological intervention with oral agents have a very high micro- and macrovascular event rate at this late stage of the disease. The Veterans Affairs Co-operative Studies Program has approved a long-term trial to explore the benefits and risks of intensive glycaemic control in this group [73–75].

It is increasingly clear that the benefits of intensified insulin therapy to diminish the incidence and retard the progression of diabetic microangiopathy are among the most impressive that any intervention in modern medicine can deliver and, further, that if this therapeutic regimen was generally implemented the microvascular complications of diabetes would become uncommon [63, 77].

9.6   GLYCAEMIC RE-ENTRY

In type 1 diabetes a consistent finding, replicated in most but not all studies [76], is of an acute transient deterioration in the extent of retinopathy following the tightening of glycaemic control [1, 52, 78–81]. In the DCCT study, the initial deterioration occurred over the first 3–6 months of intensified control and was most obvious in those with more advanced retinopathy at baseline [1, 81]. Fortunately this initial deterioration is usually transient. In the longer term, improvement and a reduced rate of retinopathy progression was observed in most studies. In some reports, however, there has been relentless and irreversible progression of the microangiopathic process, with progressively increasing severity of retinopathy and, rarely, visual loss [82, 83]. Progression of retinopathy has been correlated with the degree of blood glucose lowering [79, 80, 82, 83].

Recent evidence from some but not all studies [76] suggests that the same phenomenon is seen in type 2 diabetes [84, 85]. The most recent study [86] concludes that while hyperglycaemia was a risk factor for the progression of retinopathy in all patients, change of treatment from oral hypoglycaemic medication to insulin was associated with a 100% increased risk of retinopathy progression and a threefold increased risk of blindness/visual impairment [86] (Figure 9.8). The group who

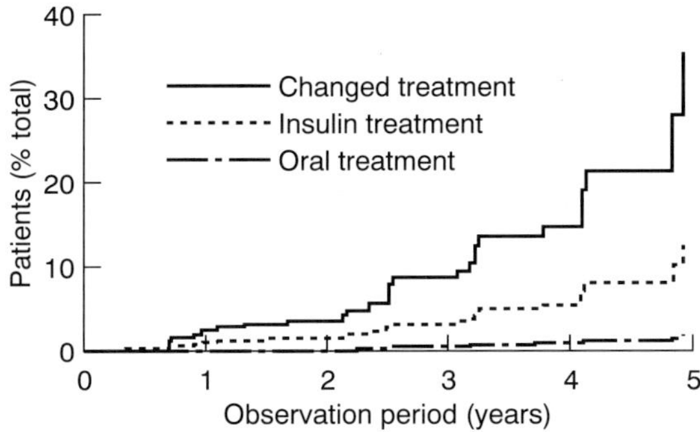

Figure 9.8 The prevalence of blindness following change of therapy to insulin in non-insulin dependent diabetes. Modified from [86].

changed therapy had the highest average HbA1c values during the study period, more advanced retinopathy at baseline and again, progression was related to the baseline glycaemic level. Significant retinal micro-angiopathy was therefore most advanced in the group who progressed and the deterioration may be largely attributable to 'glycaemic memory', perhaps accelerated by the precipitate and significant improvements in glycaemic control achieved on commencing insulin. Certainly insulin therapy *per se* did not emerge as an independent risk factor for progression of retinopathy in multivariate analysis. The authors concluded that change of therapy from oral agents to insulin, poor glycaemic control and retinopathy at first examination were the most important predictors of progression of diabetic retinopathy, reaffirming the need to strive for normoglycaemia in type 2 diabetes from diagnosis, but also emphasizing the need for careful ophthalmological supervision when treatment is intensified in type 2 diabetes.

What pathophysiological processes contribute to 'glycaemic re-entry' or the 'normoglycaemic re-entry phenomenon'? The transient progression of retinal microangiopathy may be a consequence of impaired autoregulation within the retinal microcirculation, resulting in direct end-organ (retinal) exposure to the

haemodynamic consequences of sudden relative glucose deprivation, key amongst which will be a fall in retinal perfusion. Autoregulation, the capacity of the microcirculation to maintain constant flow in the face of a changing pressure head, fails in patients with diabetes of moderate duration [87–89] and inability to maintain retinal perfusion particularly with the rapid attainment of near normoglycaemia after prolonged hyperglycaemia has been thought to be a principal mechanism. This hypothesis is supported by the 20% reduction in retinal blood flow demonstrated when blood glucose concentrations are reduced from 15 mmol/l to 8 mmol/l [90, 91].

If the glucose deprivation is absolute rather than relative, and an increased frequency of severe hypoglycaemia is a common though not inevitable consequence of tight glycaemic control, the haemodynamic stress is further increased [1, 92]. With autoregulatory failure, increased systemic pressure will be transmitted to the microvascular bed, increasing capillary pressure and accelerating vascular damage. The retina, which has an intrinsically high metabolic rate usually closely matched to its nutrient supply, is especially vulnerable to autoregulatory failure. A sudden reduction in glucose supply would seriously compromise retinal metabolism until adaptive changes had occurred [92]. The possible role of hypoglycaemia in the potentiation of microangiopathy is considered further below.

Another potential mechanism for worsening retinopathy associated with intensification of treatment incriminates growth factors in general, and insulin-like growth factor 1 (IGF-1) in particular, in the flare of retinopathy [93]. In poorly controlled insulinopenic patients with type 1 diabetes, plasma IGF-1 concentrations are low. In severely undertreated type 1 diabetes associated with growth and sexual retardation (Mauriac's syndrome), institution of intensive insulin therapy and tight glycaemic control has been

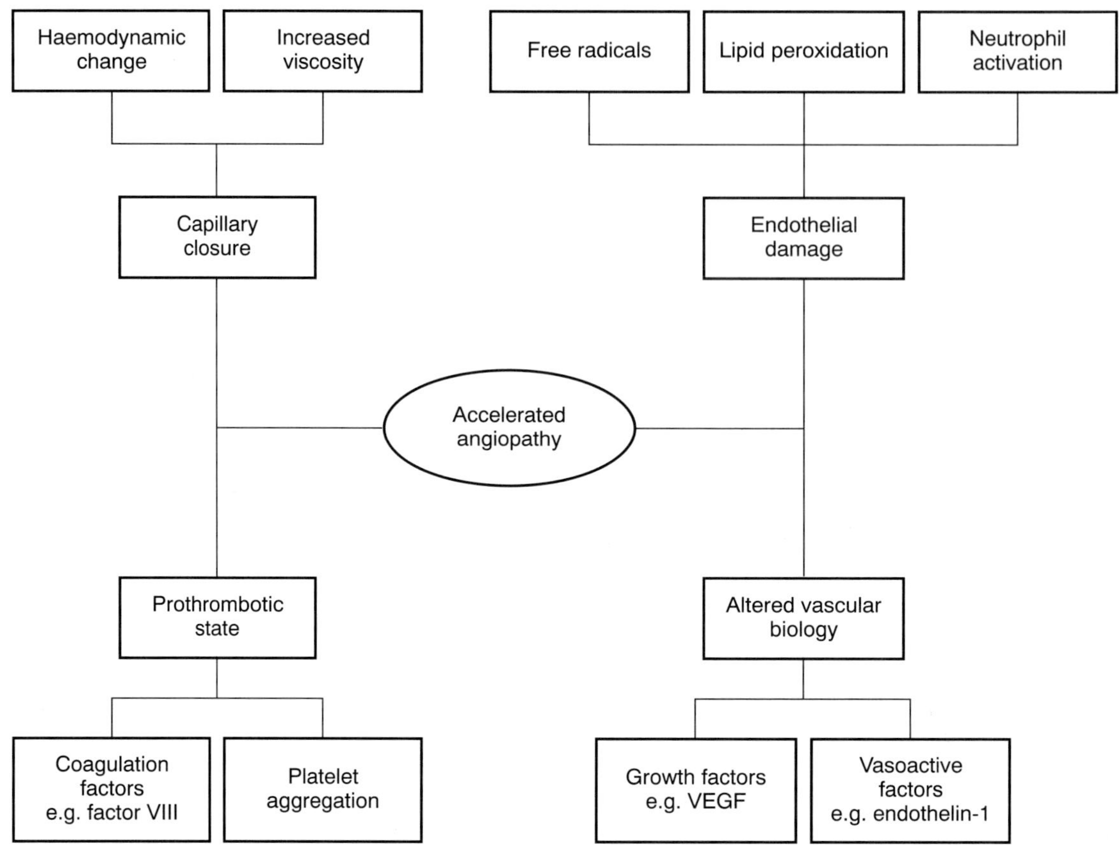

Figure 9.9 Potential mechanisms by which hypoglycaemia may contribute to microangiopathy. Modified from [99].

associated with the development of proliferative retinopathy and a large acute rise in plasma concentrations of IGF-1 [93]. In other less extreme cases, a rapid rise of IGF-1 from low to normal levels has been described in association with progression of retinopathy and tightening of glycaemic control [94]. An increasing body of circumstantial clinical and direct experimental evidence supports a role for IGF-1 in the pathogenesis of normoglycaemic re-entry. Thus puberty and pregnancy, physiological states associated with increasing IGF-1 concentrations, are periods of increased susceptibility for progression of retinopathy whereas pituitary ablation and the associated reduction in IGF-1 have been associated with improvements in proliferative

retinopathy [95]. In addition, direct intravitreal injection of IGF-1 induces vasodilatation, microaneurysm formation and neovascularization [96], infusion of recombinant IGF-1 resulted in intraretinal microangiopathic abnormalities [97] and lowering IGF-1 concentrations with a somatostatin analogue reduced neovascularization in ischaemic mice by about one-third [98].

9.7 HYPOGLYCAEMIA AND MICROANGIOPATHY

Many similarities exist between the metabolic and hormonal milieu that characterize the chronic hyperglycaemia of poorly controlled diabetes, and the maximal counter-regulatory hormonal response to acute hypoglycaemia [99]. Acute hypoglycaemia is, however, a transient phenomenon in human diabetes and we have seen that the microangiopathic complications take years to develop. It has been postulated that the profound haemodynamic and haemorrheologic consequences of acute hypoglycaemia may precipitate local changes in nutritional flow that accelerate microangiopathy in those with established microvascular disease [91].

The haemodynamic consequences of hypoglycaemia include hypertension and regional redistribution of blood flow to preserve fuel supply to critical organs, notably the brain. These haemodynamic changes may involve significant ischaemic stress and cause slow-flow-related intravascular coagulation, accelerating capillary closure. In the kidney, for example, acute hypoglycaemia has been shown to reduce renal plasma flow and glomerular filtration in normoalbuminuric patients with type 1 diabetes [100]. A similar effect in patients with incipient or established nephropathy would potentially have more detrimental effects. In the eye, hypoglycaemia is associated with a sudden fall in intraocular pressure [101], potentially increasing shear stress on retinal new vessels thereby precipitating vitreous haemorrhage, which has been described by diabetic patients following severe nocturnal hypoglycaemia [102].

The haemorrheological consequences of hypoglycaemia include increased blood viscosity, increased release of factor VIII and von Willebrand factor, and increased platelet and neutrophil activation factors contributing to a hypercoagulable state [103–107]. This, together with increased free-radical activation [108] and increased secretion of the potent vasoconstrictor endothelin-1 [109], may all contribute to an acceleration of microangiopathy secondary to acute glucose deprivation (Figure 9.9).

More direct evidence for an effect of hypoglycaemia on microangiopathic processes comes from studies of growth factor production. Vascular endothelial growth factor/ vascular permeability factor (VEGF/VPF) is a potent vascular endothelial cell mitogen which is mainly upregulated by hypoxia and is closely associated with the development and the progression of diabetic retinopathy [110]. Basal production of VEGF is significantly greater from cultured retinal pigment epithelial cells (RPE) than from retinal endothelial cells or pericytes and is significantly elevated by long-term (10 days) but not short-term (1–3 days) exposure to hyperglycaemia (16.5 mmol/l glucose compared to 5.5 mmol/l) [111]. VEGF production from RPE is significantly upregulated (57% over baseline) by a hypoglycaemic stimulus (fall in glucose concentration in medium from 5.5 mmol/l to 0.5 mmol/l) but is not induced by rapid normalization of high glucose concentrations (from 33 or 16.5 to 5.5 mmol/l glucose). These data suggest that hypoglycaemia may contribute to the worsening of diabetic retinopathy by up-regulating intraocular VEGF production. Exposure to a high progesterone concentration (but still within the normal physiological range for pregnancy) is also associated with increased VEGF production from RPE cells and synergy between the effects of hypoglycaemia and pregnancy may explain the deterioration of retinopathy occasionally seen during pregnancy [111, 112].

9.8 MORE THAN GLUCOSE: THE MISSING LINKS?

Although these studies clearly demonstrate the pivotal role for disturbances in glucose homeostasis in general and chronic hyperglycaemia in particular, much remains unexplained in the development and progression of microangiopathy. The clinical conundrum of patients who maintain poor glycaemic control and yet see the dire predictions of their diabetologists go unfulfilled as they remain mystifyingly free from the ravages of micro-angiopathy are as puzzling as the few patients who progress with significant micro-angiopathy despite near optimal glycaemic control. Furthermore, the observation that only a proportion of those patients with hyperglycaemia develop microvascular com-plications hints at the presence in some at least, of other non-glucose factors, promoting or protecting against microangiopathy.

Thus the role of chronic hyperglycaemia is pivotal in the development and progression of microangiopathy, but in order to explain the variability in disease expression in those with consistent hyperglycaemia, it is neces-sary to a invoke a role for numerous other factors in the evolution of microangiopathy in diabetes. Several other factors have been implicated or proposed. These include age, age of onset of diabetes, sex, race, hyper-tension, hyperlipidaemia, smoking and heter-ogeneity in a range of candidate cardiovascular and metabolic genes.

Until better and earlier markers of suscepti-bility to the complications of diabetes are available, the optimal glycaemic control that an individual patient can achieve and live with remains a central goal of therapy in the successful management of diabetes.

REFERENCES

1. The Diabetes Control and Complications Trial Research Group. The effect of intensive treatment of diabetes on the development and progression of long-term complications in insulin-dependent diabetes mellitus. *N. Engl. J. Med.*, 1993, **329**, 977–86.
2. National Diabetes Data Group. Classification and diagnosis of diabetes and other cate-gories of glucose intolerance. *Diabetes*, 1979, **28**, 1039–57.
3. Nathan, D.M. The pathophysiology of dia-betic complications: How much does the glu-cose hypothesis explain? *Ann. Intern. Med.*, 1996, **124**, 86–9.
4. Pirart, J. Diabetes mellitus and its degen-erative complications: a prospective study of 4400 patients observed between 1947 and 1973. *Diabetes Care*, 1978, **1**, 168–88.
5. Davis, M.D, Kern, T.S. and Rand, L.I. Dia-betic retinopathy, In *International Textbook of Diabetes Mellitus*, 2nd edn, (eds K.G.M. Alberti, P. Zimmet and R.A. DeFronzo), Wiley, Chichester, 1997, pp. 1413–46.
6. Osterby, R. Early phases in the development of diabetic glomerulopathy. *Acta Med. Scand.*, 1985, **574**, 3–82.
7. Tesfaye, S., Malik, R. and Ward, J.D. Vascular factors in diabetic neuropathy. *Diabetologia*, 1994, **37**, 847–54.
8. Jarrett, R.J. and Keen, H. Hyperglycaemia and diabetes mellitus. *Lancet*, 1976, **ii**, 1009–12.
9. Pettitt, D.J., Knowler, W.C., Lisse, J.R. and Bennett, P.H. Development of retinopathy and proteinuria in relation to plasma-glucose concentrations in Pima Indians. *Lancet*, 1980, **ii**, 1050–52.
10. Klein, B., Klein, S.E. and Moss, S.E. The Wis-consin epidemiological study of retinopathy: a review. *Diabet. Metab. Rev.*, 1989, **5**, 559–70.
11. Klein, R., Barrett-Connor, E.L., Blunt, B.A. and Wingard, D.L.Visual impairment and retinopathy in people with normal glucose tolerance, impaired glucose tolerance, and newly diagnosed NIDDM. *Diabetes Care*, 1991, **14**, 914–18.
12. U.K. Prospective Diabetes Study 6. Compli-cations in newly diagnosed type 2 diabetic patients and their association with different clinical and biochemical risk factors. *Diabetes Res.*, 1990, **13**, 1–11.
13. Damsgaard, E.M. and Mogensen, C.E. Micro-albuminuria in elderly hyperlgycaemic patients and controls. *Diabet. Med.*, 1986, **3**, 430–5.
14. Olivarius, N. de F., Andreasen, A.H., Keiding, N. and Mogensen, C.E. Epidemiology of renal involvement in newly-diagnosed mid-dle-aged and elderly diabetic patients. Cross-sectional data from the population-based study 'Diabetes Care in General Practice', Denmark. *Diabetologia*, 1993, **36**, 1007–16.
15. Haffner, S.M., Gonzales, C., Valdez, R.A., Mykkanen, L., Hazuda, H.P., Mitchell, B.D. *et al.* Is microalbuminuria part of the predia-betic state? The Mexico City Diabetes Study. *Diabetologia*, 1993, **36**, 1002–6.

16. Mykkanen, L., Haffner, S.M., Kuusisto, J., Pyorala, K. and Laakso, M. Microalbuminuria precedes the development of NIDDM. *Diabetes,* 1994, **43,** 552–7.

17. Keen, H., Chluoverakis, C., Fuller, J.H. and Jarrett, R.J. The concomitants of raised blood sugar: studies in newly-detected hyperglycemics. II.Urinary albumin excretion, blood pressure and their relationship to bloodsugar levels. *Guy's Hosp. Rep.,* 1969, **118,** 247–54.

18. Collins, V.R., Dowse, G.K., Finch, C.F., Zimmett, P.Z. and Linane, A.W. Prevalence and risk factors for micro- and macroalbuminuria in diabetic subjects and entire population of Nauru. *Diabetes,* 1989, **38,** 1602–10.

19. Nelson, R.G., Knowler, W.C., Pettitt, D.J., Saad, M.F., Charles, M.A. and Bennett, P.H. Assessment of risk of overt nephropathy in diabetic patients from albumin excretion in untimed urine specimens. *Arch. Intern. Med.,* 1991, **151,** 1761–5.

20. Wingard, D.L., Barrett-Connor, E.L., Scheidt-Nave, C. and McPhillips, J.B. Prevalence of cardiovascular and renal complications in older adults with normal or impaired glucose tolerance or NIDDM. A population-based study. *Diabetes Care,* 1993, **16,** 1022–5.

21. Franklyn, B.M., Kahn, L.B., Baxter, J., Marshal, J.A. and Hamman, R.F. Sensory neuropathy in non-insulin dependent diabetes mellitus: the San LuisValley Diabetes Study. *Am. J. Epidemiol.,* 1990, **131,** 633–43.

22. Matschinsky, F.M., Liang, Y., Kesavan, P. *et al.* Glucokinase as pancreatic beta cell glucose sensor and diabetes gene. *J. Clin. Invest.,* 1993, **92,** 2092–8.

23. Froguel, P., Zouali, H., Vionnet, N. *et al.* Familial hyperglycaemia due to mutations in glucokinase. Definition of a new type of diabetes mellitus. *N. Engl. J. Med.,* 1993, **928,** 697–702.

24. Hattersley, A.T. and Turner, R.C. Mutations of the glucokinase gene and type 2 diabetes. *Q. J. Med.,* 1993, **86,** 227–32.

25. Page, R.C., Hattersley, A.T., Levy, J.C. *et al.* Clinical characteristics of patients with a missense mutation in glucokinase. *Diabet. Med.,* 1995, **12,** 209–17.

26. Hatterlsey, A.T. Maturity-onset diabetes of the young. *Ballière's Clin. Paediat.,* 1996, **4,** 663–80.

27. Yamagata, K., Oda, N., Kaisaki, P.J. *et al.* Mutations in the hepatic nuclear factor 1 alpha gene in maturity-onset diabetes of the young (MODY3). *Nature,* 1996, **384,** 455–8.

28. Yamagata, K., Furuta, H., Oda, N. *et al.* Mutations in the hepatocyte nuclear factor 4 alpha gene in maturity-onset diabetes of the young (MODY1). *Nature,* 1996, **384,** 458–60.

29. Hatterlsey, A.T. Maturity-onset diabetes of the young. *Bailliere's Clin. Paediatr.* 1996, **4,** 663–79.

30. Chase, H.P., Jackson, W.E., Hoops, S.L., Cockerham, R.S., Archer, P.G. and O'Brien, D. Glucose control and the renal and retinal complications of insulin-dependent diabetes. *J. Am. Med. Assoc.,* 1989, **261,** 1155–60.

31. Norgaard, K., Storm, B., Graae, M. and Feldt-Rasmussen, B. Elevated albumin excretion and retinal changes in children with type I diabetes are related to long-term poor glucose control. *Diabet. Med.,* 1989, **6,** 325–8.

32. Johnsson, S. Retinopathy and nephropathy in diabetes mellitus: comparison of the effects of two modes of treatment. *Diabetes,* 1960, **9,** 128.

33. Lawrence, R.D. Treatment of 90 severe diabetics with soluble insulin for 20–40 years. Effect of diabetic control on complications. *Br. Med. J.,* 1963, **II,** 1624–5.

34. Palmberg, P., Smith, M., Waltman, S. *et al.* The natural history of retinopathy in insulin-dependent juvenile onset diabetes. *Ophthalmology,* 1981, **88,** 613–18.

35. Klein, R., Klein, B.E.K., Moss, S.E. *et al.* The Wisconsin Epidemiologic Study of Diabetic Retinopathy when age at diagnosis is less than 30 years. *Arch. Ophthalmol.,* 1984, **102,** 520–6.

36. Rand, L.I., Prud' homme, G.J., Ederer, F. *et al.* Diabetic retinopathy Study group. Factors influencing the development of visual loss in advanced diabetic retinopathy: Diabetic Retinopathy Study (DRS) report no. 10. *Invest. Ophthalmol. Vis. Sci.,* 1985, **26,** 983–91.

37. Krolewski, A.S., Warram, J.H., Rand, L.I. *et al.* Risk of proliferative retinopathy in juvenile-onset type 1 diabetes: a 40 year follow-up study. *Diabetes Care,* 1986, **9,** 443–52.

38. Rand, L.I., Krolewski, A.S., Aieloo, L.M. *et al.* Multiple factors in the prediction of risk of proliferative diabetic retinopathy. *N. Engl. J. Med.,* 1985, **313,** 1433–8.

39. Janka, H.U., Warram, J.H., Rand, L.I. *et al.* Risk factors for progression of background

retinopathy in long-standing IDDM. *Diabetes,* 1989, **38,** 460–4.

40. Klein, B.E.K., Moss, S.E., David, M.D. and Devets, D.L. Glycosylated hemoglobin predicts the incidence and progression of diabetic retinopathy. *J. Am. Med. Assoc.,* 1988, **260,** 2864–71.

41. Krolewski, A.S., Warram, J.H., Christlieb, A.R. *et al.* The changing natural history of nephropathy in type 1 diabetes. *Am. J. Med.,* 1985, **78,** 785–94.

42. Andersen, A.R., Christiansen, J.S., Andersen, J.K. *et al.* Diabetic nephropathy in Type 1 (insulin-dependent) diabetes: an epidemiological study. *Diabetologia,* 1983, **25,** 496–501.

43. Deckert, T., Poulsen, J.E. and Larsen, M. Prognosis of diabetes with diabetes onset before the age of thirty-one. II. Factors influencing the prognosis. *Diabetologia,* 1978, **14,** 371–7.

44. Cohen, A.J., McGill, P.D., Rossetti, R.G., Guberski, D.K. and Like, A.A. Glomerulopathy in spontaneously diabetic rat: impact of glycaemic control. *Diabetes,* 1987, **36,** 944–51.

45. Engerman, R.L. and Kern, T.S. Progression of incipient retinopathy during good glycaemic control. *Diabetes,* 1987, **36,** 808–12.

46. Kern, T.S. and Engerman, R.L. Arrest of glomerulopathy in spontaneously diabetic dogs by improved glycaemic control. *Diabetologia,* 1990, **33,** 522–5.

47. Lee, C.S., Mauer, S.M., Sutherland, D.E.R., Najarian, J.S. and Michael, A.F. Renal transplantation in diabetes mellitus in rats. *J. Exp. Med.,* 1974, **139,** 793–800.

48. Mauer, S.M., Steffes, M.W., Sutherland, D.E.R., Najarian, J.S., Michael, A.F. and Brown, D.M. Studies of the rate of regression of the glomerular lesions in diabetic rats treated with pancreatic transplantation. *Diabetes,* 1975, **24,** 280–5.

49. The Kroc Collaborative Study Group. Blood glucose control and the evolution of diabetic retinopathy and albuminuria: a preliminary multicenter trial. *N. Engl. J. Med.,* 1984, **311,** 428–32,365–72.

50. The Kroc Collaborative Study Group. Diabetic retinopathy after two years of intensified insulin treatment. *J. Am. Med. Assoc.,* 1988, **260,** 37–41.

51. Lauritzen, T., Larsen, K.F., Larsen, H.W., Deckert, T. and the Steno Study Group. Effect of one year of near-normal blood glucose levels on retinopathy in insulin-dependent diabetes. *Lancet,* 1983, **i,** 200–4.

52. Lauritzen, T., Larsen, K.F., Larsen, H.W. and Deckert, T. Steno Study Group. Two year experience with continuous subcutaneous insulin infusion in relation to retinopathy and neuropathy. *Diabetes,* 1985, **34** (suppl 3), 74–9.

53. Dahl-Jørgensen, K., Brinchmann-Hansen, O., Hanssen, K.F., Sandvic, L. and Aegenaes, O. Rapid tightening of blood glucose control leads to transient deterioration of retinopathy in insulin dependent diabetes mellitus. The Oslo Study. *Br. Med. J.,* 1985, **290,** 811–15.

54. Dahl-Jørgensen, K., Brinchmann-Hansen, O., Hanssen, K.F., Ganes, T., Kierulf, P., Smelund, E., Sandvik, K.F. and Aegenaes, O. Effects of near normoglycaemia for two years on progression of early diabetic retinopathy, nephropathy and neuropathy: the Oslo Study. *Br. Med. J.,* 1986, **293,** 1195–9.

55. Brinchmann-Hansen, O., Dahl-Jørgensen, K., Hanssen, K.F. and Sandvik, L. Oslo Study Group. Effects of intensified insulin therapy on various lesions of diabetic retinopathy. *Arch. Opthalmol.,* 1985, **100,** 644–53.

56. Brinchmann-Hansen, O., Dahl-Jørgensen, K., Hanssen, K.F. and Sandvik, L. The response of diabetic retinopathy to 41 months of multiple insulin injections, insulin pumps and conventional insulin therapy. *Arch. Opthalmol.,* 1988, **106,** 1242–6.

57. Verrillo, A., de Teresa, A., Martino, C. *et al.* Long-term correction of hyperglycaemia and progression of retinopathy in insulin-dependent diabetes. A five year randomized prospective study. *Diabetes Res.,* 1988, **8,** 71–6.

58. Reichard, P., Berglund, B., Britz, A., Cars, I., Nilsson, B.Y. and Rosenqvist, U. Intensified conventional insulin treatment retards the microvascular complications of insulin-dependent diabetes mellitus (IDDM): the Stockholm Diabetes Intervention Study (SDIS) after 5 years. *J. Intern. Med.,* 1991, **230,** 101–8.

59. Reichard, P., Nilsson, B.Y. and Rosenqvist, U. The effect of long-term intensified insulin therapy on the development of microvascular complications in insulin-dependent diabetes mellitus. *N. Engl. J. Med.,* 1993, **329,** 304–9.

60. Wang, P.H., Lau, J. and Chalmers, T.C. Meta-analysis of effects of intensive blood-glucose control on late complications of type 1 diabetes. *Lancet*, 1993, **341**, 1306–9.

61. Ramsay, R.C., Goetz, F.C., Sutherland, D.E.R., Mauer, S.M., Robson, L.L., Cantrill H.I., Knobloch, W.H. and Najarian, J.S. Progression of diabetic retinopathy after pancreas transplantation for insulin-dependent diabetes. *N. Engl. J. Med.*, 1988, **318**, 208–14.

62. Fioretto, P., Mauer, S.M., Bilous, R.W., Goetz, F.C., Sutherland, D.E. and Steffes, M.W. Effects of pancreatic transplantation on glomerular structure in insulin-dependent diabetic patients with their own kidneys. *Lancet*, 1993, **342**, 1193–6.

63. Reichard, P., Pihl, M., Rosenqvist, U. and Sule, J. Complications in IDDM are caused by elevated blood glucose level: The Stockholm Diabetes Intervention Study (SDIS) at 10-year follow-up. *Diabetologia*, 1996, **39**, 1483–8.

64. Klein, R. Hyperglycaemia and microvascular and macrovascular disease in diabetes. *Diabetes Care*, 1995, **18**, 258–71.

65. Klein, R., Klein, B.E.K. and Moss, S.E. Epidemiology of proliferative diabetic retinopathy. *Diabetes Care*, 1992, **15**, 1875–91.

66. Stamler, J., Vacarro, O., Neaton, J.D. and Wentworth, D. Diabetes, other risk factors, and the 12-yr cardiovascular mortality for men screened in the Multiple Risk Factor Intervention Trial. *Diabetes Care*, 1993, **16**, 434–44.

67. Klein, R., Klein, B.E.K., Moss, S.E. and Cruikshanks, K.J. Relationship of hyperglycaemia to the long-term incidence and progression of diabetic retinopathy. *Arch. Intern. Med.*, 1994, **154**, 2109–78.

68. Ohkubo, Y., Kishikawa, H., Araki, E., Miyata, T., Isami, S., Motoyoshi, S., Kojima, Y., Furuyoshi, N. and Shichiri, M. Intensive insulin therapy prevents the progression of diabetic microvascular complications in Japanese patients with non-insulin dependent diabetes. *Diabetes Res. Clin. Pract.*, 1995, **25**, 103–17.

69. Knatterud, G.L., Klimt, C.R., Levin, M.E., Jacobson, M.E. and Goldner M.G. Effects of hypoglycaemic agents on vascular complications in patients with adult onset diabetes. VII. Mortality and selected non-fatal events with insulin treatment. *J. Am. Med. Assoc.*, 1978, **240**, 37–42.

70. Kilo, C., Miller, J.P. and Williamson, J.R. The crux of the UGDP. *Diabetologia*, 1980, **18**, 179–85.

71. U.K. Prospective Diabetes Study Group. U.K. Prospective Diabetes Study 16. Overview of 6 years' therapy of type II diabetes: a progressive disease. *Diabetes*, 1995, **44**, 1249–58.

72. U.K. Prospective Diabetes Study 17; A nine-year update of a randomised controlled trial on the effect of the improved metabolic control and complications in non-insulin dependent diabetes mellitus. *Ann. Intern. Med.*, 1997, **124**, 136–45.

73. Colwell, J.A. The feasibility of intensive insulin management in non-insulin dependent diabetes mellitus. *Ann. Intern. Med.*, 1996, **124**, 131–5.

74. Colwell, J.A. Should we use intensive insulin therapy after oral agent failure in Type II diabetes? *Diabetes Care*, 1996, **19**, 896–8.

75. Abraira, C., Colwell, J.A., Nuttal, F.Q., Sawin, C.T., Nagel, N.J., Comstock, J.P., Emanuele, N.V., Levin, S.R., Henderson, W. and Lee, H.S. VACSDM Study Group. Veterans Affairs Cooperative Study on glycaemic control and complications in type II diabetes (VACSDM): results of the feasibility trial. *Diabetes Care*, 1995, **18**, 1113–23.

76. Emanuele, N., Klein, R., Abraira, C., Colwell, J., Comstock, J., Henderson, W., Levin, S., Nuttall, F., Sawin, C., Silbert, C., Lee, H.S.L. and Johnson-Nagel, N. VACSDM Study Group. Evaluations of retinopathy in the VA co-operative study on glycemic control and complications in type 2 diabetes (VACSDM). *Diabetes Care*, 1996, **19**, 1375–81.

77. Dahl-Jørgensen, K., Brinchman-Hansen, O., Bangstad, H.J. and Hannsen, K.F. Blood glucose control and microvascular complications – what do we know now? *Diabetologia*, 1994, **37**, 1172–7.

78. Dahl-Jørgensen, K., Hanssen, K.F., Kierulf, P., Bjoro, T., Sandvik, L. and Aegenaes, O. Reduction of urinary albumin excretion after 4 years of continuous subcutaneous insulin infusion in insulin-dependent diabetes mellitus. *Acta Endocrinol.*, 1988, **117**, 19–25.

79. Brinchmann-Hansen, O. and Dähl-Jorgensen, K. Blood glucose concentrations and progression of diabetic retinopathy: the seven year results of the Oslo study. *Br. Med. J.*, 1992, **304**, 19–22.

80. The Kroc Collaborative Study Group. 1994.

81. The Diabetes Control and Complications Trial Research Group. The effect of intensive diabetes treatment on the progression of diabetic retinopathy in insulin-dependent diabetes mellitus. *Arch. Opthalmol.*, 1995, **113**, 36–49.

82. Agardh, C.D., Eckert, B. and Agardh, E. Irreversible progression of severe retinopathy in young type 1 insulin-dependent diabetes mellitus patients after improved metabolic control. *J. Diabetes Complications*, 1992, **6**, 96–100.

83. Moskalets, E., Galstyan, G., Starositna, E., Antsiferov, M. and Chanteleau, E. Association of blindness to intensification of glycaemic control in insulin-dependent diabetes mellitus. *J. Diabetes Complications*, 1994, **98**, 45–50.

84. Roysarkar, T.K., Gupta, A., Dash, R.J. and Dogra, M.R. Effect of insulin therapy on progression of retinopathy in non-insulin dependent diabetes mellitus. *Am. J. Ophthalmol.*, 1993, **115**, 569–74.

85. Henricsson, M., Janzon, L. and Groop, L. Progression of retinopathy after change of treatment from oral antihyperglycemic agents to insulin in patients with NIDDM. *Diabetes Care*, 1995, **18**, 1571–6.

86. Henricsson, M., Nilsson, A., Lanzon, L. and Groop, L. The effect of glycaemic control and the introduction of insulin therapy on retinopathy in non-insulin dependent diabetes mellitus. *Diabet. Med.*, 1997, **14**, 123–31.

87. Grunwald, J.E., Riva, C.E., Sinclair, S.H. and Bucker, A.V. Alters retinal vascular response to 100% O_2 breathing in diabetes. *Microvasc. Res.*, 1983, **25**, 236 (abstract 35).

88. Parving, H.H., Kastrup, H., Smidt, U.M., Andersen, A.R., Feldt-Rasmussen, B.F. and Sandahl Chrsitiansen, J. Impaired acute regulation of glomerular filtration rate in Type 1 (insulin-dependent) diabetic patients with nephropathy. *Diabetologia*, 1984, **27**, 247–52.

89. Faris, I., Van Nielsen, H., Henriksen, O., Parving, H.H. and Lassen, N.A. Impaired autoregulation of blood flow in skeletal muscle and subcutaneous tissues in long-term Type 1 (insulin-dependent) diabetic patients with microangiopathy. *Diabetologia*, 1983, **25**, 486–8.

90. Grunwald, J.E., Riva, C.E., Martin, D.B., Quint, A.R. and Epstein, A. Effect of insulin induced decrease in blood glucose on the human diabetic retinal circulation. *Ophthalmology*, 1987, **94**, 1614–20.

91. Kohner, E.M. Diabetic retinopathy. *Br. Med. J.*, 1993, **307**, 1195–9.

92. Frier, B.M. and Hilsted, J. Does hypoglycaemia aggravate complications of diabetes? *Lancet*, 1985, **ii**, 1175–7.

93. Chanteleau, E. and Kohner, E.M. Why some cases of retinopathy worsen when diabetic control improves. *Br. Med. J.*, 1997, **315**, 1105–6.

94. Chanteleau, E. and Eggert, H. Acceleration of diabetic retinopathy following improved glycaemic control; a report of 13 cases. *Diabetologia*, 1997, **40** (suppl 1), A501 (abstract).

95. Sharp, P.S., Fallon, T.J., Brazier, O.J., Sandler, L., Joplin, G.F. and Kohner, E.M. Long-term follow-up of patients who underwent yttrium-90 pituitary implantation for treatment of proliferative retinopathy. *Diabetologia*, 1987, **30**, 199–207.

96. Grant, M.B., Mames, R.N., Fitzgerald, C., Ellsi, E.A., Aboufriekha, M. and Guy, J. Insulin-like growth factor-1 acts as an angiogenic agent in rabbit cornea and retina: comparative studies with basic fibroblast growth factor. *Diabetologia*, 1993, **36**, 282–91.

97. Hussain, M.A., Studer, K., Messmer, E.P. and Froesch, E.R. Treatment with insulin-like growth factor 1 alters capillary permeability in skin and retina. *Diabetes*, 1995, **44**, 1209–12.

98. Smith, L.E.H., Kopchick, J.J., Chen, W., Knapp, J., Kinose, F., Daley, D. *et al.* Essential role of growth hormone in ischaemia induced retinal neovascularisation. *Science*, 1997, **276**, 1706–8.

99. Fisher, B.M. and Frier, B.M. Effect of hypoglycaemia on vascular disease. In *Hypoglycaemia and Diabetes: Clinical and Physiological Aspects*, (eds B.M. Frier and B.M. Fisher), Edward Arnold, London, 1993, pp. 353–361.

100. Patrick, A.W., Hepburn, D.A., Swainson, C.P. and Frier, B.M. Changes in renal function during insulin-induced hypoglycaemia in patients with Type 1 diabetes. *Diabet. Med.*, 1992, **9**, 150–5.

101. Frier, B.M., Hepburn, D.A., Fisher, B.M. and Barrie, T. Fall in intraocular pressure during acute hypoglycaemia in patients with insulin dependent diabetes. *Br. Med. J.*, 1987, **294**, 610–11.

102. Kohner, E.M., McLeod, D. and Marshall, J. Diabetic eye disease. In *Complications of Diabetes*, (eds H. Keen and J. Jarrett), Edward Arnold, London, 1982, pp. 99–108.

103. Corrall, R.J.M., Webber, R.G. and Frier, B.M. Increase in coagulation factor VIII activity in man following acute hypoglycaemia: mediation via an adrenergic mechanism. *Br. J. Haematol.*, 1980, **44**, 301–5.

104. Frier, B.M., Corrall, R.J.M., Davidson, N.McD., Webber, R.G., Dewar, A. and French, E.B. Peripheral blood cell changes in response to acute hypoglycaemia in man. *Eur. J. Clin. Invest.*, 1983, **13**, 33–9.

105. Collier, A., Patrick, A.W., Hepburn, D.A., Bell, D., Jackson, M., Dawes, J. and Frier, B.M. Leucocyte mobilization and release of neutrophil elastase following acute insulin-induced hypoglycaemia in normal humans. *Diabet. Med.*, 1990, **7**, 506–9.

106. Fisher, B.M., Quin, J.D., Rumley, A., Lennie, S.E., Small, M., MacCuish, A.C. and Lowe, G.D.O. Effects of acute insulin-induced hypoglycaemia on haemostasis, fibrinolysis, and haemorrheology in insulin-dependent diabetic patients and control subjects. *Clin. Sci.*, 1991, **800**, 521–31.

107. Wieczorek, I., Pell, A.C.H., McIver, B., Macgregor, I.R., Ludlam, C.A. and Frier, B.M. Coagulation and fibrinolytic systems in Type 1 diabetes: effects of venous occlusion and insulin-induced hypoglycaemia. *Clin. Sci.*, 1993, **84**, 79–86.

108. Collier, A., Rumley, A., Fisher, B.M., Quin, J.D., MacCuish, A.C. and Small, M. Insulin-induced hypoglycaemia increases free radical activity in insulin-dependent diabetic patients. *Diabetologia*, 1991, **34** (suppl 2), A187 (abstract).

109. MacLeod, K.M., Perros, P., Webb, D.J. and Frier, B.M. Plasma endothelin responses to acute hypoglycaemia in insulin-dependent diabetes mellitus (IDDM). *Diabetologia*, 1997, **40** (suppl 1), A242 (abstract).

110. Aiello, L.P., Avery, R.l., Arrigg, P.G., Keyt, B.A., Jampel, H.D., Shaha, S.T. *et al.* Vascular endothelial growth factor in ocular fluid of patients with diabetic retinopathy and other retinal disorders. *N. Engl. J. Med.*, 1994, **331**, 1480–7.

111. Sone, H., Okuda, Y., Kawakami, Y., Kondo, S., Hanatani, Y., Matsuo, K., Suzuki, H. and Yamashita, Y. Induction of vascular endothelial growth factor (VEGF) production by progesterone in cultured retinal pigment epithelial cells. *Life Sci.*, 1996, **59**, 21–5.

112. Sone, H., Kawakami, Y., Okuda, A., Kondo, S., Hanatani, M., Suzuki, H. and Yamashira, K. Vascular endothelial growth factor (VEGF) is induced by chronic high glucose concentration and upregulated by acute glucose deprivation in cultured bovine retinal pigment epithelial cells. *Biochem. Biophys. Res. Commun.*, 1996, **221**, 193–8.

Joseph R. Williamson and Yasuo Ido

While the pathogenesis of diabetic complications is clearly multifactorial and complex, the single most important risk factor is generally acknowledged to be hyperglycaemia. The Diabetes Control and Complications Trial [1] firmly established the importance of the severity and duration of hyperglycaemia in the development and progression of diabetic microvascular complications in subjects with insulin-requiring diabetes. Nevertheless, the nature of the metabolic imbalances induced by hyperglycaemia in vascular cells and/or in contiguous non-vascular parenchymal cells, and their interactions that result in vascular dysfunction and pathology, remain unclear.

A full understanding of the natural history and pathogenesis of diabetic vascular disease requires elucidation of the very earliest manifestation(s) of vascular dysfunction induced by elevated glucose levels and identification of the metabolic imbalances that cause them. To this end, the discussion in this chapter will focus attention on vascular dysfunction and associated metabolic imbalances induced by acute hyperglycaemia in non-diabetic rats and corresponding vascular dysfunction and metabolic imbalances early after the onset of streptozotocin-induced diabetes in rats. As will become evident, metabolic imbalances and increased production/levels of growth factors linked to development of vascular dysfunction early after the onset of diabetes also are implicated in the pathogenesis of occlusive and proliferative vascular changes characteristic of end-stage diabetic vascular disease. Indeed, most of the metabolic imbalances implicated in the pathogenesis of early vascular dysfunction and late vascular structural changes induced by diabetes appear to be causally linked by a cascade of interacting reactions initiated by a hypoxia-like metabolic imbalance which develops within a few hours after the onset of hyperglycaemia.

10.1 FUNCTIONAL AND STRUCTURAL VASCULAR RESPONSES TO HYPERGLYCAEMIA

10.1.1 EARLY VASCULAR DYSFUNCTION INDUCED BY ACUTE HYPERGLYCAEMIA IN NON-DIABETIC HUMANS AND RATS

There is general agreement that acute hyperglycaemia of only a few hours duration increases blood flow in retina and kidney and increases glomerular filtration rate (GFR) in the kidney in non-diabetic humans and animals [2, 3] (refs 28, 29 in [3–5]). These haemodynamic and filtration changes are the earliest readily quantifiable consequences of elevated glucose levels. In rats infused intravenously with glucose at a rate sufficient to achieve plasma glucose levels comparable to those in diabetic rats, endoneurial and epineurial sciatic nerve blood flow as well as ocular (retinal, anterior uveal, posterior uveal and optic nerve) and renal blood flow are increased within five hours after beginning the infusion (refs 20, 21 in [4]). After this relatively brief duration of hyperglycaemia vascular albumin permeation in these same tissues is unchanged. Thus, increased blood flow induced by elevated glucose levels precedes increased vascular albumin permeation.

10.1.2   EARLY VASCULAR DYSFUNCTION IN DIABETIC HUMANS AND IN ANIMALS WITH SPONTANEOUS OR EXPERIMENTALLY INDUCED DIABETES

Haemodynamic changes

Renal blood flow and GFR are initially increased in diabetic humans and in rats (that are not severely ketotic or cachectic) with experimentally induced diabetes [3, 5]. The nature of the earliest retinal blood flow changes in diabetic humans and animals, i.e. whether blood flow is increased, unchanged or decreased, is much less clear [2, 4]. Methodological differences and problems, together with differences in severity and duration of diabetes, may account for much of the discordance in reports on retinal blood flow changes in diabetic humans and animals.

In our own studies (using the reference sample microsphere method with ^{3}H-desmethylimiprimine, a low molecular weight plasma soluble tracer, or with particulate microspheres), diabetes increases blood flow in the retina and sciatic nerve as well as in the kidney [5–8]. These increased blood flows are transient in nature [9]; the time of onset and duration of increased blood flow depends on the severity of diabetes and may vary in different tissues. In rats with moderately severe non-ketotic diabetes, increased blood flows are evident within two to three weeks and persist for six to eight weeks or longer; in rats with very mild diabetes (weight gain is normal), the onset of vascular dysfunction is delayed [10]. Reports that peripheral (sciatic) nerve blood flow is decreased in diabetic rats are based largely on assessments of blood flow in surgically exposed nerves and may reflect impaired neurogenically mediated hyperaemic responses to surgical trauma

(rather than blood flow in undisturbed nerves) [7] consistent with diabetes-induced impaired neurogenic vascular responses to a variety of other stimuli including hyperthermia, vasoactive agents, and trauma [7, 11]. Although sciatic nerve blood flow has been reported to be decreased in diabetic rats when assessed with tracers that do not require prior exposure of the nerve (iodoantipyrine and butanol) [7], these observations may be explained by: (1) the severity of diabetes and poor physiological condition of the rats, (2) the nerves were in fact exposed in some studies, and (3) differential inhibitory effects of iodoantipyrine on prostaglandin synthesis in control and diabetic rats [7].

As already noted, impaired or blunted vascular responses to vasoactive agents and trauma are well documented in diabetic humans and animals; these blunted responses are demonstrable relatively early after the onset of diabetes in animals. Evidence that the hyperaemic response to mild surgical trauma is demonstrable in sciatic nerve of normal rats within two to five minutes after simple surgical exposure of the nerve [7] suggests that the hyperaemia is mediated by neurogenic mechanisms and is consistent with evidence that sciatic nerve levels of neuropeptide mediators of neurogenic hyperaemia are decreased in diabetic rats [12].

Impaired vascular barrier function

Increased vascular permeation by iodinated rat albumin is evident in retina, nerve and aorta in diabetic rats within two to three weeks after the onset of diabetes and, in contrast to increased blood flows, remains elevated as long as the animals survive [9]. Urinary excretion of endogenous albumin also is evident within two to three weeks of the onset of diabetes and tends to become more pronounced with longer duration of diabetes [3, 9].

In contrast, vascular permeation by low molecular weight tracers such as ^{14}C-sucrose has been reported to be increased in the retina only after several months of diabetes [13]. As the filtration surface area (the functional equivalent of pores through endothelial cells and intercellular junctions between endothelial cells) available for permeation of low molecular weight tracers (such as sucrose) across the vessel wall is several orders of magnitude larger than that for albumin, a small increase in the number and/or dimension of pores/junctions that can be permeated by albumin will cause a marked percentage increase in albumin permeation without a detectable increase in permeation by low molecular weight tracers such a sucrose.

The very long circulation times (~60 min) used in the studies with sucrose as a tracer raise the possibility that the increased retinal sucrose content in rats with diabetes of several months duration may be explained by a larger extravascular (interstitial) space available to the tracer rather than an increased rate of sucrose permeation; the finding that sucrose permeation was not increased in rats with diabetes of short duration may simply indicate that the extravascular space was not increased. This view is supported by our own studies with radiolabelled rat albumin and sucrose. Thus, the retinal content of radiolabelled albumin (after correction for intravascular albumin) is higher in diabetic rats than in controls when the tracer is allowed to circulate for ~10 min, but does not differ in controls and diabetic subjects when the tracer is allowed to circulate for longer times comparable to those employed by Lightman *et al.* for sucrose. This may be explained by a relatively small extravascular space in the retina in which tracer concentration will equilibrate relatively rapidly with intravascular tracer. Since sucrose is a much smaller molecule than albumin, the filtration surface area for sucrose permeation is much greater than for albumin; therefore sucrose in the extravascular space would equilibrate with intravascular sucrose much more rapidly than albumin. These same caveats apply to the use of low molecular

weight versus macromolecular tracers for assessment of diabetes-induced changes in vascular barrier function in other tissues such as peripheral nerve.

10.1.3 VASCULAR STRUCTURAL CHANGES

Thickening of capillary basement membranes is perhaps the earliest readily quantifiable microvascular structural change observed in virtually all tissues affected by microvascular disease in humans and animals [14]. Only after several months of diabetes are vascular structural changes demonstrable in rats. Thickening of capillary basement membranes is associated with pericyte degeneration and with acellular and non-perfused capillaries in the retina and in skeletal muscle [15–17]. After a year or more of diabetes, early proliferative vascular changes are observed in the retina [15, 16]. Thickening of capillary basement membranes in peripheral nerve also is associated with pericyte degeneration and with axonal atrophy and dystrophic changes in neurones and Schwann cells [18, 19]. In the kidney, mesangial expansion develops in addition to thickening of glomerular capillary basement membranes [9, 20]. Mesangial expansion is the glomerular structural change which correlates best with renal failure [20].

10.2 PATHOPHYSIOLOGICAL SIGNIFICANCE OF INCREASED BLOOD FLOW AND LOSS OF VASCULAR BARRIER FUNCTIONAL INTEGRITY: RELATIONSHIP TO VASCULAR STRUCTURAL CHANGES

The selective increased blood flows in retina (and other ocular tissues), sciatic nerve, and kidney in the absence of any change in systemic blood pressure indicates that the tone of smooth muscle cells in resistance arterioles must be relaxed to permit the increased blood flow. This will allow transmission of systemic blood pressure further downstream in the microvasculature resulting in microvascular hypertension (despite normal arterial blood pressure). The rationale for the haemodynamic hypothesis for the pathogenesis of microvascular complications of diabetes is that microvascular hypertension increases vascular permeability and initiates vascular sclerosis resulting in occlusive microvascular changes causing ischaemia in retina and nerve and decreased glomerular filtration surface area in the kidney (refs 2, 4 in [3]). The resulting ischaemia in the retina is postulated to increase production/levels of growth factors such as vascular endothelial growth factor (VEGF, also referred to as vascular permeability factor) leading to proliferative retinopathy. The decreased filtration surface area in the kidney limits excretion of waste products resulting in renal failure.

Microvascular hypertension, independent of an increase in the number and/or dimensions of endothelial pores/junctions, will increase hydraulic conductance (permeation) of plasma water and low molecular weight constituents small enough to enter existing pores/junctions. If microvascular pressure is increased sufficiently, increased vascular wall tension may also increase the number and size of endothelial pores/junctions resulting in increased permeation of larger plasma macromolecules across the vessel wall.

Although the mechanism(s) suggested for the vascular changes outlined above are plausible, alternative interpretations for the pathogenesis of some of these vascular changes are equally (if not more) credible. Evidence that increases in blood flow are transient, whereas impaired vascular barrier functional integrity persists and progresses with longer duration of diabetes, suggests that the permeability changes are independent of increased blood flow and associated microvascular hypertension. Thus, increased blood flow, impaired vascular barrier function and vascular structural changes induced by diabetes may not be causally linked. Each of these vascular changes may be independent manifestations of metabolic imbalances and cellular dysfunction induced by the diabetic milieu. For example, VEGF increases blood flow and vascular albumin leakage in addition to stimulating endothelial cell proliferation and angiogenesis [21]. VEGF mRNA and protein levels are: (1) increased in cultured cells by elevated glucose levels independent of oxygen tension [22, 23], and (2) demonstrable in retinas of diabetic humans and animals at sites remote from evidence of vascular occlusive and/or proliferative changes [24, 25].

When blood flow is increased in a tissue in response to metabolic imbalances induced by hyperglycaemia, further increases in blood flow by vasodilating agents and other conditions may appear to be blunted when expressed as percentage change in blood flow or vessel diameter and compared to corresponding percentage changes in control subjects. Nevertheless, absolute blood flow (basal or after exposure to a vasodilating agent) in the diabetic subject may be comparable to that in control subjects or even higher. Without quantitative measures of blood flow (more importantly vascular conductance to correct for any differences in blood pressure) before addition of vasoactive agents, it is difficult if not impossible to make meaningful comparisons of blood flow and vascular tone in diabetic subjects versus controls and the effects of diabetes on vascular responses to vasoactive agents.

10.3 METABOLIC IMBALANCES IMPLICATED IN MEDIATING VASCULAR CHANGES INDUCED BY HYPERGLYCAEMIA AND THE DIABETIC MILIEU

Although the Diabetes Control and Complications Trial [1] established the importance of the severity and duration of hyperglycaemia in the onset and progression of diabetic retinopathy, neuropathy and nephropathy, it did not address the nature of the metabolic imbalances that mediate the effects of elevated glucose levels on vascular and neural tissue. The apparent predilection of tissues in which glucose uptake is insulin-independent to develop complications suggests an important role for metabolic imbalances resulting from increased intracellular glucose levels. On the other hand, metabolic imbalances induced by increased intracellular glucose levels must vary considerably in different tissues as susceptibility to development of vascular and neural complications differs greatly even among tissues in which glucose uptake is insulin-independent. Thus, vascular changes are much more pronounced in retina and peripheral nerve than in the brain.

Metabolic imbalances implicated in the pathogenesis of early vascular dysfunction and structural changes in animal models of diabetes include sequelae of increased metabolism of glucose via the sorbitol pathway, non-enzymatic glycation reactions, carnitine depletion, oxidative stress, reductive stress and activation of protein kinase C [4, 5, 9, 26–34]. The two most extensively studied metabolic imbalances linked to vascular changes in animal models of diabetes are increased sorbitol pathway metabolism and non-enzymatic glycation and their sequelae. While non-enzymatic glycation reactions do not appear to be rapid enough to account for vascular dysfunction induced by acute hyperglycaemia of a few hours' duration, they may contribute to vascular dysfunction relatively early after the onset of diabetes and in the pathogenesis of early as well as late vascular structural changes.

Numerous investigations have provided strong evidence linking increased metabolism of glucose via the sorbitol pathway to vascular and neural dysfunction in animal models of diabetes [28, 31, 35] (refs 2, 4 in [35]). Negative results reported by some investigators appear to be attributable largely to incomplete inhibition of the sorbitol pathway, i.e. administration of aldose reductase inhibitors at doses that markedly reduce or normalize sorbitol levels but that do not normalize fructose levels. The same may be true for disappointing results of clinical trials with aldose reductase inhibitors [36], although, in addition, the duration of these trials also may not have been long enough in view of the length of time required to demonstrate beneficial effects of improved glucose control in the Diabetes Control and Complications Trial and other clinical trials [1].

In the first step of the sorbitol pathway, glucose is reduced to sorbitol by aldose reductase coupled to oxidation of the co-factor nicotine adenine dinucleotide phosphate (from its reduced form, NADPH, to $NADP^+$). In the second step of the pathway sorbitol is oxidized to fructose by sorbitol dehydrogenase coupled to reduction of the co-factor nicotine adenine dinucleotide (from its oxidized form, NAD^+, to NADH). Alterations in the levels of both co-factors as well as sorbitol and fructose have been postulated to mediate vascular and neural changes associated with increased sorbitol pathway metabolism. These include: (1) accumulation of sorbitol resulting in osmotic stress and intracellular oedema [31], (2) sequelae of osmotic stress including *myo*-inositol depletion and decreased levels of free radical scavenging osmolites such as taurine [28, 35, 37] (refs 2, 4, 7 in [35]), (3) speculation that levels of NADPH might be decreased sufficiently to limit the activity of: (a) glutathione reductase (resulting in decreased levels of reduced glutathione, an important antioxidant) and (b) nitric oxide synthase activity (resulting in decreased blood flow and tissue hypoxia [5, 6, 38, 39, 40], and (4) an increased ratio of cytosolic free $NADH/NAD^+$ (resulting from increased oxidation of sorbitol to fructose) which impacts on the activity of numerous dehydrogenase enzymes, several of which have been implicated in the pathogenesis of diabetic complications [3–5, 35].

To the extent that vascular changes in diabetic humans and animals are mediated by these same or corresponding metabolic imbalance(s), elucidation of the roles of these metabolic imbalances in mediating hyperglycaemia-induced vascular changes in animal models may yield important insights for understanding the pathogenesis of diabetic vascular disease and for development of new approaches for preventing and treating complications. Of the metabolic imbalances implicated in the pathogenesis of diabetic complications, the one most closely linked to the development of early vascular dysfunction (increased blood flow) in animal models of diabetes is the increased ratio of cytosolic free $NADH/NAD^+$ resulting from increased oxidation of sorbitol to fructose.

10.4   CYTOSOLIC FREE $NADH/NAD^+$ AND REDUCTIVE STRESS, ENERGY METABOLISM AND REGULATION OF BLOOD FLOW

In several different animal models, the earliest metabolic imbalance linked to increased blood flow induced by acute hyperglycaemia is cytosolic reductive stress, a redox change like that induced by hypoxia, i.e. an increased ratio of cytosolic free $NADH/NAD^+$. Because

of the near-equilibrium established between cytosolic free $NADH/NAD^+$ and lactate/pyruvate ratios established by lactate dehydrogenase [41], an increase in the ratio of one will be manifested by a corresponding increase in the other (Figure 10.1). Thus reduction of pyruvate to lactate is coupled to oxidation of NADH to NAD^+ by lactate dehydrogenase and vice versa. A caveat to the use of tissue lactate/pyruvate ratios as a parameter of cytosolic free $NADH/NAD^+$ is that the equilibrium between the two ratios is pH-sensitive [41]. Thus, at low pH an increased lactate/pyruvate ratio may not indicate an increase in $NADH/NAD^+$. In perfused hearts from diabetic rats the increased lactate/pyruvate ratio is not associated with a decrease in pH which indicates that cytosolic free $NADH/NAD^+$ is increased [42]. Whether or not the increased ratio of lactate/pyruvate (and other redox-sensitive metabolite couples such as glycerol-3-phosphate dehydrogenase/dihydroxyacetone phosphate) reflect changes in $NADH/NAD^+$ or in pH, the altered metabolite levels (i.e. pyruvate and

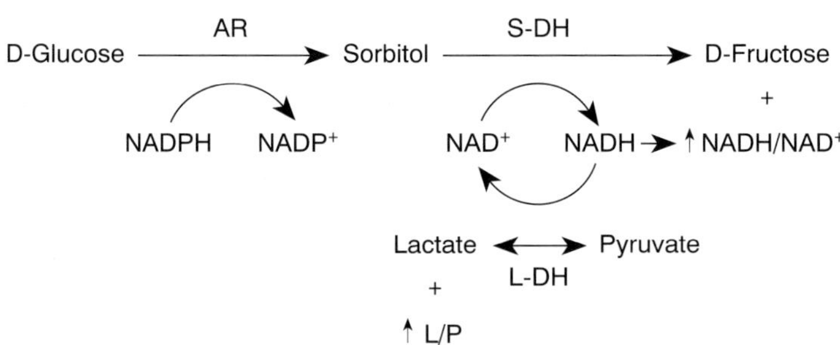

Figure 10.1 Links between oxidation of sorbitol to fructose and ratios of cytosolic $NADH/NAD^+$ and lactate/pyruvate (L/P) established by lactate dehydrogenase (L-DH). In the first step of the sorbitol pathway, glucose is reduced to sorbitol coupled to oxidation of NADPH to $NADP^+$ by aldose reductase (AR). In the second step of the pathway sorbitol is oxidized to fructose coupled to reduction of NAD^+ to NADH by sorbitol dehydrogenase (S-DH). Increased oxidation of sorbitol to fructose results in an increased ratio of $NADH/NAD^+$. The increased availability of NADH drives reduction of pyruvate to lactate coupled to oxidation of NADH to NAD^+ by lactate dehydrogenase. Because of the near-equilibrium established between $NADH/NAD^+$ and lactate/pyruvate by lactate dehydrogenase, an increased ratio of $NADH/NAD^+$ is associated with an increased lactate/pyruvate ratio.

glycerol phosphate) may contribute to metabolic imbalances associated with diabetic complications.

An increased lactate/pyruvate ratio (cytosolic reductive stress) is observed in lens, retina and nerve of diabetic rats [4, 35, 43–45] (ref. 2 in [35], ref. 30 in [4]) and is demonstrable in nerve early (10 days) after the onset of diabetes (when blood flow is increased) in the absence of evidence of mitochondrial reductive stress [44]. Lactate/pyruvate ratios also are increased in these same tissues (as well as in isolated glomeruli from normal rats) and in human erythrocytes after incubation at elevated glucose levels for only one to two hours or less [3–5, 35] (refs 35–38 in [4]).

In animal models of diabetes and in human erythrocytes exposed to elevated glucose levels, this redox change develops because the increased rate of reduction of NAD^+ to NADH by sorbitol dehydrogenase exceeds the rate of reoxidation of cytosolic NADH to NAD^+ (Figure 10.2). Flux of glucose via the sorbitol pathway even at normal glucose levels impacts on cytosolic $NADH/NAD^+$; sorbitol pathway inhibitors decrease cytosolic $NADH/NAD^+$ and tissue sorbitol and fructose levels [4] in retina and nerve incubated at normal glucose levels. In addition, zopolrestat (an inhibitor of aldose reductase) decreases myocardial lactate/pyruvate ratios in control as well as in diabetic rats [42].

In hypoxic tissues this same redox imbalance results from impaired mitochondrial oxidation of NADH to NAD^+ by the electron transport chain (Figure 10.3). This, in turn, limits transport of cytosolically generated reducing equivalents, i.e. electrons and hydrogens (H) of NADH, into the mitochondria by the glycerol phosphate and/or malate aspartate shuttles for oxidation by the electron transport chain. As different mechanisms mediate the increased cytosolic ratio of free $NADH/NAD^+$ caused by hypoxia and by hyperglycaemia, their effects on reductive stress and its sequelae should be additive.

This prediction is supported by observations that hypoxic injury to hepatocytes is accentuated by metabolism of substrates that is coupled to reduction of NAD^+ to NADH (sorbitol, xylitol, ethanol and β-hydroxybutyrate) and is attenuated by metabolism of substrates that is coupled to oxidation of NADH to NAD^+ (pyruvate, fructose, oxaloacetate, acetoacetate, acetaldehyde) [46, 47].

The glycerol phosphate and malate aspartate shuttles have a limited capacity to transport cytosolically generated reducing equivalents into mitochondria [48]. The maximum rate of myocardial glucose utilization via glycolysis is the same in anoxia and in (aerobic) working hearts and is limited by the rate of oxidation of cytosolic NADH [48]. Under these conditions, oxidation of triose phosphates by glyceraldehyde 3-phosphate dehydrogenase is limited by availability of the co-factor NAD^+ and this reaction becomes the rate-limiting step in glycolysis. This is because as the rate of oxidation of triose phosphates by glyceraldehyde 3-phosphate dehydrogenase increases during aerobic work or anoxia, NAD^+ is reduced to NADH at a faster rate than NADH can be transported into the mitochondria by the shuttles (or oxidized by other pathways in the cytosol). Thus, under these stressful conditions, availability of NAD^+ can limit the rate of glycolysis and associated cytosolic ATP synthesis and production of pyruvate for mitochondrial ATP synthesis. Such observations suggest that tissues of diabetic animals experiencing reductive stress due to increased flux of glucose via the sorbitol pathway may be more susceptible to injury by superimposed reductive stress from other mechanisms such as hypoxia or ethanol intoxication as observed in the liver [47].

Although increased flux of glucose via the sorbitol pathway appears to be largely responsible for cytosolic reductive stress in non-ketotic diabetic rats and in acutely hyperglycaemic non-diabetic rats, other metabolic

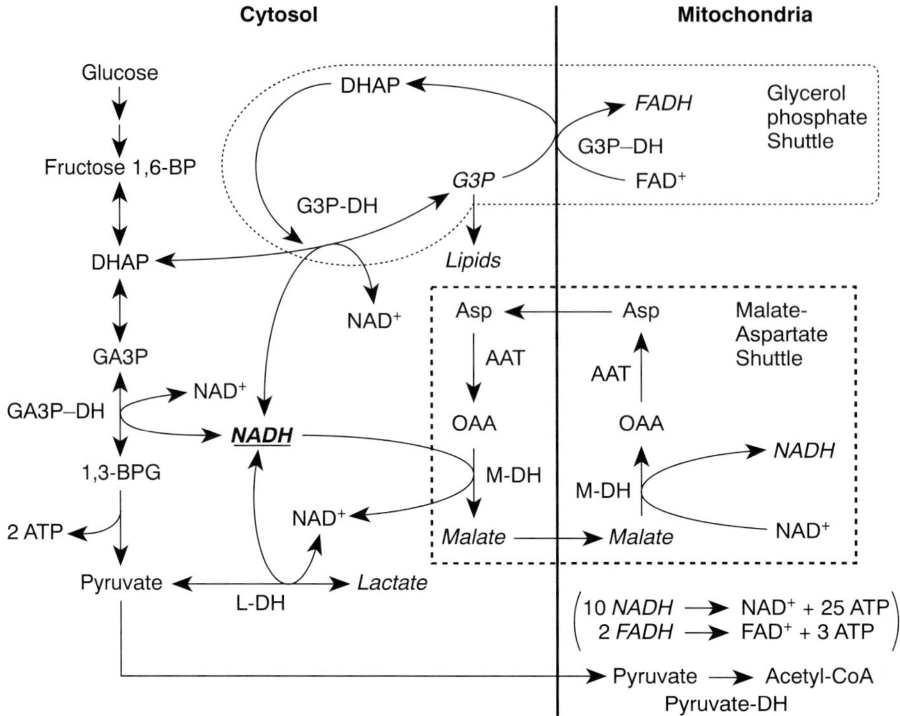

Figure 10.2 Oxidation of cytosolic NADH (modified from Figure 4 in [48] with permission of the authors and publisher). Cytosolic NADH produced by glyceraldehyde 3-phosphate dehydrogenase (GAP-DH) (as well as sorbitol dehydrogenase, see Figure 10.1) is oxidized to $NAD(^+)$ by lactate dehydrogenase, the malate aspartate shuttle and the glycerol phosphate shuttle. Pyruvate utilized for mitochondrial oxidative phosphorylation is not available for cytosolic oxidation of NADH (by lactate dehydrogenase) which must be reoxidized by the shuttles in order to maintain GAP-DH activity for cytosolic ATP synthesis and pyruvate for mitochondrial ATP synthesis. In the heart, oxidation of cytosolic NADH is rate-limiting for maximum glycolysis and ATP synthesis from glucose under conditions of hypoxia as well as aerobic work [48]. AAT, aspartate aminotransferase; acetyl-CoA, acetyl co-enzyme A; Asp, aspartate; ATP, adenosine triphosphate; 1,3-BPG, 1,3-bisphosphoglycerate; DHAP, dihydroxyacetone phosphate; FAD, flavin adenine dinucleotide; fructose 1,6-BP, fructose 1,6-bisphosphate; G3P, glycerol 3-phosphate; G3P-DH, glycerol 3-phosphate dehydrogenase; GA3P, glyceraldehyde 3-phosphate; GAP-DH, glyceraldehyde dehydrogenase; L-DH, lactate dehydrogenase; M-DH, malate dehydrogenase; NAD^+, nicotinamide adenine dinucleotide (oxidized form); NADH, nicotinamide adenine dinucleotide (reduced form); $NADP^+$, nicotinamide adenine dinucleotide phosphate (oxidized form); NADPH, nicotinamide adenine dinucleotide phosphate (reduced form); OAA, oxaloacetate; pruvate-DH, pyruvate dehydrogenase.

imbalances associated with the diabetic milieu may contribute to reductive stress in non-ketotic diabetic humans and in humans and animals with ketoacidosis. Evidence consistent with increased metabolism of glucose via the glucuronic acid pathway has been reported in diabetic humans [49]; metabolism of glucose via this pathway generates 3 moles of NADH per mole of glucose compared with only 1 mole of NADH per mole of glucose metabolized via the sorbitol pathway. Increased oxidation of fatty acids and ketones increases mitochondrial NADH/NAD$^+$ [5, 50–54] which may, like mitochondrial reductive stress induced by hypoxia, slow the transport of cytosolic reducing equivalents into the mitochondria (Figure 10.3) enough to cause cytosolic reductive stress.

The importance of changes in the cytosolic ratio of free NADH/NAD$^+$ is the central role of redox cycling of NAD(H) in normal glucose, lipid and energy metabolism (ATP synthesis). Redox cycling of NAD(H) is essential for ATP synthesis in the cytosol as well as in the mitochondria. In addition, altered activities of several dehydrogenase enzymes that utilize NAD(H) as a co-factor are linked to imbalances in glucose and lipid metabolism and to the pathogenesis of diabetic complications [5]. Furthermore, an increased cytosolic ratio of NADH/NAD$^+$ (apparently regardless of the cause) is associated with increased blood flow in the affected tissue [5]. To appreciate the potential of changes in cytosolic NADH/NAD$^+$ to mediate many of the metabolic imbalances implicated in diabetic vascular (and neural) dysfunction, it is insightful to briefly consider the nature of the basic role of NAD(H) cycling in energy metabolism and the concept that cytosolic NADH/NAD$^+$ coordinates physiological blood flow and energy metabolism.

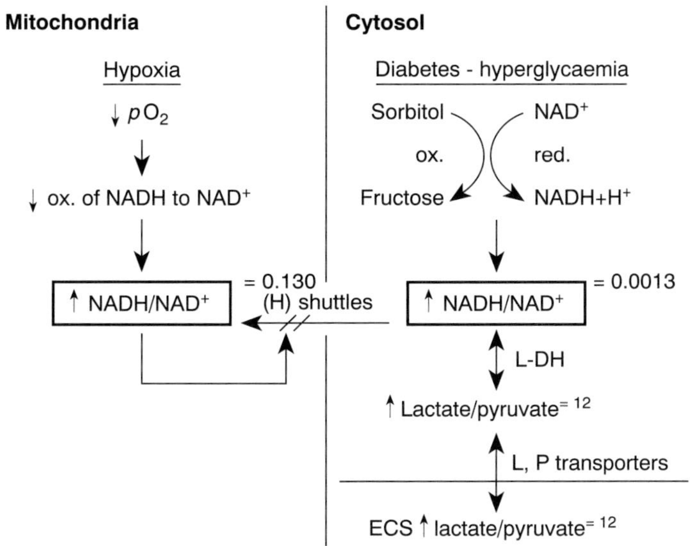

Figure 10.3 Links between mitochondrial and cytosolic free NADH/NAD$^+$ and cytosolic and extracellular space (ECS) lactate/pyruvate ratio in hypoxia and diabetes. The approximate ratios of cytosolic and mitochondrial free NADH/NAD$^+$ (0.0013 versus 0.130) and of lactate/pyruvate in the cytosol and extracellular space (~12 for each) are based on published values for the liver [41]. Impaired oxidation of NADH to NAD$^+$ by the electron transport chain during hypoxia limits transport of reducing equivalents from the cytoplasm into the mitochondria resulting in an increased ratio of cytosolic free NADH/NAD$^+$ even without any change in the rate of cytosolic reduction of NAD$^+$ to NADH. Because of the equilibrium between cytosolic free NADH/NAD$^+$ and lactate/pyruvate ratios established by lactate dehydrogenase, the cytosolic lactate/pyruvate ratio will also be increased. This in turn will increase the extracellular lactate/pyruvate ratio by the activity of plasma membrane lactate and pyruvate transporters. L-DH, lactate dehydrogenase; L, lactate; P, pyruvate; NAD$^+$, nicotinamide adenine dinucleotide (oxidized form); NADH, nicotinamide adenine dinucleotide (reduced form); ox., oxidation; red., reduction.

10.4.1 REDOX CYCLING OF NAD(H) AND ATP SYNTHESIS

Oxidation of glucose and its metabolites for synthesis of ATP is dependent on redox cycling of NAD(H), i.e. reduction of NAD^+ to NADH and reoxidation of NADH to NAD^+, in the cytoplasm and in the mitochondria. In the cytoplasm oxidation of glyceraldehyde 3-phosphate to 1,3-bisphosphoglycerate by glyceraldehyde 3-phosphate dehydrogenase is coupled to reduction of NAD^+ to NADH (Figure 10.2). Subsequent metabolism of 1,3-bisphosphoglycerate to pyruvate yields 2 moles of ATP from ADP coupled to dephosphorylation of 1,3-bisphosphoglycerate to 3-phosphoglycerate by phosphoglycerate kinase and dephosphorylation of 2-phosphoglycerate to pyruvate by pyruvate kinase. Continued cytosolic ATP synthesis by these reactions is dependent on reoxidation of cytosolic NADH to NAD^+ for use by glyceraldehyde 3-phosphate dehydrogenase (Figure 10.2). Under anaerobic conditions NADH is reoxidized to NAD^+ by lactate dehydrogenase coupled to reduction of pyruvate to lactate (Figure 10.2).

Under aerobic conditions pyruvate transported into the mitochondria for oxidative metabolism is unavailable for reoxidation of cytosolic NADH (by lactate dehydrogenase) produced by glyceraldehyde 3-phosphate dehydrogenase. This NADH can be reoxidized to NAD^+ coupled to reduction of dihydroxyacetone phosphate to glycerol 3-phosphate by cytosolic glycerol 3-phosphate dehydrogenase. This is the first step in one pathway for *de novo* synthesis of diacylglycerol (a natural activator of protein kinase C) from triose phosphates (Figures 10.2 and 10.4). Alternatively, glycerol 3-phosphate produced by this reaction can be utilized by the glycerol phosphate shuttle (for transfer of cytosolic H and electrons into mitochondria); cytosolic glycerol 3-phosphate diffuses into the intermembranous space of mitochondria where it is oxidized to dihydroxyacetone phosphate coupled to reduction of flavin adenine dinucleotide from FAD^+ to FADH by mitochondrial glycerol 3-phosphate dehydrogenase which is associated with the outer surface of the inner membrane. FADH is then reoxidized to FAD^+ coupled to reduction of NAD^+ to NADH which is reoxidized by the electron transport chain coupled to synthesis of ATP and reduction of oxygen to water. Cytosolic NAD(H) and electrons also can be transported into the mitochondrial matrix by the malate aspartate shuttle for reoxidation and ATP synthesis by the electron transport chain except that mitochondrial NAD^+ is utilized rather than FAD^+ as the electron acceptor (Figure 10.2).

In addition to the central role of NAD(H) (and the $NADH/NAD^+$ ratio) in cytosolic and mitochondrial ATP synthesis, several lines of evidence suggest that cytosolic free $NADH/NAD^+$ also plays an important role in co-ordinating blood flow with energy metabolism and work. As noted above an increase in cytosolic free $NADH/NAD^+$, regardless of the cause, is associated with increased blood flow; conversely, pharmacological interventions that normalize cytosolic $NADH/NAD^+$ normalize (reduce) blood flow. Normalization of blood flow by pharmacological interventions that do not prevent reductive stress appears to be attributable to blocking the sequelae of reductive stress.

We hypothesize that an increase in cytosolic free $NADH/NAD^+$ signals the need for increased blood flow to provide more oxygen and/or substrates for ATP synthesis, and/or to remove products of energy metabolism including lactate and CO_2. Thus, blood flow is increased when cytosolic free $NADH/NAD^+$ is increased due to increased: (1) production of reducing equivalents in the cytoplasm (i.e. by oxidation of sorbitol to fructose or of ethanol to acetaldehyde by their respective dehydrogenases), (2) mitochondrial $NADH/NAD^+$ caused by hypoxia or cyanide poisoning and (3) work-induced glycolysis.

Increased glycolysis causes cytosolic reductive stress by two mechanisms: (1) lactate production is increased which elevates intra- and extracellular lactate levels thereby increasing intracellular lactate/pyruvate ratios and cytosolic $NADH/NAD^+$ via lactate dehydrogenase (Figure 10.3) and (2) increased reduction of NAD^+ to NADH by glyceraldehyde 3-phosphate dehydrogenase at a faster rate than NADH reducing equivalents can be transported into the mitochondria by the shuttles (Figure 10.2).

As predicted by the relationships between intra- and extracellular lactate/pyruvate ratio and cytosolic $NADH/NAD^+$ (Figure 10.3), co-infusion of pyruvate prevents increased retinal, sciatic nerve and renal blood flow induced by infusion of glucose or lactate, and sorbitol pathway inhibitors prevent cytosolic reductive stress and increased blood flow induced by hyperglycaemia and diabetes [4, 5, 21, 35, 55–57] (refs 20, 21 in [4], unpublished observations). We hypothesize that while an increased cytosolic ratio of free $NADH/NAD^+$ is 'sensed' as hypoxia and initiates a cascade of events that increase tissue blood flow, reductive stress that is not due to hypoxia (i.e. increased sorbitol pathway activity, hyperlactataemia and work) may not be normalized and blood flow will remain elevated as long as the metabolic change/imbalance responsible for reductive stress persists (or is compensated for by some other mechanism(s). This hypothesis is supported by evidence that, in response to various kinds of work, increased tissue blood flow: (1) delivers much more oxygen than is utilized for energy metabolism and (2) glucose uptake and lactate production and levels are increased despite tissue hyperoxia [58–60].

The signalling cascade implicated in mediating increased blood flow induced by elevated glucose levels in non-diabetic rats and in rats with diabetes of short duration is shown in Figure 10.4. This tentative scenario is supported by observations in several different animal models, however, it does not exclude potentially important roles for other mediators and vasoactive agents. Reductive stress increases superoxide formation by several different mechanisms discussed in the following section. Superoxide increases intracellular calcium which activates the constitutive isoform of nitric oxide synthase resulting in increased blood flow [61–63]. With longer duration of diabetes the rate of production of free radicals such as superoxide may exceed the relatively slow rate of nitric oxide formation by the constitutive isoform with the result that blood flow returns to normal or may even be decreased.

10.5 NADPH: CO-FACTOR FOR ALDOSE REDUCTASE, NITRIC OXIDE SYNTHASE AND GLUTATHIONE REDUCTASE

While the pyridine nucleotide co-factor NAD^+ is reduced to NADH coupled to oxidation of sorbitol to fructose by sorbitol dehydrogenase, the co-factor NADPH is oxidized to $NADP^+$ coupled to reduction of glucose to sorbitol by aldose reductase in the first step of the pathway (Figure 10.1). The functions of these two co-factors, the normal ratios of their reduced to oxidized forms and the mechanisms that regulate their redox state differ considerably. The primary function of NAD(H) is as an electron carrier for ATP synthesis. During the oxidation of substrates for ATP synthesis NAD^+ accepts two electrons and a hydrogen ion. In contrast NADP(H) is utilized as an electron donor/hydrogen carrier for a variety of reductive biosynthetic reactions including synthesis of fatty acids, cholesterol, glutathione, and nucleotides and nucleic acids. The ratio of cytosolic free $NADH/NAD^+$ is several orders of magnitude lower than that of $NADPH/NADP^+$ (0.002 versus 62) [43]. The reactions involved in redox cycling of NAD(H) have been discussed above and are essentially independent of those for NADP(H). $NADP^+$

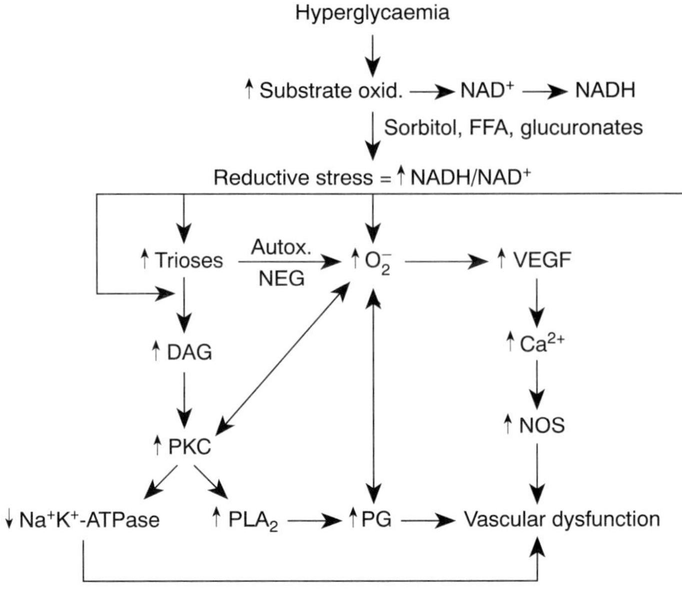

Figure 10.4 Tentative scenario for inter-relationships between metabolic imbalances induced by diabetes-mediated cytosolic reductive stress. Increased oxidation of substrates coupled to reduction of the co-factor NAD^+ to NADH (at a rate faster than NADH can be reoxidized) results in an increased cytosolic ratio of free $NADH/NAD^+$. This favours accumulation of triose phosphates (trioses) which undergo autoxidation with production of superoxide and which also increase *de novo* synthesis of diacylglycerol (DAG), a natural activator of protein kinase C (PKC). PKC activity is associated with production of superoxide (and its activity is modulated by superoxide), inhibition of Na^+,K^+-ATPase activation of phospholipase A_2 (PLA_2), and activation of vascular endothelial growth factor (VEGF). Activation of PLA_2 releases arachidonic acid which increases synthesis of prostaglandins (PG) which is associated with superoxide production. Superoxide alters prostaglandin synthesis, increases VEGF levels, and increases intracellular calcium which activates the constitutive isoform of nitric oxide synthase (NOS). Vascular function is modulated by nitric oxide, prostaglandins, VEGF and Na^+,K^+-ATPase activity as well as numerous other vasoactive agents (i.e. endothelins) which may be altered by hyperglycaemia. FFA, free fatty acids (non-esterified fatty acids); NEG, non-enzymatic glycation; O_2^-, superoxide.

generated from NADPH in reductive synthetic reactions is reduced to NADPH via the pentose phosphate pathway and the pyruvate/malate cycle.

As the enzymes nitric oxide synthase, glutathione reductase and aldose reductase all utilize the co-factor NADPH as the hydrogen donor, it has been speculated that (in diabetes) increased utilization of NADPH by aldose reductase for reduction of glucose to sorbitol might limit availability of NADPH for synthesis of nitric oxide and for maintenance of reduced glutathione [28, 38–40].

The predicted consequences would be vasoconstriction due to impaired nitric oxide synthesis (resulting in tissue hypoxia) and increased susceptibility to effects of oxidative stress due to decreased levels of glutathione. The speculation that NADPH levels are decreased and limiting to synthesis of nitric oxide and glutathione is not supported by measurements of $NADPH/NADP^+$. $NADPH/NADP^+$ ratios in sciatic nerve at 10 days and four months after the onset of diabetes are increased about twofold at both time points and these increases are prevented by inhibitors of the sorbitol pathway [43–45]. In cultured human endothelial cells exposed to 33 mM glucose for 5–7 days (compared with 5.5 mM), NADPH levels are not decreased (total NAD^+ and NADH also were not altered, however, cytosolic $NADH/NAD^+$ was not reported) [64].

Providing that the sum of NADPH + $NADP^+$ is not decreased, the more reduced $NADPH/NADP^+$ ratio in sciatic nerve of diabetic rats would favour increased nitric oxide synthesis and is consistent with our observations that blood flow is increased early after the onset of diabetes. Interestingly, cytosolic free $NADH/NAD^+$ was increased at these same time points whereas mitochondrial reductive stress was not evident at 10 days but was present at four months. At both time points, sorbitol pathway inhibitors also prevented the increased $NADH/NAD^+$ ratios in the cytosol but not in mitochondria in the four-month study [43–45]. These observations support the likelihood that mitochondrial reductive stress in these diabetic rats reflects increased oxidation of ketones or fatty acids rather than hypoxia. The finding in the four-month study that impaired nerve conduction in diabetic rats was normalized by sorbitol pathway inhibitors supports the importance of cytosolic reductive stress, independent of mitochondrial reductive stress, in mediating electrophysiological dysfunction.

In some reports implicating decreased nitric oxide production as the cause of decreased blood flow, impaired Na^+,K^+-ATPase activity and electrophysiological dysfunction in peripheral nerve of diabetic rats, the investigators used non-selective inhibitors of nitric oxide synthase at doses that caused arterial hypertension in control as well as in diabetic rats [38, 40]. The development of hypertension in these rats suggests inhibition of constitutive nitric oxide synthase activity with widespread constriction of resistance arterioles, possibly involving peripheral nerve causing neural ischaemia. This could cause the functional abnormalities observed,

independent of the diabetic milieu. Thus, these studies do not provide insight into the actual mechanisms that mediate corresponding functional abnormalities in diabetic rats as hypoxia causes neural dysmetabolism and dysfunction similar to that induced by diabetes [5, 28, 65, 66]. Although impaired production of nitric oxide and decreased levels of glutathione may contribute to vascular dysfunction and structure at some point in the pathogenesis of diabetic vascular disease, there is no evidence at the present time to suggest that they are the consequence of decreased availability of NADPH.

The physiological importance of nitric oxide, as well as pathological consequences of excess nitric oxide are well recognized; however, only the pathological consequences of excess superoxide and other free radicals are widely appreciated. An increasing body of evidence indicates that free radicals also play important roles in normal signal transduction and physiological regulation of cellular metabolism and function [5, 67–70]. Small increases in superoxide production/levels appear to play an important role in signalling the physiological need for increased blood flow associated with increased energy metabolism. On the other hand, even small increases in free radical levels/production, if sustained, constitute oxidative stress [5, 26] and may lead to pathological consequences via signal transduction mechanisms discussed below.

10.6 METABOLIC CONSEQUENCES OF CYTOSOLIC REDUCTIVE STRESS

10.6.1 CYTOSOLIC REDUCTIVE STRESS, OXIDATIVE STRESS, NON-ENZYMATIC GLYCATION, AND EXTRACELLULAR MATRIX CHANGES

An increase in cytosolic free $NADH/NAD^+$ favours reduction of 1,3-phosphoglycerate to glyceraldehyde 3-phosphate by glyceraldehyde 3-phosphate dehydrogenase. Because of the equilibrium between glyceraldehyde 3-phosphate, dihydroxyacetone phosphate and fructose 1,6-bisphosphate (Figure 10.2), all three of these glycolytic metabolites (referred to collectively as triose phosphates) will accumulate. Accumulation of triose phosphates is well documented for reductive stress induced by hypoxia as well as by elevated glucose levels [3, 4, 71, 72] (refs 29, 35–38 in [4]); the increase in triose phosphates induced by elevated glucose levels, but not that by hypoxia, is prevented by sorbitol pathway inhibitors (refs 36, 37 in [4]). Triose phosphates are highly reactive compounds which readily undergo autoxidation/glycation reactions coupled to production of superoxide (Figure 10.4). Thus accumulation of triose phosphates due to reductive stress may play an important role in intracellular glycation and oxidative damage to DNA, proteins and polyunsaturated membrane lipids [9, 34]. Triose phosphates also are substrates for synthesis of methylglyoxal, a highly toxic compound also postulated to contribute to the pathogenesis of diabetic complications [73].

Non-enzymatic glycation (by glucose) of extracellular tissue constituents and plasma membranes and of intracellular constituents in cells that do not require insulin for glucose uptake, i.e. haemoglobin, is also well documented and the function of some of these glycated constituents appears to be impaired (superoxide dismutase, Na^+,K^+-ATPase, Ca^{2+}-ATPase [74–76]. In addition, autoxidation of glycated products is associated with production of free radicals and reactive aldehydes and dicarbonyls which cause further damage to membrane proteins and polyunsaturated phospholipids [9, 34]. Even early glycation products undergo autoxidation with release of free radicals [9]. Autoxidation of early glycation products is not prevented by aminoguanidine (which does prevent cross-linking reactions between glycated and non-glycated constituents) [9]. Thus the beneficial effects of aminoguanidine in attenuating sequelae of (intra- as well as extracellular) non-enzymatic glycation appear to be attributable primarily to its action as a chain-breaking scavenger of reactive aldehyde products of autoxidation of glycation products.

As aminoguanidine also inhibits nitric oxide synthase (the cytokine-inducible isoform is preferentially inhibited) [77–79], it is unclear to what extent prevention of vascular and neural dysfunction by aminoguanidine is due to inhibition of nitric oxide synthase versus its effects on non-enzymatic glycation reactions. Increased granulation tissue blood flow and vascular albumin permeation induced by glycated rat albumin, like vascular dysfunction induced by elevated glucose levels, is prevented by nitric oxide synthase inhibitors as well as by free radical scavengers such as probucol and superoxide dismutase [5, 29, 80] (unpublished observations). The failure of aminoguanidine in some studies to prevent vascular and neural dysfunction in chronically diabetic rats raises the possibility that these changes are mediated by: (1) early glycation reactions and autoxidation reactions that are not affected by aminoguanidine or (2) metabolic imbalances independent of non-enzymatic glycation reactions [9].

An increased ratio of $NADH/NAD^+$ favours production of reactive oxygen species (ROS) by several mechanisms independent of triose phosphate accumulation and autoxidation of glucose and glycation products. Many of these mechanisms are also implicated in the generation of ROS during reperfusion following ischaemia/hypoxia during which the ratio of $NADH/NAD^+$ is markedly increased, i.e. more NAD^+ is reduced to NADH [5, 47, 70]. A microsomal cytochrome b_5 NADH oxidase which has been demonstrated in endothelial and vascular smooth muscle cells from pulmonary and coronary arteries may be a particularly important source of NADH-induced superoxide production [70]. Additional mechanisms of increased ROS production favoured by an increased NADH/NAD$^+$ ratio include: (1) stimulation of cyclo-oxygenase activity which is associated with ROS production [5, 70], (2) release of Fe^{2+} from ferritin which will catalyse production of ROS via the Fenton reaction [5, 47, 70] and (3) increased oxidation of the substrates xanthine and hypoxanthine by xanthine oxidase (versus xanthine dehydrogenase) which produces much more superoxide than xanthine dehydrogenase (which utilizes NAD$^+$ in preference to oxygen as the electron acceptor) [81]. Reductive stress induced by elevated glucose levels is not nearly as marked as that caused by severe ischaemia/hypoxia and, because it develops in the presence of oxygen, associated ROS production is continuous at a rate corresponding to the rate of production (levels) of reducing equivalents.

The plausibility of the hypothesis that increased ROS resulting from reductive stress contribute to vascular changes induced by the diabetic milieu is supported by evidence that: (1) corresponding vascular changes are induced by ROS alone and (2) antioxidants as well as agents that prevent reductive stress prevent vascular changes induced by diabetes. The effects of ROS on vascular metabolism and function are dose-dependent, i.e. processes that are activated by small elevations in ROS may be inhibited by higher levels. Thus ROS: (1) modulate extracellular matrix production (induce gene expression and synthesis of type 1 collagen in human fibroblasts) [82, 83] and preferentially inhibit glomerular heparin sulphate proteoglycan synthesis versus type IV collagen and laminin [84], (2) increase VEGF mRNA and protein levels [85], (3) modulate production/levels of vasoactive agents, i.e. VEGF, nitric oxide and prostaglandins [5, 70, 85], (4) increase intracellular calcium, pH and arachidonate release [61–63, 68] (which has been linked to protein kinase C-mediated activation of VEGF, cytosolic phospholipase A$_2$ and inhibition of Na$^+$,K$^+$-ATPase [70, 86]), (5) activate protein kinase C [87], (6) activate transcription factors including NF-kB [88, 89], (7) increase protein kinase C-dependent expression of c-*fos*, c-*jun*, and c-*myc* proto-oncogene mRNA levels [88, 90], (8) stimulate vascular smooth muscle cell proliferation (protein kinase C-independent) [90, 91], (9) inhibit DNA synthesis in endothelial cells and fibroblasts [90], (10) stimulate human fibroblast proliferation [92], (11) reduce Na$^+$,K$^+$-ATPase activity [93], (12) mediate post-ischaemic myocardial stunning [94] and (13) inactivate pyruvate dehydrogenase [95].

The linkage between many of these phenomena to reductive stress-induced ROS due to increased sorbitol pathway metabolism, and their role in mediating diabetes induced glomerular dysfunction, is supported by evidence that hyperglycaemia-induced increases in diacylglycerol, protein kinase C, phospholipase A$_2$ and prostaglandin production as well as glomerular dysfunction are prevented by inhibitors of aldose reductase as well as by inhibitors of protein kinase C [5, 96, 97] (refs 13, 65, 67, 89, 93 in [5]). Possible relationships between these imbalances are suggested in Figure 10.4.

10.6.2 CYTOSOLIC REDUCTIVE STRESS AND VASCULAR ENDOTHELIAL GROWTH FACTOR

A potentially important role for VEGF in mediating proliferative retinopathy is supported by several recent investigations [21–25, 85, 98]. The importance of hypoxia as a stimulus for increasing VEGF mRNA and protein levels is well documented. However, the mechanism(s) by which hypoxia increases VEGF is not well understood. Evidence that elevated glucose levels also increase VEGF mRNA and protein levels (independent of hypoxia) in cultured human aortic vascular smooth muscle cells (mediated by protein kinase C) and in retinal pigment epithelial cells [22, 23] raises the possibility that: (1) increased VEGF mRNA and protein levels induced by hypoxia and by elevated glucose levels may be mediated by increased cytosolic free $NADH/NAD^+$ and (2) increased VEGF may play a role in mediating vascular dysfunction induced by hyperglycaemia *per se* early after the onset of diabetes (in the absence of vascular occlusive disease and hypoxia). The plausibility of this hypothesis is supported by observations (in the skin chamber granulation tissue model) that increased granulation tissue blood flow and vascular albumin permeation induced by elevated glucose levels (and by elevated sorbitol levels at normal glucose levels) in non-diabetic rats are markedly attenuated or prevented by: (1) interventions that decrease cytosolic free $NADH/NAD^+$, i.e. inhibitors of sorbitol pathway metabolism or administration of pyruvate [21, 57, 99], and (2) antibodies to VEGF [21].

The likelihood that ROS mediate hypoxia and hyperglycaemia-stimulated increased VEGF levels is supported by evidence that a superoxide-generating system (xanthine oxidase + hypoxanthine) increases VEGF mRNA and protein levels in cultured cells [85], causes cytoplasmic alkalinization which has been linked to initiation of DNA synthesis by growth factors [68, 90] and increases blood flow and vascular albumin permeation (in skin chamber granulation tissue) to the same extent as that caused by elevated glucose levels [21]. These vascular changes, like those induced by elevated glucose and sorbitol levels, are prevented by VEGF antibodies as well as by inhibitors of nitric oxide synthase, and by superoxide dismutase [21] (unpublished observations). All of these observations are consistent with evidence that vascular dysfunction caused by VEGF is mediated by nitric oxide [100–102]. Both VEGF and superoxide increase intracellular calcium levels which activate the constitutive isoform of nitric oxide synthase [21, 61–63].

10.6.3   CYTOSOLIC REDUCTIVE STRESS, *DE NOVO* SYNTHESIS OF DIACYLGLYCEROL, AND ACTIVATION OF PROTEIN KINASE C

Activation of protein kinase C (PKC), particularly the β-isoform, has been demonstrated in cultured vascular cells exposed to elevated glucose levels and in several tissues (retina, heart, kidney and aorta) of diabetic rats [23, 32, 97, 98]. VEGF also activates PKC (and PKC-dependent phospholipase D) in cultured cells [103, 104]. Inhibitors of PKC or sequelae of PKC activation prevent vascular dysfunction in these same tissues [96, 105]. They also attenuate or prevent vascular dysfunction induced by elevated glucose levels in the granulation tissue model [99, 105] (unpublished observations with LY333531, a selective inhibitor of the β-isoform of PKC).

Cytosolic reductive stress induced by elevated glucose levels may activate PKC by at least three mechanisms. Evidence considered above suggests that PKC can be activated by VEGF (increased levels of which may be mediated by superoxide generated by reductive stress). Increased free $NADH/NAD^+$ also favours reduction of dihydroxyacetone phosphate (a triose phosphate) to glycerol 3-phosphate coupled to oxidation of NADH to NAD^+ by glucose-3-phosphate dehydrogenase (Figure 10.2), the first step in one pathway for *de novo* synthesis of diacylglycerol, a natural activator of PKC [99]. *De novo* synthesis of diacylglycerol also can occur by direct acylation of dihydroxyacetone phosphate followed by reduction of carbon 2 (using the cofactor NADPH as the hydrogen donor) to form lysophosphatidic acid which is then acylated to form phosphatidate and dephosphorylated to yield diacylglycerol [99]. Although this synthetic pathway would be favoured by an increased ratio of $NADPH/NADP^+$ as observed in nerve noted earlier, peripheral nerve is one tissue in which diacylglycerol levels are not increased by diabetes [5, 26] and the role of activation of protein kinase C in mediating diabetic neuropathy is unclear. Nevertheless, inhibitors of protein kinase C normalize peripheral nerve Na$^+$,K$^+$-ATPase activity in diabetic mice [106]. Despite evidence that diacylglycerol levels are not increased in peripheral nerve of diabetic rats, normalization of electrophysiological dysfunction is associated with a significant decrease in diacylglcerol [26]. The potential importance of these mechanisms of *de novo* diacylglycerol synthesis (and associated activation of PKC) in other tissues, however, is supported by evidence that elevated glucose levels stimulate *de novo* synthesis of diacylglycerol in glomeruli as well as in cultured vascular cells and that diacylglycerol levels are increased in several tissues of diabetic rats and in granulation tissue (in non-diabetic rats) exposed to elevated glucose levels [5, 32, 97, 99] (refs 65, 67 in [5]).

10.6.4 VASCULAR CONSEQUENCES OF CYTOSOLIC REDUCTIVE STRESS IN NON-VASCULAR VERSUS VASCULAR CELLS

Vascular consequences of hyperglycaemia-induced cytosolic reductive stress may be mediated by reductive stress in non-vascular parenchymal cells as well as in vascular cells *per se*. VEGF mRNA and protein levels are increased in: (1) cultured RPE cells (as well as in human aortic smooth muscle cells) exposed to elevated glucose levels noted earlier [22, 23] and (2) neural and glial cells remote from areas of vascular occlusion (potentially hypoxic areas) and angiogenesis in retinas from diabetic humans and animals [24, 25]. These observations suggest a potentially important role for increased production of growth factors, induced by hypoxia-like reductive stress in non-vascular cells, in the pathogenesis of retinal vascular dysfunction and angiogenesis.

The inability of Thomas *et al.* to demonstrate increased lactate/pyruvate ratios in cultured retinal pigment epithelial cells exposed to elevated glucose levels [107] may be due to any one of several effects of the *in vitro* milieu including marked changes in glucose metabolism and oxidative stress when cells are cultured in media equilibrated with 20% oxygen [108]. In the report of Thomas *et al.*, lactate/pyruvate ratios in cells grown in media containing 5 mM glucose were over 100 in contrast to lactate/pyruvate ratios of 20 to 30 in whole retinas incubated in 5 mM glucose and comparable or slightly lower lactate/pyruvate ratios in freshly removed retinas [4] (refs 36, 37, 58 in [4]). Gilles *et al.* also reported that elevated glucose levels had no effect on lactate/pyruvate ratios in cultured bovine retinal capillary endothelial cells [109]; lactate/pyruvate ratios in their experiments were ~9 for cells grown in 5 or 30 mM glucose. These remarkably low ratios raise questions regarding the conditions of these experiments, including the lactate and pyruvate content of the medium and the metabolic state of the cells. The experimental conditions for demonstration of cytosolic reductive stress are very critical, not only for cultured cells, but also for incubated tissues and for tissues *in vivo*. Extraordinary care and attention to detail are required for rapid tissue sampling as well as for extraction and measurement of lactate and pyruvate in order to obtain reliable data. Even when these precautions are observed, because of changes in glucose metabolism in cultured cells in general and the oxidative stress cells experience under standard culture conditions, cultured cells may not be a reliable paradigm for investigating effects of elevated glucose levels on cytosolic reductive stress or oxidative stress. To the extent that observations in cultured cells and incubated tissues are discordant with *in vivo* data, clearly the relevance of the *in vitro* data to the *in vivo* milieu is questionable.

Observations in transgenic mice overexpressing GLUT 1 transporters exclusively in skeletal muscle also attest to the impact of sorbitol pathway-mediated cytosolic reductive stress in non-vascular cells on vascular function. In these mice, plasma glucose levels are slightly lower than in control mice and plasma insulin levels are normal but intracellular free glucose levels in skeletal muscle are elevated fourfold [110]. Skeletal muscle blood flow is selectively increased in these transgenic mice compared with controls. The increased blood flow and markedly increased muscle sorbitol levels are reversed by inhibitors of aldose reductase [111]. These findings support the importance of sorbitol pathway-mediated reductive stress, induced by elevated intracellular glucose levels (despite normal or slightly lower than normal extracellular glucose levels), in non-vascular (muscle) cells on blood flow.

10.6.5   CYTOSOLIC REDUCTIVE STRESS, PARADOXICAL RESPONSES TO ISCHAEMIC INJURY, AND METABOLIC SUPPRESSION

Since mechanisms of reductive stress induced by hypoxia and by hyperglycaemia are different and their effects are additive, hypoxia/ischaemia may cause more severe vascular and neural dysfunction and injury in cells and tissues experiencing hyperglycaemia-induced reductive stress than in non-diabetic subjects. This prediction appears to be confirmed in some tissues and conditions. However, paradoxical findings are observed in others. While basal electrophysiological function (nerve conduction velocity) is impaired by diabetes in retina and peripheral nerve, these same tissues are more resistant to ischaemia-induced electrophysiological dysfunction [28, 66, 112]; in peripheral nerve both of these phenomena are prevented by aldose reductase inhibitors [28]. On the other hand, more extensive ischaemic structural damage develops in peripheral nerve in diabetic versus control rats following injection of microspheres or topical application of endothelin 1, a potent vasoconstrictor peptide (refs. 28, 50 in [7]).

Basal myocardial contractile function is impaired in diabetic rats and global ischaemia-induced contractile dysfunction develops more rapidly than in control hearts whereas, during reperfusion, recovery of ischaemia-induced myocyte and vascular smooth muscle cell contractile function is improved in hearts from diabetic versus control rats. In contrast, although basal endothelial barrier function does not differ in perfused hearts from controls and diabetic subjects prior to global ischaemia, vascular albumin permeation during reperfusion is two- to threefold higher in hearts from diabetic subjects compared with controls. These paradoxical observations on the effects of diabetes on basal versus post-ischaemic myocyte and vascular smooth muscle cell contractile function and endothelial cell barrier function have been linked to impaired activity of ATPase-dependent enzymes involved in ion transport (Na^+, K^+, Ca^{2+} and H^+) and contractile function [5, 113–115]. Myocardial ATP and phosphocreatine levels have been reported to be unchanged or decreased in hearts from diabetic animals [113, 114, 116]; the discordance in these observations may be related to differences in duration and/or severity of diabetes, tissue sampling procedures, etc. It is noteworthy that most measurements of myocardial ATP and phosphocreatine in diabetic animals have been obtained after *in vitro* perfusion with media containing much lower glucose levels that the plasma glucose levels of the donors.

ATP levels are normal in peripheral nerve and retina of diabetic rats although ouabain-sensitive ATPase (Na^+,K^+-ATPase) is decreased in both tissues [30, 117, 118]. In the retina Ca^{2+},Mg^{2+}-ATPase also is reduced, but not ouabain-insensitive ATPase [117], whereas ouabain-insensitive ATPase activity also is decreased in the nerve [30]. In sciatic nerve of diabetic rabbits, oxygen consumption and ATP production are decreased ~30% although ATP and phosphocreatine levels are normal [119]. In diabetic rabbits Na^+,K^+-ATPase activity is decreased in retinal pigment epithelial (RPE) cells and in selected layers of the neural retina, Na^+ is increased in RPE cells (indicative of impaired Na^+,K^+-ATPase activity) and sorbitol levels are increased whereas *myo*-inositol levels are decreased [120]. Corresponding changes in peripheral nerve in diabetic rats are largely prevented by inhibitors of aldose reductase [28].

These observations in non-ischaemic heart, nerve and retina demonstrate that diabetes: (1) decreases the activity of ATPases (required to support work, i.e. mechanical, electrophysiological and maintenance of transmembrane ionic gradients) and ATP synthesis (as well as oxygen consumption) whereas ATP levels remain normal and (2) impairs resting (basal) contractile and electrophysiological function of cells. These findings indicate that ATP utilization is impaired by diabetes and are consistent with the concept of 'metabolic suppression' [121], i.e. a coordinated decrease in: (1) utilization of ATP by ATPases for work and (2) consumption of oxygen and substrates for ATP synthesis. Metabolic suppression is postulated to be a defence mechanism which increases resistance to hypoxia and hypothermia-induced cellular dysfunction and injury by slowing the rate of depletion of ATP (and accumulation of toxic levels of products of energy metabolism, i.e. lactate and H^+) needed to maintain critical membrane ionic gradients.

Thus, many of the metabolic imbalances and functional impairments induced by the diabetic milieu may be explained by mild chronic metabolic suppression caused by hypoxia-like cytosolic reductive stress. This hypothesis is supported by the correspondence between the effects of diabetes and of hypoxic preconditioning or stunning, both of which cause: (1) mild impairment of cellular function, (2) resistance to ischaemia/hypoxia-induced dysfunction, (3) improved recovery of dysfunction during reperfusion following ischaemia/hypoxia and (4) translocation (activation) of protein kinase C [122–124].

10.7 CONCLUSIONS

Observations in several animal models of diabetes attest to an important role for cytosolic reductive stress, i.e. a hypoxia-like increased cytosolic ratio of free $NADH/NAD^+$, in the pathogenesis of early vascular dysfunction as well as vascular structural changes induced by diabetes. Although this redox change in animal models of diabetes and in human erythrocytes is mediated largely by increased flux of glucose via the sorbitol pathway, other mechanisms may be equally or more important in mediating reductive stress in tissues prone to development of vascular disease in human diabetic subjects. The potentially important implication of these findings is that pharmacological interventions which prevent cytosolic reductive stress (i.e. prevent pathophysiological increases in the rate of reduction of NAD^+ to NADH or promote increased oxidation of NADH to NAD^+) or its sequelae could be efficacious in the prevention and treatment of complications of diabetes. Pharmacological agents of this genre also may be useful in the prevention and treatment of other conditions associated with reductive stress of diverse origins.

REFERENCES

1. Diabetes Control and Complications Trial. The relationship of glycemic exposure (HbA1c) to the risk of development and progression of retinopathy in the Diabetes Control and Complications Trial. *Diabetes*, 1995, **44**, 968–83.
2. Kohner, E.M., Patel, V. and Rassam, S.M.B. Role of blood flow and impaired autoregulation in the pathogenesis of diabetic retinopathy. *Diabetes*, 1995, **44**, 603–7.
3. Tilton, R.G., Baier, L.D., Harlow, J.E., Smith, S.R., Ostrow, E. and Williamson, J.R. Diabetes-induced glomerular dysfunction: Links to a more reduced cytosolic ratio of $NADH/NAD^+$. *Kidney Int.*, 1992, **41**, 78–88.
4. Van den Enden, M.K., Nyengaard, J.R., Ostrow, E., Burgan, J.H. and Williamson, J.R. Elevated glucose levels increase retinal glycolysis and sorbitol pathway metabolism:

Implications for diabetic retinopathy. *Investigative Ophthalmol. Vis. Sci.*, 1995, **36,** 1675–85.

5. Williamson, J.R., Chang, K., Frangos, M., Hasan, K.S., Ido, Y., Kawamura, T., Nyengaard, J.R., Van den Enden, M., Kilo, C. and Tilton, R. G. Hyperglycemic pseudohypoxia and diabetic complications. *Diabetes*, 1993, **42,** 801–13.

6. Chang, K., Ido, Y., LeJeune, W., Williamson, J.R. and Tilton, R. G. Increased sciatic nerve blood flow in diabetic rats: assessment by 'molecular' vs. particulate microspheres. *Am. J. Physiol.*, 1997, **273,** E164–173.

7. Ido, Y., Chang, K., LeJeune, W., Tilton, R.G., Monafo, W.W. and Williamson, J.R. Diabetes impairs sciatic nerve hyperaemia induced by surgical trauma: Implications for diabetic neuropathy. *Am. J. Physiol.*, 1997, **273,** E174–184.

8. Tilton, R.G., Chang, K., Allison, W. and Williamson, J.R. Comparable diabetes induced increases in retinal blood flow assessed with conventional vs "molecular" (^{3}H-desmethylimiprimine) microspheres (Abstract). *Invest. Ophthalmol. Vis. Sci.*, 1992, **33,** 1048 (abstract).

9. Nyengaard, J.R., Chang, K., Berhorst, S., Reiser, K.M., Williamson, J.R. and Tilton, R.G. Discordant effects of guanidines on renal structure and function and on regional vascular dysfunction and collagen changes in diabetic rats. *Diabetes*, 1997, **46,** 94–106.

10. Pugliese, G., Tilton, R.G., Speedy, A., Chang, K., Santarelli, E., Province, M.A., Eades, D., Sherman, W.R. and Williamson, J.R. Effects of very mild versus overt diabetes on vascular haemodynamics and barrier function in rats. *Diabetologia*, 1989, **32,** 845–57.

11. Tooke, J.E. Microvascular function in human diabetes. A physiological perspective. *Diabetes*, 1995, **44,** 721–6.

12. Diemel, L.T., Stevens, E.J., Willars, G. and Tomlinson, D.R. Depletion of substance P and calcitonin gene-related peptide in sciatic nerve of rats with experimental diabetes: effects of insulin and aldose reductase inhibition. *Neurosci. Lett.*, 1992, **137,** 253–6.

13. Lightman, S., Pinter, G., Yuen, L. and Bradbury, M. Permeability changes at blood-retinal barrier in diabetes and effect of aldose reductase inhibition. *Am. J. Physiol.*, 1990, **259,** R601–R605.

14. Williamson, J.R., Hoffmann, P.L., Kohrt, W.M., Spina, R.J., Coggan, A.R. and Holloszy, J.O. Endurance exercise training decreases capillary basement membrane width in older non-diabetic and diabetic adults. *J. Appl. Physiol.*, 1996, **80,** 747–53.

15. Engerman, R.L. Pathogenesis of diabetic retinopathy. *Diabetes*, 1989, 38, 1203–6.

16. Robison, W.G., Jr., McCaleb, M.L., Feld, L.G., Michaelis, O.E.I., Laver, N. and Mercandetti, M. Degenerated intramural pericytes ('ghost cells') in the retinal capillaries of diabetic rats. *Curr. Eye Res.*, 1991, **10,** 339–50.

17. Tilton, R.G., Faller, A.M., Burkhardt, J. K., Hoffmann, P.L., Kilo, C. and Williamson, J.R. Pericyte degeneration and acellular capillaries are increased in the feet of human diabetics. *Diabetologia*, 1985, **28,** 895–900.

18. Giannini, C. and Dyck, P.J. Basement membrane reduplication and pericyte degeneration precede development of diabetic polyneuropathy and are associated with its severity. *Ann. Neurol.*, 1995, **37,** 498–504.

19. Yagihashi, S. Pathology and pathogenetic mechanisms of diabetic neuropathy. *Diabetes Metab. Rev.*, 1995, **11,** 193–225.

20. Mauer, S.M., Steffes, M.W., Ellis, E.N., Sutherland, D.E.R., Brown, D.M. and Goetz, F.C. Structural–functional relationships in diabetic nephropathy. *J. Clin. Invest.*, 1984, **74,** 1143–55.

21. Tilton, R.G., Kawamura, T., Chang, K.C., Ido, Y., Bjercke, R.J., Stephan, C.C., Brock, T.A. and Williamson, J.R. Vascular dysfunction induced by elevated glucose levels in rats is mediated by vascular endothelial growth factor. *J. Clin. Invest.*, 1997, **99,** 2192–202.

22. Sone, S., Kawakami, Y., Okuda, Y., Kondo, S., Hanatani, M., Suzuki, H. and Yamashita, K. Vascular endothelial growth factor is induced by long-term high glucose concentration and up-regulated by acute glucose deprivation in cultured bovine retinal pigmented epithelial cells. *Biochem. Biophys. Res. Commun.*, 1996, **221,** 193–8.

23. Williams, B., Gallacher, B., Patel, H. and Orme, C. Glucose-induced protein kinase C activation regulates vascular permeability factor mRNA expression and peptide production by human vascular smooth muscle cells, *in vitro. Diabetes*, 1997, **46,** 1497–503.

24. Amin, R.H., Frank, R.N., Kennedy, A., Eliott, D., Puklin, J.E. and Abrams, G.W. Vascular

endothelial growth factor is present in glial cells of the retina and optic nerve of human subjects with nonproliferative diabetic retinopathy. Investigative *Ophthalmol. Vis. Sci.*, 1997, **38**, 36–47.

25. Murata, T., Nakagawa, K., Kahlil, A., Ishibashi, T., Inomata, H. and Sueishi, K. The relation between expression of vascular endothelial growth factor and breakdown of the blood-retinal barrier in diabetic rat retinas. *Lab. Invest.*, 1996, **74**, 819–25.

26. Baynes, J.W. Role of oxidative stress in development of complications in diabetes. *Diabetes*, 1991, **40**, 405–12.

27. Brownlee, M. Glycation and diabetic complications. *Diabetes*, 1994, **43**, 836–41.

28. Cameron, N.E. and Cotter, M.A. The relationship of vascular changes to metabolic factors in diabetes mellitus and their role in the development of peripheral nerve complications. *Diabetes Metab. Rev.*, 1994, **10**, 189–224.

29. Ido, Y., Kilo, C. and Williamson, J.R. Interactions between the sorbitol pathway, non-enzymatic glycation, and diabetic vascular dysfunction. *Nephrol. Dial. Transpl.*, 1996, **11**, (suppl 5), 72–5.

30. Ido, Y., McHowat, J., Chang, K.C., Arrigoni-Martelli, E., Orfalian, Z., Kilo, C., Corr, P.B. and Williamson, J.R. Neural dysfunction and metabolic imbalances in diabetic rats. Prevention by acetyl-L-carnitine. *Diabetes*, 1994, **43**, 1469–77.

31. Kinoshita, J.H. and Nishimura, C. The involvement of aldose reductase in diabetic complications. *Diabetes Metab. Rev.*, 1988, **4**, 323–37.

32. Lee, T.S., Saltsman, K.A., Ohashi, H. and King, G.L. Activation of protein kinase C by elevation of glucose concentration. Proposal for a mechanism in the development of diabetic vascular complications. *Proc. Natl Acad. Sci. U.S.A.*, 1989, **86**, 5141–5.

33. Soulis-Liparota, T., Cooper, M.E., Dunlop, M. and Jerums, G. The relative roles of advanced glycation, oxidation and aldose reductase inhibition in the development of experimental diabetic nephropathy in the Sprague-Dawley rat. *Diabetologia*, 1995, **38**, 387–94.

34. Vlassara, H., Bucala, R. and Striker, L. Biology of disease: Pathogenic effects of advanced glycosylation: Biochemical, biologic, and clinical implications for diabetes and aging. *Lab. Invest.*, 1994, **70**, 138–51.

35. Tilton, R.G., Chang, K., Nyengaard, J.R., Van den Enden, M., Ido, Y. and Williamson, J.R. Inhibition of sorbitol dehydrogenase. Effects on vascular and neural dysfunction in streptozocin-induced diabetic rats. *Diabetes*, 1995, **44**, 234–42.

36. Frank, R.N. The aldose reductase controversy. *Diabetes*, 1994, **43**, 169–72.

37. Stevens, M.J., Lattimer, S.A., Kamijo, M., Van Huysen, C., Sima, A.A.F. and Greene, D.A. Osmotically-induced nerve taurine depletion and the compatible osmolyte hypothesis in experimental diabetic neuropathy in the rat. *Diabetologia*, 1993, **36**, 608–14.

38. Cameron, N.E., Cotter, M.A., Dines, K.C. and Maxfield, E.K. Pharmacological manipulation of vascular endothelium function in non-diabetic and streptozotocin-diabetic rats: effects on nerve conduction, hypoxic resistance and endoneurial capillarization. *Diabetologia*, 1993, **36**, 516–22.

39. Nagamatsu, M., Nickander, K.K., Schmelzer, J.D., Raya, A., Wittrock, D.A., Tritschler, H. and Low, P.A. Lipoic acid improves nerve blood flow, reduces oxidative stress, and improves distal nerve conduction in experimental diabetic neuropathy. *Diabetes Care*, 1995, **18**, 1160–7.

40. Stevens, M.J., Dananberg, J., Feldman, E.L., Lattimer, S.A., Kamijo, M., Thomas, T.P., Shindo, H., Sima, A.A. and Greene, D.A. The linked roles of nitric oxide, aldose reductase and, (Na^+,K^+)-ATPase in the slowing of nerve conduction in the streptozotocin diabetic rat. *J. Clin. Invest.*, 1994, **94**, 853–9.

41. Williamson, D.H., Lund, P. and Krebs, H.A. The redox state of free nicotinamide-adenine dinucleotide in the cytoplasm and mitochondria of rat liver. *Biochem. J.*, 1967, **103**, 514–27.

42. Ramasamy, R., Oates, P.J. and Schaefer, S. Aldose reductase inhibition protects diabetic and nondiabetic rat hearts from ischemic injury. *Diabetes*,1997, **46**, 292–300.

43. Ido, Y., Ostrow, E., Mylari, B.L., Oates, P.J. and Williamson, J. R. Decreased motor nerve conduction velocity (MNCV) in diabetic rats is linked to cytosolic reductive stress. *Diabetologia*, 1997, **40** (suppl. 2), 5115–17.

44. Obrosova, I., Faller, A., Burgan, J. and Williamson, J.R. Mitochondrial redox state of NAD-couples and energy metabolism in sciatic nerve of rats with short-term diabetes

and galactosaemia. Effect of an aldose reductase inhibitor. *Diabetes*, 1996, **45,** (suppl 2), 191A (abstract).

45. Obrosova, I., Marvel, J., Faller, A.M. and Williamson, J.R. Reductive stress is a very early metabolic imbalance in sciatic nerve in diabetic and galactose-fed rats. *Diabetologia*, 1995, **38,** (suppl 1), A8.

46. Anundi, I., King, J., Owen, D.A., Schneider, H., Lemasters, J.J. and Thurman, R.G. Fructose prevents hypoxic cell death in liver. *Am. J. Physiol.*, 1987, **253,** G390–G396.

47. Khan, S. and O'Brien, P.J. Modulating hypoxia-induced hepatocyte injury by affecting intracellular redox state. *Biochim. Biophys. Acta*, 1995, **1269,** 153–61.

48. Kobayashi, K. and Neely, J.R. Control of maximum rates of glycolysis in rat cardiac muscle. *Circulation Res.*, 1979, **44,** 166–75.

49. Winegrad, A.I. and Burden, C.L. L-Xylulose metabolism in diabetes mellitus. *N. Engl. J. Med.*, 1966, **274,** 298–305.

50. Kim, D.K., Heineman, F.W. and Balaban, R.S. Effects of β-hydroxybutyrate on oxidative metabolism and phosphorylation potential in canine heart *in vivo*. *Am. J. Physiol.*, 1991, **260,** H1767–H1773.

51. Neely, J.R., Whitmer, K.M. and Mochizuki, S. Effects of mechanical activity and hormones on myocardial glucose and fatty acid utilization. *Circulation Res.*, 1976, **38** (suppl 1), 122–30.

52. Sato, K., Kashiwaya, Y., Keon, C.A., Tsukchiya, N., King, M.T., Radda, G.K., Chance, B., Clarke, K. and Veech, R.L. Insulin, ketone bodies, and mitochondrial energy transduction. *FASEB J.*, 1995, **9,** 651–58.

53. Williamson, J.R. Glycolytic control mechanisms. II. Kinetics of intermediate changes during the aerobic-anoxic transition in perfused rat heart. *J. Biol. Chem.*, 1966, **241,** 5026–36.

54. Williamson, J.R., Kreisberg, R.A. and Felts, P.W. Mechanism for the stimulation of gluconeogenesis by fatty acids in perfused rat liver. *Proc. Natl Acad. Sci. U.S.A.*, 1966, **56,** 247–54.

55. Ido, Y., LeJeune, W.S., Chang, K. and Williamson, J.R. Cytosolic reductive stress and increased superoxide and nitric oxide production mediate increased blood flow induced by lactate. *Diabetes*, 1997, **46** (suppl 1), 235A (abstract).

56. Williamson, J.R., Chang, K. and Ido, Y. The role of reductive stress in mediating increased retinal and sciatic nerve blood flow induced by diabetes. *Diabetologia*, 1995, **38** (suppl 1), A276 (abstract).

57. Williamson, J.R., Ostrow, E., Eades, D.M., Chang, K., Allison, W., Kilo, C. and Sherman, W.R. Glucose-induced microvascular functional changes in nondiabetic rats are stereospecific and are prevented by an aldose reductase inhibitor. *J. Clin. Invest.*, 1990, **85,** 1167–72.

58. Brooks, G.A. Lactate production under fully aerobic conditions: the lactate shuttle during rest and exercise. *Fed. Proc.*, 1986, **45,** 2924–9.

59. Fox, P.T., Raichle, M.E., Mintun, M.A. and Dence, C. Nonoxidative glucose consumption during focal physiologic neural activity. *Science*, 1988, **241,** 462–4.

60. Ueki, M., Linn, F. and Hossmann, K.A. Functional activation of cerebral blood flow and metabolism before and after global ischemia of rat brain. *J. Cerebral Blood Flow Metab.*, **8,** 486–94.

61. Franceschi, D., Graham, D., Sarasua, M. and Zollinger, R.M. Mechanisms of oxygen free radical-induced calcium overload in endothelial cells. *Surgery*, 1990, **108,** 292–7.

62. Ikebuchi, Y., Masumoto, N., Tasaka, K., Koike, K. and Kasahara, K. Superoxide anion increases intracellular pH, intracellular free calcium, and arachidonate release in human amnion cells. *J. Biol. Chem.*, 1991, **266,** 13233–7.

63. Masumoto, N., Tasaka, K., Miyake, A. and Tanizawa, O. Superoxide anion increases intracellular free calcium in human myometrial cells. *J. Biol. Chem.*, 1990, **265,** 22533–6.

64. Asahina, T., Kashiwagi, A., Yoshihiko, N., Ikebuchi, M., Harada, N., Tanaka, Y., Takagi, Y., Saeki, Y., Kikkawa, R. and Shigeta, Y. Impaired activtion of glucose oxidation and NADPH supply in human endothelial cells exposed to H_2O_2 in high-glucose medium. *Diabetes*, 1995, **44,** 520–6.

65. Hotta, N., Koh, N., Sakakibara, F., Nakamura, J., Hamada, Y., Hara, T., Mori, K., Nakashima, E., Naruse, K., Fukasawa, H., Kakuta, H. and Sakamoto, N. Effects of Beraprost sodium and insulin on the electroretinogram, nerve conduction, and nerve blood flow in

rats with streptozotocin-induced diabetes. *Diabetes*, 1996, **45,** 361–6.

66. Tesfaye, S., Malik, R. and Ward, J.D. Vascular factors in diabetic neuropathy. *Diabetologia*, 1994, **37,** 847–54.

67. Heinecke, J.W. and Shapiro, B.M. The respiratory burst oxidase of fertilization. A physiological target for regulation by protein kinase C. *J. Biol. Chem.*, 1992, **267,** 7959–62.

68. Shibanuma, M., Kuroki, T. and Nose, K. Superoxide as a signal for increase in intracellular pH. *J. Cell. Physiol.*, 1988, **136,** 379–83.

69. Sundaresan, M., Yu, Z.-X., Ferrans, V. J., Irani, K. and Finkel, T. Requirement for generation of H_2O_2 for platelet-derived growth factor signal transduction. *Science*, 1995, **270,** 296–9.

70. Wolin, M.S. Reactive oxygen species and vascular signal transduction mechanisms. *Microcirculation*, 1996, **3,** 1–17.

71. Hems, D.A. and Brosnan, J.T. Effects of ischaemia on content of metabolites in rat liver and kidney *in vivo*. *Biochem. J.*, 1970, **120,** 105–11.

72. Lowry, O.H., Passonneau, J.V., Hasselberger, F.X. and Schulz, D.W. Effect of ischaemia on known substrates and co-factors of the glycolytic pathway in brain. *J. Biol. Chem.*, 1964, **239,** 18–30.

73. Vander Jag, D.L., Robinson, B., Taylor, K.K. and Hunsaker, L. A. Reduction of trioses by NADPH-dependent aldo-keto reductases. Aldose reductase, methylglyoxal, and diabetic complications. *J. Biol. Chem.*, 1992, **267,** 4364–9.

74. González Flecha, F.L., Bermúdez, M.C., Cédola, N.V., Gagliardino, J.J. and Rossi, J.P.F.C. Decreased Ca^{2+}-ATPase activity after glycosylation of erythrocyte membranes *in vivo* and *in vitro*. *Diabetes,* 1990, **39,** 7–11.

75. Kawamura, N., Ookawara, T., Suzuki, K, Konishi, K., Mino, M. and Taniguchi, N. Increased glycated Cu,Zn-superoxide dismutase levels in erythrocytes of patients with insulin-dependent diabetes mellitus. *J. Clin. Endocrinol. Metab.*, 1992, **74,** 1352–4.

76. Tehrani, S.T., Yamamoto, J.J. and Garner, M.H. Na^+,K^+-ATPase and changes in ATP hydrolysis, monovalent cation affinity, and K^+ occlusion in diabetic and galactosemic rats. *Diabetes*, 1990, **39,** 1472–8.

77. Corbett, J.A., Tilton, R.G., Chang, K., Hasan, K.S., Ido, Y., Wang, J.L., Sweetland, M.A., Lancaster, J.R., Jr., Williamson, J.R. and McDaniel, M.L. Aminoguanidine, a novel inhibitor of nitric oxide formation prevents diabetic vascular dysfunction. *Diabetes*, 1992, **41,** 552–6.

78. Misko, T.P., Moore, W.M., Kasten, T.P., Nickols, G.A., Corbett, J.A., Tilton, R.G., McDaniel, M.L., Williamson, J.R. and Currie, M.G. Selective inhibition of the inducible nitric oxide synthase by aminoguanidine. *Eur. J. Pharmacol.*, 1993, **233,** 119–25.

79. Tilton, R.G., Chang, K., Hasan, K.S., Smith, S., Petrash, J.M., Misko, T.P., Moore, W.M., Currie, M.G., Corbett, J.A., McDaniel, M.L. and Williamson, J.R. Prevention of diabetic vascular dysfunction by guanidines: Inhibition of nitric oxide synthase versus advanced glycation end product formation. *Diabetes*, 1993, **42,** 221–32.

80. Tilton, R.G., Chang, K. and Faller, A.M. Probucol prevents vascular protein leakage induced by diabetes, glucose and glycated proteins. *Diabetes*, 1993, **42** (suppl 1), 89A (abstract).

81. Nishino, T. and Tamura, I. The mechanism of conversion of xanthine dehydrogenase to oxidase and the role of the enzyme in reperfusion injury. *Adv. Exp. Med. Biol.*, 1991, **309A,** 135–8.

82. Chandrakasan, G. and Bhatnagar, R.S. Stimulation of collagen synthesis in fibroblast cultures by superoxide. *Cell. Mol. Biol.*, 1991, **37,** 751–5.

83. Chojkier, M., Houglum, K., Solis-Herruzo, J. and Brenner, D.A. Stimulation of collagen gene expression by ascorbic acid in cultured human fibroblasts. *J. Biol. Chem.*, 1989, **264,** 16957–62.

84. Kashihara, N., Watanabe, Y., Makino, H., Wallner, E.I. and Kanwar, Y. S. Selective decreased *de novo* synthesis of glomerular proteoglycans under the influence of reactive oxygen species. *Proc. Natl Acad. Sci. U.S.A.*, 1992, **89,** 6309–13.

85. Kuroki, M., Voest, E.E., Amano, S., Beerepoot, L.V., Takashima, S., Tolentino, M., Kim, R.Y., Rohan, R.M., Colby, K.A., Yeo, K.T. and Adamis, A.P. Reactive oxygen intermediates increase vascular endothelial growth factor expression *in vitro* and *in vivo*. *J. Clin. Invest.*, 1996, **98,** 1667–75.

86. Xia, P., Kramer, R.M. and King, G.L. Identification of the mechanism for the inhibition of Na$^+$, K$^+$-adenosine triphosphatase by hyperglycemia involving activation of protein kinase C and cytosotic phospholipase A$_2$. *J. Clin. Invest.*, 1995, **96**, 733–40.

87. Brawn, M.K. and Chiou, W.J. Oxidant-induced activation of protein kinase C in UC11MG cells. *Free Radical Res.*, 1995, **22**, 23–37.

88. Sies, H. Strategies of antioxidant defense. *Eur. J. Biochem.*, 1993, **215**, 213–19.

89. Storz, G., Tartaglia, L.A. and Ames, B.N. Transcriptional regulator of oxidative stress-inducible genes: direct activation by oxidation. *Science,* 1990, **248**, 189–94.

90. Rao, G.N. and Berk, B.C. Active oxygen species stimulate vascular smooth muscle cell growth and protooncogene expression. *Circulation Res.*, 1992, **70**, 593–9.

91. Baas, A.S. and Berk, B.C. Differential activation of mitogen-activated protein kinases by H$_2$O$_2$ and O$_2$- in vascular smooth muscle cells. *Circulation Res.*, 1995, **77**, 29–36.

92. Murrell, G.A.C., Francis, M.J.O. and Bromley, L. Modulation of fibroblast proliferation by oxygen free radicals. *Biochem. J.*, 1990, **265**, 659–65.

93. Kim, M.S. and Akera, T. O$_2$ free radicals: cause of ischaemia-reperfusion injury to cardiac Na$^+$,K$^+$-ATPase. *Am. J. Physiol.*, 1987, **252**, H252–H257.

94. Bolli, R. Oxygen-derived free radicals and myocardial reperfusion injury. An overview. *Cardiovasc. Drugs Ther.*, 1991, **5**, 249–68.

95. Tabatabaie, T., Potts, J.D. and Floyd, R.A. Reactive oxygen species-mediated inactivation of pyruvate dehydrogenase. *Arch. Biochem. Biophys.*, 1996, **336**, 290–6.

96. Ishii, H., Jirousek, M.R., Koya, D., Takagi, C., Xia, P., Clermont, A., Bursell, S.E., Kern, T.S., Bassas, L.M., Heath, W.F., Stramm, L.E., Feener, E.P. and King, G.L. Amelioration of vascular dysfunctions in diabetic rats by an oral PKC β inhibitor. *Science*, 1996, **272**, 728–31.

97. Keogh, R.J., Dunlop, M.E. and Larkins, R.G. Effect of inhibition of aldose reductase on glucose flux, diacylglycerol formation, protein kinase C, and phospholipase A2 activation. *Metabolism*, 1997, **46**, 41–7.

98. Takagi, H., King, G.L. and Aiello, L.P. Identification and characterization of vascular endothelial growth factor receptor (Flt) in bovine retinal pericytes. *Diabetes*, 1996, **45**, 1016–23.

99. Wolf, B.A, Williamson, J.R., Easom, R.A., Chang, K., Sherman, W.R. and Turk, J. Diacylglycerol accumulation and microvascular abnormalities induced by elevated glucose levels. *J. Clin. Invest.*, 1990, **87**, 31–8.

100. Ku, D.D., Zaleski, J.K., Liu, S. and Brock, T.A. Vascular endothelial growth factor induces EDRF-dependent relaxation in coronary arteries. *Am. J. Physiol.*, 1993, **265**, H586–H592.

101. Ramírez, M.M., Kim, D.D. and Durán, W.N. Protein kinase C modulates microvascular permeabililty through nitric oxide synthase. *Am. J. Physiol.*, 1996, **271**, H1702–H1705.

102. Yang, R., Thomas, G.R., Bunting, S., Ko, A., Ferrara, N., Keyt, B., Ross, J. and Jin, H. Effects of vascular endothelial growth factor on hemodynamics and cardiac performance. *J. Cardiovasc. Cardiol.*, 1996, **27**, 838–44.

103. Seymour, L.W., Shoaibi, M.A., Martin, A., Ahmed, A., Elvin, P., Kerr, D.J. and Wakelam, M.J.O. Vascular endothelial growth factor stimulates protein kinase C-dependent phospholipase D activity in endothelial cells. *Lab. Invest.*, 1996, **75**, 427–37.

104. Xia, P., Aiello, L.P., Ishii, H., Jiang, Z.Y., Park, D.J., Robinson, G.S., Takagi, H., Newsome, W.P., Jirousek, M.R. and King, G.L. Characterization of vascular endothelial growth factor's effect on the activation of protein kinase C, its isoforms, and endothelial cell growth. *J. Clin. Invest.*, 1996, **98**, 2018–26.

105. Birch, K.A., Heath, W.F., Hermeling, R.N., Johnston, C.M., Stramm, L., Dell, C., Smith, C., Williamson, J.R. and Reifel-Miller, A. LY290181, an inhibitor of diabetes-induced vascular dysfunction, blocks protein kinase C-stimulated transcriptional activation through inhibition of transcription factor binding to a phorbol response element. *Diabetes*, 1996, **45**, 642–50.

106. Hermenegildo, C., Felipo, V., Miñana, M.D., Romero, F.J. and Grisolia, S. Sustained recovery of Na$^+$,K$^+$-ATPase activity in sciatic nerve of diabetic mice by administration of H7 or Calphostin C, inhibitors of PKC. *Diabetes*, 1993, **42**, 257–62.

107. Thomas, T.P., Porcellati, F., Kato, K., Stevens, M.J., Sherman, W.R. and Greene, D.A. Effects of glucose on sorbitol pathway activation,

cellular redox, and metabolism of myo-inositol, phosphoinositide, and diacylglycerol in cultured human retinal pigment epithelial cells. *J. Clin. Invest.*, 1994, **93**, 2718–24.

108. Akeo, K., Curran, S.A. and Dorey, C.K. Superoxide dismutase activity and growth of retinal pigment epithelial cells are suppressed by 20% oxygen *in vitro. Curr. Eye Res.*, 1988, **7**, 961–6.

109. Gillies, M.C., Su, T., Stayt, J., Simpson, J.M., Naidoo, D. and Salonikas, C. Effect of high glucose on permeability of retinal capillary endothelium *in vitro. Invest. Ophthalmol. Vis. Sci.*, 1997, **38**, 635–42.

110. Ren, J.M., Marshall, B.A., Gulve, E.A., Gao, J. Johnson, D.W., Holloszy, J.O. and Mueckler, M. Evidence from transgenic mice that glucose transport is rate-limiting for glycogen deposition and glycolysis in skeletal muscle. *J. Biol. Chem.*, 1993, **268**, 16113–15.

111. Williamson, J.R., Ido, Y., Ostrow, E., Chang, K., Ensor, N., Marshall, B.A. and Mueckler, M.M. Increased blood flow in murine skeletal muscle overexpressing GLUT-1 is mediated by increased sorbitol pathway metabolism. *Diabetes*, 1997, **46** (suppl 1), 228A (abstract).

112. Rimmer, T. and Linsenmeier, R.A. Resistance of diabetic rat electroretinogram to hypoxaemia. *Invest. Ophthalmol. Vis. Sci.*, 1993, **34**, 3246–52.

113. Tahiliani, A.G. and McNeill, J.H. Diabetes-induced abnormalities in the myocardium. *Life Sci.*, 1986, **38**, 959–74.

114. Tani, M. and Neely, J.R. Hearts from diabetic rats are more resistant to *in vitro* ischaemia. Possible role of altered Ca^{2+} metabolism. *Circulation Res.*, 1988, **62**, 931–40.

115. Tilton, R.G., Daugherty, A., Sutera, S.P., Larson, K.B., Land, M.P., Rateri, D.L., Kilo, C. and Williamson, J.R. Myocyte contracture, vascular resistance, and vascular permeability after global ischaemia in isolated hearts from alloxan-diabetic rabbits. *Diabetes*, 1989, **38**, 1484–91.

116. Mokhtar, N., Rousseau-Migneron, S., Tancrède, G. and Nadeau, A. Physical training attenuates phosphocreatine and long-chain acyl-CoA alterations in diabetic rat heart. *J. Appl. Physiol.*, 1993, **74**, 1785–90.

117. Kern, T.S., Kowluru, R.A. and Engerman, R.L. Abnormalities of retinal metabolism in diabetes or galactosaemia: ATPases and glutathione. *Invest. Ophthalmol. Vis. Sci.*, 1994, **35**, 2962–7.

118. Thurston, J.H., McDougal, D.B., Jr., Hauhart, R.E. and Schulz, D.W. Effects of acute, subacute, and chronic diabetes on carbohydrate and energy metabolism in rat sciatic nerve. *Diabetes*, 1995, **44**, 190–5.

119. Greene, D.A. and Winegrad, A.I. Effects of acute experimental diabetes on composite energy metabolism in peripheral nerve axons and Schwann cells. *Diabetes*, 1981, **30**, 967–74.

120. Marano, C.W. and Matschinsky, F.M. Biochemical manifestations of diabetes mellitus in microscopic layers of the cornea and retina. *Diabetes Metab. Rev.*, 1989, **5**, 1–15.

121. Hochachka, P.W. Defense strategies against hypoxia and hypothermia. Science, 1986, **231**, 234–41.

122. Kida, M., Fujiwara, H., Ishida, M., Kawai, C., Ohura, M., Miura, I. and Yabuuchi, Y. Ischemic preconditioning preserves creatine phosphate and intracellular pH. *Circulation*, 1991, **84**, 2495–503.

123. Liu, Y., Ytrehus, K. and Downey, J.M. Evidence that translocation of protein kinase C is a key event during ischemic preconditioning of rabbit myocardium. *J. Mol. Cell. Cardiol.*, 1994, **26**, 661–8.

124. Schaper, W. Molecular mechanisms in 'stunned' myocardium. *Cardiovasc. Drugs Ther.*, 1991, **5**, 925–32.

A PATHOPHYSIOLOGICAL FRAMEWORK FOR THE PATHOGENESIS OF DIABETIC MICROANGIOPATHY

John E. Tooke

11.1 INTRODUCTION

Since the development of the concept that the origin of many of the late complications of diabetes resided in disease or malfunction of the microvessels of the afflicted organs, innumerable theories have been advanced to explain the origins of such microangiopathy. It has long been recognized that retinopathy and nephropathy represented small vessel damage and yet the pathogenesis remains a subject of debate. However, obtaining reliable human scientific data on a part of the circulation that is both minute, and for the large part inaccessible, has proven technically daunting. Furthermore, resort to animal experimentation does not overcome the problem as there are no perfect animal models of diabetic microangiopathic complications which faithfully reproduce the human condition in its entirety.

With the dawn of new molecular biological techniques, the array of potential cellular mechanisms has been amplified further. However, rather than dismissing the need for an understanding of the pathophysiology of small vessels in the diabetic state, such technology has heightened the need for knowledge against which the legitimacy of candidate mechanisms can be judged and the significance of the abnormality in terms of the functioning of the whole organ and the health of the individual appreciated. Increasingly it has come to be acknowledged that the exploitation of information concerning the functioning of subcellular processes needs to be integrated with an understanding of physiology as a whole.

Knowledge of the pathophysiology of diabetic microangiopathy, which in turn is bedded in an understanding of the normal functioning of the microcirculation, would allow the generation of plausible candidate cellular and molecular mechanisms; plausible in the sense that their disturbance would effect changes compatible with the physiological facts. The principal function of the microcirculation is the exchange of nutrients and metabolites between blood and tissue fluid. It has subsidiary functions, including tissue defence and repair and a variety of specialized functions in different organ beds, e.g. excretion by the kidney, heat dissipation by the skin. The physical parameters defining these transport and exchange functions comprise flow and its spatial distribution, capillary pressure and the intrinsic permeability of the capillary wall and the surface area available for exchange. It is only in the last two decades that techniques have been developed to measure some of these variables in a severely restricted number of vascular beds in man [1].

Before going on to summarize the knowledge describing disturbances of microvascular function in diabetes, it is important to appreciate that, although given a single generic term, microangiopathy, the microvascular abnormalities that occur evolve through stages [2]. Early, partially or completely reversible abnormalities are succeeded by structural adaptation modifying function further; ultimately microvascular function fails, an event that may involve capillary closure or extinction. Even then the microangiopathic process may not be complete. Misplaced, potentially damaging reparative mechanisms may be induced, most notably the neovascularization that may follow retinal underperfusion. Clearly, the functional response of the microvasculature may differ according to the stage, and different organs and individuals will progress along this continuum at differing rates. Indeed intrinsic susceptibility to complications may, according to this analysis, operate through several different mechanisms determining the progression from one stage to another. This makes it highly unlikely that one genetic factor alone will determine such propensity.

Even within the same microvascular bed one component may be more susceptible than another. Although evidence is lacking, it is possible that such localization represents the imperfect geometry of the microvascular bed which dictates that functional characteristics such as pressure, and flow cannot be uniformly distributed. Such a scheme is analogous with the localization of atheroma and its precursors in arteries at the point of turbulence and altered shear stress. Alternatively, maldistribution may represent a primary malfunction of those intrinsic microvascular compensatory mechanisms that serve to ensure homogeneity of distribution over time and space to overcome geometric asymmetry.

11.2 INDIRECT EVIDENCE FOR MICROVASCULAR MALFUNCTION IN DIABETES

The evidence for haemodynamic disturbance at a microvascular level has been slow to accumulate and, until the development of direct techniques, was reliant on inference from non-specific findings, clinical observation and extrapolation from whole organ blood flow studies.

First to emerge were observations suggesting that maximum perfusion to the extremities might be limited. Megibow *et al.* described reduction in toe arterial inflow following release of all sympathetic tonus in a group of diabetic patients all under the age of 45 years, lacking evidence of large vessel disease. They interpreted this finding as evidence of small vessel occlusion [3]. In the same year, Mendlowitz failed to confirm such findings using the indirect technique of calorimetry [4], whereas Barany was able to demonstrate a lower clearance rate of intradermal radioactive sodium after nerve blockade from the sole of the foot from a group of diabetic subjects under the age of 30 years and thus regarded as free from macroangiopathy [5]. In interpreting his findings, Barany was one of the first to consider the hypothesis of shunting of blood away from certain capillary areas via arteriovenous anastomoses, which are prevalent in the extremities to aid thermoregulation. Contemporary investigations involving the measurement of venous oxygen tension [6], Doppler waveforms [7] and radioactive macroaggregate partitioning [8] have supported the concept of increased arteriovenous shunt flow in the extremities, particularly in patients with neuropathy, although whether or not this results in a microvascular 'steal' of blood away from the nutritive capillary bed remains debatable (Chapter 18).

In contrast to this fragmentary early evidence suggesting that microvascular perfusion might be limited under conditions designed to maximize flow, plethysmographic studies of limb blood flow (deriving estimates of total arterial inflow) under *resting* conditions suggested that during poor glycaemic control, flow was paradoxically increased in the forearm and skin [9].

Studies of blood flow to less accessible but arguably more relevant organs support the concept that in early diabetes resting flow might be increased, whereas with disease progression maximum hyperaemia might be attenuated. Early observations on the retinal circulation using the transit time of fluorescent dyes as a measure of flow rate suggested that insulin-dependent diabetes mellitus (IDDM) was characterized by increased retinal flow in early stages of the condition [10], flow falling as diabetes duration and retinopathy advanced. In the kidney, insulin-dependent diabetes mellitus IDDM is characterized by an early (control-related) increase in renal plasma flow and glomerular filtration rate1 [1] which falls with the development of advanced nephropathy.

11.3 THE HAEMODYNAMIC HYPOTHESIS OF DIABETIC MICROANGIOPATHY

Parving *et al.* were the first to collate these various blood flow observations and formulate what has come to be termed the haemodynamic hypothesis of the pathogenesis of diabetic microangiopathy [12]. It was suggested that it was likely that microvascular blood flow and pressure were increased early in diabetic life and that this haemodynamic stress resulted in basement membrane thickening of capillary walls which ultimately reduced the vasodilatory capacity of the microvessels, as well as their ability to modify their diameter in the face of a change of perfusion pressure (i.e. autoregulate). These innovative concepts for the first time provided a physiological framework for the evolution of microangiopathy (Figure 11.1) although, in the absence of unambiguous measurements of microvascular pressure and flow, many of the assertions were necessarily assumptive.

In clinical support of the hypothesis were the anecdotal observations that unilateral carotid [13] and renal artery stenosis [14] appeared to protect against the development

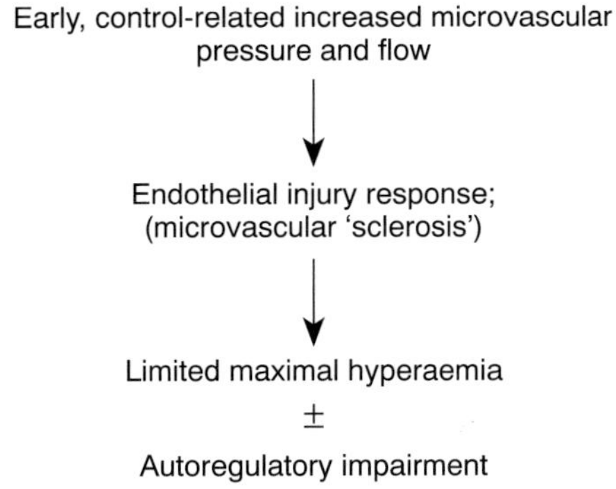

Figure 11.1 The haemodynamic hypothesis of the pathogenesis of diabetic microangiopathy.

of ipsilateral retinopathy and nephropathy, respectively. The concept that increased capillary hydrostatic pressure could trigger capillary basement thickening found further support in the observations that capillary basement membrane width was greater in subjects with congestive cardiac failure in whom venous pressure and hence presumably capillary pressure was elevated [15]. Furthermore in both animals [16] and man [17] capillary basement membrane thickness appears to be greater the further below the heart from which a tissue sample was taken, presumably in response to the capillary hydrostatic pressure which increases (in the upright posture) from the trunk to the foot. Infants fail to exhibit this graduation in basement membrane width before they start to walk [18], i.e. before their lower extremities are exposed to higher intravascular pressures.

That capillary pressure or some other correlate of a hyperaemic state might be an important stimulus to basement membrane thickening is not in doubt; what was less certain at the time that the haemodynamic hypothesis was formulated was the assertion that capillary pressure was raised. It might simplistically be assumed (and indeed it often was) that increased organ flow necessarily implies increased microvascular pressure. Capillary pressure in a simple in-series circuit, however, is a function of both pre- and post-capillary resistance. If both pre- and post-capillary resistance fall, flow will increase whereas mean capillary pressure may remain normal. An increase in capillary pressure signifies a relative increase in the post- to pre-capillary resistance ratio. The importance of this concept is that it emphasizes the need to consider the control of the post-capillary or venular segment and its disturbance by the diabetic state. This part of the microvasculature has been largely neglected in pathogenetic terms, other than in the significance of the altered balance of efferent and afferent arteriolar tone in the glomerulus.

In organ beds where there are microvascular networks in parallel, i.e. shunts between arteries and veins exist, the assumption that increased flow necessarily implies increased nutritive capillary pressure may be even less secure.

A further assertion of the haemodynamic hypothesis that bears further analysis is the concept that capillary wall thickening acts as a major determinant of microvascular resistance. In support of this concept, recent physiological studies suggest that capillary calibre is much more variable than once imagined. Nonetheless, it is generally accepted that the arteriole is the greatest determinant of pre-capillary resistance. Furthermore, histological studies demonstrate the widespread alteration of arterioles and small arteries by the diabetic process with the accumulation of periodic acid–Schiff (PAS)-stain-positive material in the intima [19], the chemical nature of which is akin to basement membrane, comprising principally type IV collagen. It is the presence of this material that has been correlated with the impairment of autoregulatory capacity observed in foot skin microvessels. According to this analysis, capillary basement membrane thickening may be a surrogate marker for more important upstream changes which have a greater bearing on resistance control.

11.3.1   DIRECT SUPPORT FOR THE HAEMODYNAMIC HYPOTHESIS

Direct support for the haemodynamic hypothesis has come with the development of techniques for directly measuring microvascular pressure and flow in humans. Although estimates of glomerular capillary pressure in diabetic rat models suggested glomerular hypertension [20], the first human evidence for capillary hypertension relied on the development of an electronic technique for measuring pressure in nail-fold capillaries by direct cannulation. Using this methodology Sandeman *et al.* demonstrated that mean capillary pressure at heart level in 45 patients with IDDM was elevated compared with values obtained in age- and sex-matched controls [21]. Furthermore, in the diabetic patients, capillary pressure was directly correlated with the glycated haemoglobin percentage at the time of pressure measurement and elevated capillary pressure in subjects with a short disease duration could be reduced by a three-month period of improved glycaemic control.

Although such observations are supportive of the haemodynamic hypothesis, to be regarded as a prime-moving pathogenetic mechanism it is reasonable to expect the abnormality to conform to certain key epidemiological and clinical facts, in addition to an association with glycaemic control alluded to above. Perhaps most important is that pressure should be more elevated (for a given degree of glycaemic control) in subjects at high risk of microangiopathy than those who are not. The presence of microalbuminuria in IDDM carries an increased risk of many other microvascular complications as well as nephropathy, whereas patients who avoid microalbuminuria after a long disease duration have a more benign prognosis. Capillary pressure is particularly elevated in patients

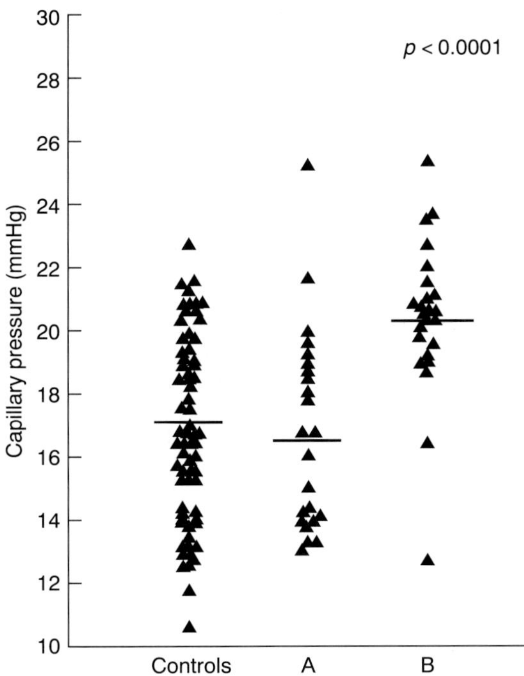

Figure 11.2 Nail-fold capillary pressure values in subjects with (A) insulin-dependent diabetes and (B) incipient nephropathy (microalbuminuria). Subjects were patients of similar disease duration who have avoided this complication matched for age, sex and glycaemic control; and healthy controls matched for age and sex.

with microalbuminuria, compared to disease duration and glycaemic control matched individuals who have avoided excessive urinary albumin leak after a long disease duration, who exhibit relatively normal capillary pressures (Figure 11.2).

11.4   REDUCED MICROVASCULAR VASODILATORY RESERVE

The haemodynamic hypothesis proposes that the capacity of microvessels to maximally dilate diminishes with increasing disease duration, representing, at least in part, a physical limitation imposed by the accumulation of extravascular matrix proteins as a consequence of haemodynamically induced

endothelial 'injury'. In the skin in adults with IDDM, it has been demonstrated that maximum microvascular hyperaemia to a thermal stimulus is diminished in the absence of evidence of large vessel disease and neuropathy. This abnormality is more marked with increasing disease duration [22] and the co-existence of clinical evidence of microangiopathy [23], particularly incipient nephropathy. The independence of this abnormality from arterial disease is illustrated by the fact that it is also demonstrable in pre-pubertal children who demonstrate a similar duration related impairment [24]. In keeping with the haemodynamic hypothesis, the degree of hyperaemic impairment correlates with the capillary basement membrane width in skin biopsies taken from the same anatomical area as flow measurements [25] although it is possible that such capillary changes are merely surrogate markers for more relevant arteriolar hyalinosis.

Human microvascular techniques have by necessity been targeted at the skin; are the findings in skin representative of other organs? In the renal vascular bed renal blood flow falls as renal failure ensues and the capacity for autoregulation becomes impaired [26]. In subcutaneous tissues, autoregulatory impairment correlates with the degree of PAS-positive staining of arterioles [27]. In the retina the proliferative phase is preceded by a reduction in retinal blood flow [28].

11.5   ALTERNATIVE PATHOPHYSIOLOGICAL CONCEPTS

11.5.1   THE ROLE OF INCREASED MICROVASCULAR PERMEABILITY

There is a pervading view that increased leakiness is a characteristic feature of diabetic microangiopathy although the direct evidence for such an assertion is far from clear. Increased flux of water (capillary filtration coefficient) and labelled albumin (transcapillary escape rate of albumin) has been demonstrated in IDDM during poor metabolic control [29], abnormalities that are corrected with restoration of good control. Both measures are increased in subjects who develop microalbuminuria [30, 31] whereas values observed in subjects who remain complication-free despite a similar (long) disease duration exhibit relatively normal values. The passage of small molecules appears to be normal early in diabetes, regardless of control [29], but increases with increasing disease duration [32].

Although changes in water and albumin flux could represent altered permeability characteristics of the capillary wall, the lack of specificity of the currently available techniques for studying microvascular permeability in man means that such conclusions can only be assumptive. The passage of water and, to a certain extent, the passage of large molecules such as albumin is dependent on the balance of Starling's forces. Of these capillary pressure is the most important, as well as the surface area available for exchange. These other variables are seldom, if ever, known at the time of permeability measurement. However with newer sophisticated plethysmographic multiple pressure step techniques, it is assumed that the increments in venous pressure imposed, that drive filtration, equate to capillary pressure [33]. Such considerations are very relevant when it is appreciated that control-related increases in capillary pressure have been demonstrated, particularly in those subjects who demonstrate increased protein and fluid flux [21].

Central importance for permeability change has been proposed as the determinant of propensity to 'malignant' microangiopathy (Figure 11.3). The 'Steno' hypothesis [34], generated by Deckert *et al.* from the Steno Hospital, proposes that changes in the endothelial layer charge barrier which occur as a consequence of underexpression of heparan

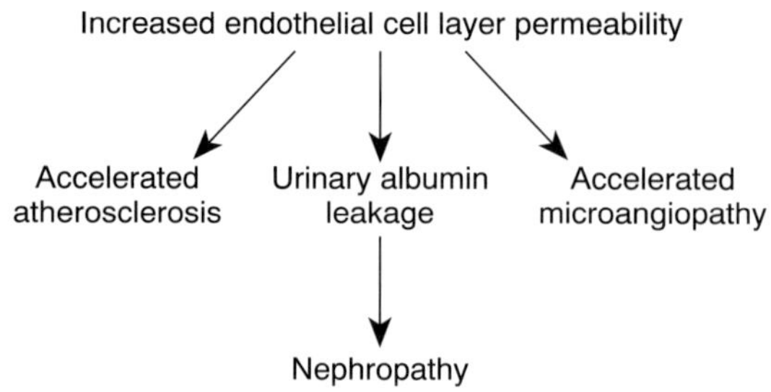

Figure 11.3 The hyperpermeability hypothesis of the pathogenesis of diabetic microangiopathy.

sulphate proteoglycan, possibly due to inherited differences in key enzymes such as D-acetylase, could explain the increased microvascular permeability in subjects with microalbuminuria, as well as the propensity to atherosclerosis due to an accelerated ingress of lipoproteins in such subjects. Although human data directly supporting this hypothesis are limited, microalbuminuria can be reduced by the infusion of heparinoids [35].

Of course increased microvascular pressure and increased microvascular permeability as physiological pathways to microangiopathy are not mutually exclusive. Indeed, they may be interrelated as there are several potential ways in which capillary pressure may influence permeability (Table 11.1). To examine these potential interactions, Klaentschi *et al.* constructed a capillary wall model which

Table 11.1 Potential ways in which microvascular pressure may influence microvascular permeability

---

Microvessel rupture
Formation of transcellular holes
Stretching of inter-endothelial cell junctional complexes
Altered expression of inter-endothelial cell junctional complex adhesion
Concentration polarization of macromolecules at the capillary wall surface – the filter cake phenomenon
Compression of basement membrane

---

allowed the manipulation of pressure in a pulsatile manner in the physiological pressure range as well as the chemical composition of the fluid and degree of glycation of dissolved albumin and reconstituted basement membrane. Pressure dependency of the passage of normal and glycated albumin was observed with glycated basement membrane appearing more permeable at higher pressures, an abnormality that was exaggerated under pulsatile conditions [36]. Given that the majority of water and albumin passes through interendothelial cell clefts, such studies need to be repeated with microvascular endothelial cell monolayers to clarify further the interrelationships between pressure and permeability. Early studies using such a system suggest that chronic exposure to slightly increased pressure can reduce the expression of interendothelial cell adhesion molecules, an effect that is exaggerated in the presence of a high glucose environment [37]. Until the availability of unambiguous techniques for measuring human microvascular permeability in a variety of microvascular beds, it is a defensible premise that propensity to microangiopathy in IDDM is characterized by early, glycaemic control-related increase in capillary pressure plus or minus inherited or acquired increases in microvascular permeability to water and albumin.

11.6 THE PATHOPHYSIOLOGY OF THE MICROCIRCULATION IN NON-INSULIN DEPENDENT DIABETES

At first sight it may appear superfluous to entertain the possibility of different pathophysiological origins of microangiopathy in non-insulin-dependent diabetes mellitus (NIDDM) compared with IDDM; retinopathy and nephropathy are common to both major types of diabetes, yet cursory examination of the presentation, nature and progression of these complications argues for greater scrutiny (Table 11.2). Unlike IDDM, where a significant duration of diabetes must elapse before clinical complications appear, such complications are commonly present at diagnosis in NIDDM [38]. Whereas it is commonly assumed that this represents the impact of years of undisclosed diabetes, an alternative hypothesis is that, in some cases at least, changes are occurring to the microvasculature in the pre-diabetic state [39].

Direct estimates of capillary pressure [40] and capillary filtration coefficient [41] in normotensive NIDDM patients have revealed values indistinguishable from age- and sex-matched controls, whereas maximum microvascular hyperaemia which declines slowly in IDDM with increasing disease duration is markedly impaired at diagnosis in patients with NIDDM [42]; the degree of abnormality

Table 11.2 Differences in the expression of vascular disease and its associates in NIDDM compared with IDDM

	NIDDM	*IDDM*
Hypertension	High prevalence ~ 40%	Relatively normal prevalence in the absence of nephropathy
Retinopathy	Maculopathy common cause of visual loss	Proliferative retinopathy common cause of visual loss
Nephropathy	Lower prevalence? slower progression?	30% afflicted
Arterial disease	Higher prevalence	Lower prevalence (in the absence of nephropathy)

observed is consistent with that observed after 18 years of IDDM. The findings have stimulated the formulation of an alternative hypothesis to explain the microvascular pathophysiology observed in NIDDM. It has been proposed that during the pre-diabetic phase there is a relative increase in arteriolar resistance that limits the rise in capillary pressure and filtration when hyperglycaemia-induced pre-capillary vasodilatation ensues, as well as contributing to the high prevalence of hypertension observed in NIDDM [43]. This increase in arteriolar resistance, resulting in a limited capacity to maximally vasodilate, could be secondary to some consequence of the insulin resistance state that commonly precedes the breakdown in glucose tolerance in such patients or it could be primary, even contributing to the genesis of diabetes itself.

To test this hypothesis, maximum microvascular hyperaemia has been assessed in subjects with fasting hyperglycaemia who exhibit a deficit similar to that observed in fully developed NIDDM [44] which is negatively correlated with calculated insulin sensitivity [45]. Capillary pressure is normal during this pre-diabetic stage [46].

11.7   A PATHOPHYSIOLOGICAL FRAMEWORK FOR DIABETIC MICROANGIOPATHY

From these various human microvascular studies it is possible to construct a pathophysiological framework for the development of diabetic microangiopathy in the two major types of diabetes, demonstrated in schematic form in Figure 11.3 [39]. In IDDM, the emergence of hyperglycaemia results in capillary hypertension due to pre-capillary vasodilatation, with changes in microvascular permeability and/or the capacity of the post-capillary segment to dilate compounding the functional consequences of this rise in susceptible individuals. Ultimately the haemodynamic stress results in microvascular sclerosis which contributes to a limitation of

perfusion under certain demands as well as impaired autoregulation. The latter may exaggerate the impairment in pressure regulation as well as flow regulation, as has been experimentally verified.

In contrast, in NIDDM (and arguably in patients with IDDM with nephropathy who exhibit more insulin resistance) the capacity of the microcirculation to dilate at arteriolar level is impaired before the emergence of glucose tolerance. This protects the microcirculation (in the absence of hypertension which can result in capillary hypertension and increased albumin flux) from the typical changes observed in IDDM but nonetheless profoundly reducing maximum perfusion.

One indirect test of this hypothesis is to examine microvascular function in genetically discrete forms of diabetes in which the metabolic characteristics are well documented. In maturity onset diabetes of the young (MODY), the primary defect is at β-cell level and despite the prefix of maturity onset and the fact that many such patients do not require insulin, insulin resistance is not a typical characteristic [47]. The pathophysiological framework proposed would suggest that such individuals would behave as mild IDDM. Such is the case, with a moderate duration-related impairment in maximum hyperaemic response being observed [48].

The value of such a pathophysiological framework is in its capacity to focus attention on key mechanistic issues, and to provide a pattern of physiological behaviour with which any proposed cellular or molecular mechanism should be consistent; the following chapters consider such candidate mechanisms.

REFERENCES

1. Tooke, J.E. Methodologies used in the study of the microcirculation in diabetes mellitus. *Diabetes Metab. Rev.*, (New York NY), **9**.
2. Tooke, J.E. Microcirculation and diabetes. *Br. Med. Bull.*, 1989, **45**, 206–23.

3. Megibow, R.S., Megibow, S.J., Pollack, H., Bookman, J.J. and Osserman, K. The mechanism of accelerated peripheral vascular sclerosis in diabetes mellitus. *Am. J. Med.*, 1953, **13**, 322–29.

4. Mendlowitz, M., Grossman, E.B. and Alpert, S. Decreased hallucal circulation, an early manifestation of vascular disease in diabetes mellitus. *Am. J. Med.*, 1953, **13**, 316–21.

5. Barany, F.R. Abnormal vascular reactions in diabetes mellitus. *Acta Med. Scand.*, 1955, suppl 304, 13.

6. Boulton, A.J.M., Scarpello, J.H.B. and Ward, J.D. Venous oxygenation in the diabetic neuropathic foot: evidence of arteriovenous shunting. *Diabetologia*, 1982, **22**, 6–8.

7. Edmonds, M.E., Roberts, V.C. and Watkins, P.J. Blood flow in the diabetic neuropathic foot. *Diabetologia*, 1982, **22**, 9–15.

8. Partsch, H. Neuropathies of the ulceromutilating types. Clinical aspects, classification, circulatory measurements. V.A.S.A., 1977, suppl 6, 1–48.

9. Mathiesen, E.R., Hilsted, J., Feldt–Rasmussen, B., Bonde Petersen, F., Christensen, N.J. and Parving, H.H. The effect of metabolic control on hemodynamics in short-term insulin-dependent diabetic patients. *Diabetes*, 1985, **34**, 1301–5.

10. Kohner, E.M. The problems of retinal blood flow in diabetes. *Diabetes*, 1976, **25** suppl 2, 839–44.

11. Christiansen, J.S., Gammelgaard, J., Frandsen, M. and Parving, H.H. Increased kidney size, glomerular filtration rate and renal plasma flow in short-term insulin-dependent diabetics. *Diabetologia*, 1981, **20**, 451–6.

12. Parving, H.H., Viberti, G.C., Keen, H., Christiansen, J.S. and Lassen, N.A. Hemodynamic factors in the genesis of diabetic microangiopathy. *Metab. Clin. Exp.* 1983, **32**, 943–9.

13. Duker, J.S., Brown, G.C., Bosley, T.M., Colt, C.A. and Reber, R. Asymmetric proliferative diabetic retinopathy and carotid artery disease. *Ophthalmology*, 1990, **97**, 869–74.

14. Berkman, J. and Rifkin, H. Unilateral nodular diabetic glomerulosclerosis (Kimmel-Steel-Wilson): report of a case. *Metabolism*, 1973, **22**, 715–22.

15. Williamson, J.R. and Kilo, C. Current status of capillary basement-membrane disease in diabetes mellitus. *Diabetes*, 1977, **26**, 65–73.

16. Williamson, J.R., Vogler, N.J. and Kilo, C. Regional variations in the width of the basement membrane of muscle capillaries in man and giraffe. *Am. J. Pathol.*, 1971, **63**, 359–67.

17. Vracko, R. Skeletal muscle capillaries in diabetics. *Circulation*, 1970, **41**, 271–83.

18. Williamson, J.R. and Kilo, C. Capillary basement membranes in diabetes. *Diabetes*, 1983, **32** suppl 2, 96–100.

19. Goldenberg, S., Alex, M., Joshi, R.A. and Blumenthal, H.T. Nonatheromatous peripheral vascular disease of the lower extremity in diabetes mellitus. *Diabetes*, 1959, **8**, 261–73.

20. Hostetter, T.H., Troy, J.L. and Brenner, B.M. Glomerular hemodynamics in experimental diabetes mellitus. *Kidney Int.*, 1981, **19**, 410–15.

21. Sandeman, D.D., Shore, A.C. and Tooke, J.E. Relation of skin capillary pressure in patients with insulin-dependent diabetes mellitus to complications and metabolic control. *N. Engl. J. Med.*, 1992, **327**, 760–4.

22. Rayman, G., Williams, S.A., Spencer, P.D., Smaje, L.H., Wise, P.H. and Tooke, J.E. Impaired microvascular hyperaemic response to minor skin trauma in type I diabetes. *Br. Med. J.*, 1986, **292**, 1295–8.

23. Walmsley, D., Wales, J.K. and Wiles, P.G. Reduced hyperaemia following skin trauma: evidence for an impaired microvascular response to injury in the diabetic foot. *Diabetologia*, 1989, **32**, 736–9.

24. Shore, A.C., Price, K.J., Sandeman, D.D., Green, E.M., Tripp, J.H. and Tooke, J.E. Impaired microvascular hyperaemic response in children with diabetes mellitus. *Diabetic Med.*, 1991, **8**, 619–23.

25. Rayman, G., Malik, R.A., Sharma, A.K. and Day, J.L. Microvascular response to tissue injury and capillary ultrastructure in the foot skin of type 1 diabetic patients. *Clin. Sci.*, 1995, **89**, 467–74.

26. Parving, H.H., Kastrup, H., Smidt, U.M., Andersen, A.R., Feldt-Rasmussen, B. and Christiansen, J.S. Impaired autoregulation of glomerular filtration rate in type 1 (insulin-dependent) diabetic patients with nephropathy. *Diabetologia*, 1984, **27**, 547–52.

27. Kastrup, J., Norgaard, T., Parving, H.H., Henriksen, O. and Lassen, N.A. Impaired autoregulation of blood flow in subcutaneous tissue of long-term type 1(insulin-dependent) diabetic patients with microangiopathy:an

index of arteriolar dysfunction. *Diabetologia,* 1985, **28,** 711–17.

28. Bresnick, G.H., de Venecia, G. and Myers, E.C. Retinal ischaemia in diabetic retinopathy. *Arch. Ophthalmol.,* 1975, **93,** 1300–10.

29. Parving, H.H., Noer, I., Deckert, T., Evrin, P.E., Nielsen, S.L., Lyngsoe, J., Mogensen, C.E., Rorth, M., Svendsen, P.A., Trap-Jensen, J. and Lassen, N.A. The effect of metabolic regulation on microvascular permeability to small and large molecules in short-term juvenile diabetics. *Diabetologia,* 1976, **12,** 161–6.

30. Jaap, A.J., Shore, A.C. and Tooke, J.E. Differences in microvascular fluid permeability between long-duration type 1 (insulin-dependent) diabetic patients with and without significant microangiopathy. *Clin. Sci.,* 1996, **90,** 113–17.

31. Feldt-Rasmussen, B. Increased transcapillary escape rate of albumin in type 1 (insulin-dependent) diabetic patients with microalbuminuria. *Diabetologia,* 1986, **29,** 282–6.

32. Trap-Jensen, J. and Lassen, N.A. Increased capillary diffusion capacity for small ions in skeletal muscle in long-term diabetics. *Scand. J. Clin. Lab. Invest.,* 1968, **21,** 116–22.

33. Gamble, J., Christ, F. and Gartside, I.B. Mercury in silastic strain gauge plethysmography for the clinical assessment of the microcirculation. *Postgrad. Med. J.,* 1992, **68** (suppl 2), S25–S33.

34. Deckert, T., Feldt-Rasmussen, B., Borch-Johnsen, K., Jensen, T. and Kofoed Enevoldsen, A. Albuminuria reflects widespread vascular damage. The Steno hypothesis. *Diabetologia,* 1989, **32,** 219–26.

35. Myrup, B., Hansen, P.M., Jensen, T., Kofoed-Enevoldsen, A., Feldt-Rasmussen, B., Gram, J., Kluft, C., Jespersen, J. and Deckert, T. Effect of low-dose heparin on urinary albumin excretion in insulin-dependent diabetes mellitus. *Lancet,* 1995, **345,** 421–2.

36. Klaentschi, K., Brown, J.A., Shore, A.C. and Tooke, J.E. Pressure-permeability relationships in basement membrane: the effects of static and dynamic pressures. *Am. J. Physiol.,* 1997, 1988, H1327–34.

37. Klaentschi, K., Shore, A.C. and Tooke, J.E. Effect of pressure and glucose on PECAM expression by microvascular endothelium cells. Medical and Scientific Section Spring meeting B.D.A., 1998.

38. UKPDS Group. UK Prospective Diabetes Study 6. Complications in newly diagnosed type 2 diabetic patients and their association with different clinical and biochemical risk factors. *Diabetes Res.,* 1990, **13,** 1–11.

39. Jaap, A.J. and Tooke, J.E. Pathophysiology of microvascular disease in non-insulin-dependent diabetes. *Clinical Sci.,* 1995, **89,** 3–12.

40. Shore, A.C., Jaap, A.J. and Tooke, J.E. Capillary pressure in patients with NIDDM. *Diabetes,* 1994, **43,** 1198–202.

41. Jaap, A.J., Shore, A.C., Gamble, J., Gartside, I.B. and Tooke, J.E. Capillary filtration coefficient in type II (non-insulin-dependent) diabetes. *J. Diabetes Complications,* 1994, **8,** 111–16.

42. Sandeman, D.D., Pym, C.A., Green, E.M., Seamark, C., Shore, A.C. and Tooke, J.E. Microvascular vasodilatation in feet of newly diagnosed non-insulin dependent diabetic patients. *Br. Med J.,* 1991, **302,** 1122–3.

43. UKPDS Group. United Kingdom Prospective Diabetes Study III. Prevalance of hypertension and hypotensive therapy in patients with new diagnosed diabetes. *Hypertension,* 1985, **7** suppl 2, 8–13.

44. Jaap, A.J., Hammersley, M.S., Shore, A.C. and Tooke, J.E. Reduced microvascular hyperaemia in subjects at risk of developing type 2 (non-insulin-dependent) diabetes mellitus. *Diabetologia,* 1994, **37,** 214–16.

45. Jaap, A.J., Shore, A.C. and Tooke, J.E. Relationship of insulin resistance to microvascular dysfunction in subjects with fasting hyperglycaemia. *Diabetologia,* 1997, **40,** 238–43.

46. Shore, A.C., Morris, S.J., Stockman, A.J. and Tooke, J.E. Capillary pressure in subjects with fasting hyperglycaemia. *Diabetologia,* 1997, **40,** suppl 1, A587.

47. Lehto, M., Tuorni, T., Mahtani, M.M., Widen, T. et al. Characterization of the MODY 3 phenotype. Early-onset diabetes caused by an insulin secretion defect. *J. Clin. Invest.,* 1997, **99,** 582–91.

48. Lee, B.C., Appleton, M., Shore, C.S., Tooke, J.E. and Hattersley, A.T. Impaired maximum microvascular hyperaemia in subjects with mutations in hepatocyte nuclear factor 1a gene (MODY 3). *Diabetologia,* 1998, (under review).

Lucilla Poston

12.1 INTRODUCTION

The last decade of vascular research has been remarkable for the extraordinary emphasis placed upon the endothelium. Vascular smooth muscle has assumed second place to this single-cell layer, now recognized to be a remarkably versatile organ. The endothelium controls vascular permeability, is essential for normal haemostasis, makes an important contribution to inflammatory responses and, through the synthesis of constrictor and dilator agonists, significantly modifies the tone of the underlying smooth muscle. In diabetes, compromised endothelial function has been implicated in microthrombus formation, ischaemia, neuropathy and increased risk of atherosclerosis and hypertension. Other chapters in this book consider various aspects of macrovascular dysfunction, particularly atherogenesis, whereas this chapter focuses upon the smaller vessels in diabetes, in which endothelial vasodilator/constrictor dysfunction may contribute to the generation of the microangiopathies.

Some of the earliest indications that the diabetic milieu could adversely affect the endothelial cell layer came from reports describing raised plasma concentrations of markers for endothelial cell disruption or activation in diabetic patients. This expanded into the description of abnormal levels of almost every known indicator of endothelial cell dysfunction. Thus in patients with insulin dependent diabetes mellitus (IDDM), raised serum or plasma concentrations of angiotensin-converting enzyme [1], tissue plasminogen activator [2], endothelin [3], plasma free N-terminal fibronectin [4], von Willebrand factor [5], vascular endothelial cell antibodies [6] and circulating cell adhesion molecules [7] have been reported (Figure 12.1). Similarly, many of these markers are raised in patients with non-insulin-dependent diabetes mellitus (NIDDM) [8, 9] and a report of a progressive rise in serum von Willebrand factor with increasing albuminuria is suggested to reflect the gradual deterioration of endothelial cell function in the glomerulus [10].

Vascular tone is under the influence of several important endothelium-derived factors. The endothelium synthesizes the constrictor agonists endothelin, thromboxane A_2 and angiotensin. Prostacyclin was recognized to be an endothelium-dependent vasodilator more than 20 years ago, and the presence of a hitherto unidentified endothelium-derived hyperpolarizing factor (EDHF) is now generally accepted [11]. However, endothelium derived nitric oxide (NO), synthesized from the conversion of L-arginine to L-citrulline, through the action of constitutive NO synthase (NOS-III) is a quantitatively more effective vasodilator and, in common with prostacyclin, is a potent antithrombotic agent which also prevents leucocyte adhesion. First recognized by Furchgott [12] as the mediator of acetylcholine-induced vasodilation, the synthesis, degradation and biological role of this free radical species has been extensively

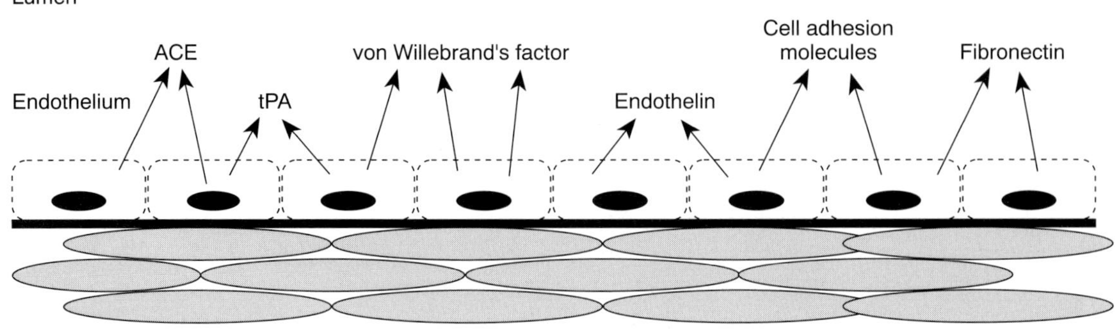

Figure 12.1 Markers of endothelial cell dysfunction reported to be raised in the plasma of patients with insulin-dependent diabetes mellitus. ACE, angiotensin converting enzyme; tPA, tissue plasminogen activator.

researched. Much of the focus on the endothelium in diabetes has been placed on the role of this well characterized L-arginine NO pathway.

Investigations of vascular endothelial NO in diabetes range from non-invasive studies of human subjects to detailed analyses of single small arteries or capillaries. Essentially there are two approaches, independent of the size of artery or vascular bed to be studied.

The first utilizes the endothelial/NO dependence of the response to acetylcholine; thus acetylcholine or, occasionally, another muscarinic agonist is infused into the patient, added to the organ bath or even suffused through the skin by iontophoresis, and vasodilator responses recorded. The NO dependence of the response can be evaluated with the use of specific inhibitors of NO synthesis, e.g. N^G-nitro-L-arginine methyl ester (LNAME) or N^G-monomethyl-L-arginine (lNMMA). Distinction between inappropriate NO release or metabolism and an abnormal response of the underlying vascular smooth muscle to NO can be made by recording dilatation to exogenous NO applied in the form of a nitrovasodilator, such as sodium nitroprusside or glyceryl trinitrate (GTN).

The second approach, less extensively used, is the investigation of flow-mediated dilation.

The shear stress which results from the flow of blood past the endothelial cell layer is, in some vascular beds, a potent stimulus to NO release [13]. This is thought to involve mechanotransduction of the signal through the cytoskeleton to the basolateral side of the cell and consequent activation of focal adhesion sites [13] which in turn leads to tyrosine phosphorylation of NO synthase [14] and calcium-independent NO synthesis [15]. Prolonged, genomic responses in which NO synthase expression is increased are also involved through increased expression of transcription factors, including nuclear factor κβ[16]. The acute responses to flow can be determined in isolated small arteries, using the technique of 'perfusion myography' or in the diabetic patient using high resolution ultrasound to 'visualize' the walls of larger vessels.

12.2 VASCULAR RESPONSES TO ACETYLCHOLINE IN DIABETES

The technique most commonly used to determine agonist-mediated endothelial function in the diabetic patient is the evaluation of forearm blood flow by venous occlusion plethysmography. This method enables functional studies of the skeletal muscle resistance arteries in the forearm, and in so doing avoids any mechanical interference from atheromatous lesions on dilation of the larger vessels.

In IDDM patients this technique has yielded some discrepancies, with some reports of normal dilatation to acetylcholine (ACh) and one recent observation of hyper-responsiveness to both ACh and sodium nitroprusside in patients with macroalbuminuria [17]. Using inhibitors of NO synthesis, others have calculated a reduced NO component of endothelium-dependent relaxation [18] or have reported reduced dilation to methacholine [19]; two reports have shown reduced basal NO release [18, 20]. Another has documented a 40% reduction of the ratio of endothelium-dependent to endothelium-independent relaxation in patients with poor glycaemic control compared with that of normal subjects or of patients with good glycaemic control [21].

In NIDDM the picture is clearer, with several observations of blunted endothelium-dependent relaxation; firstly by McVeigh *et al.* [22] who also reported blunted response to GTN, followed by Williams *et al.* [23] who, by pretreatment with aspirin, excluded any role for enhanced constrictor prostanoid synthesis in the reduced methacholine induced dilatation observed. More recently, Watts *et al.* [24] circumvented potential influences of hypoglycaemic drugs or of insulin by confining their study to NIDDM men who were treated by diet alone, and these subjects again showed reduced responses to ACh and to a nitrovasodilator. Whilst producing much useful information, venous occlusion plethysmography has some inherent technical difficulties which may explain some of the variability of results observed. In relation to diabetes, the influence of basal blood flow and the relation of blood flow to glycaemic control are particularly relevant. However, another method of measuring blood flow, using a thermodilution technique has supported the majority of observations in NIDDM patients. Steinberg *et al.* [25] have shown a 40% reduction in methacholine-induced enhancement of leg blood flow in NIDDM patients and, interestingly, a similar abnormality in obese, insulin-resistant subjects without NIDDM.

There are obvious advantages to the investigation of small arteries *in vitro* as vessels can be studied in isolation from humoral and neuronal influences and the extracellular milieu can be carefully defined. Most studies have relied upon the use of the Mulvany–Halpern myograph; effectively a scaled-down organ bath in which the vessel is fixed for isometric tension recording by two fine wires passed through the lumen and secured by small screws at either end [26].

The lack of available human material has necessarily restricted the study of *in vitro* responses in arteries from diabetic patients, but McNally *et al.* [27] have reported abnormal acetylcholine-induced dilation of small arteries dissected from gluteal subcutaneous fat biopsies obtained from patients with IDDM (Figure 12.2). In a report of small subcutaneous arteries in NIDDM, Cipolla *et al.* [28] have shown *enhanced* dilation to ACh, although this study was carried out using the more technically demanding pressure myograph in which vessels are mounted on fine glass cannulae. Interestingly, these arteries showed an enhanced constrictor response to noradrenaline which, unlike the control arteries, was not further increased by the application of a NOS inhibitor. This is a strong indication for reduced NO release in the IDDM arteries, as basal NO synthesis normally blunts noradrenaline induced constriction.

In our laboratory we have taken advantage of the high rate of caesarean sections amongst women with gestational diabetes by obtaining small sections of subcutaneous fat, with consent, at delivery. Gestational diabetes is similar in some ways to NIDDM as it is characterized by insulin resistance and abnormal glucose tolerance. Arteries dissected from the biopsy tissue showed abnormal ACh-

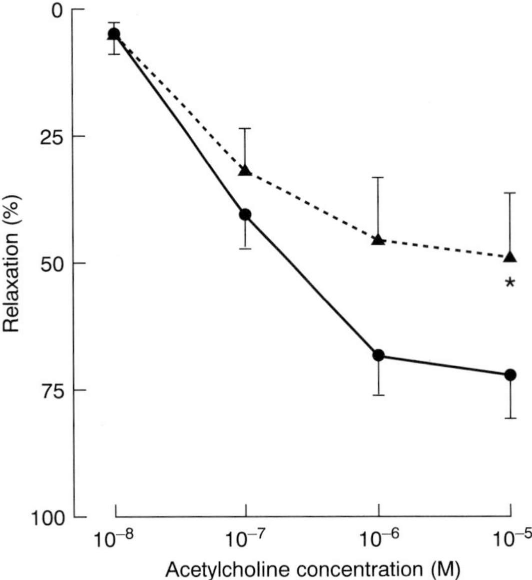

Figure 12.2 Reduced endothelium-dependent relaxation to acetylcholine in small subcutaneous arteries from patients with insulin-dependent diabetes mellitus (▲) compared with controls (●). *Significant difference ($p < 0.05$) between dose–response curves. Redrawn from [27] with permission.

induced relaxation when compared with those obtained from non-diabetic women [29]. Moving further down the vascular bed, the technique of laser Doppler perfusion imaging has been used to measure acetylcholine-induced increases in blood flow in capillaries of the forearm. In patients with fasting hyperglycaemia who have a predisposition to develop NIDDM, the local application of ACh and subsequent iontophoresis led to less of an increase in blood flow than in normal controls [30] and, in patients with established NIDDM, this was confounded by a reduced response to exogenously applied NO in the form of sodium nitroprusside [31].

The sparsity of investigations in human isolated small arteries is more than compensated by numerous reports of animal models of diabetes; principally the streptozotocin (STZ)-induced diabetic rat but also the alloxan-treated rabbit or dog, the genetic spontaneously diabetic rat (BB rat) and the Zucker fatty diabetic rat model of NIDDM (for reviews see [32, 33]). In the IDDM models, there is general, but not quite unanimous, agreement upon a defect of the ACh dilatory response. In our laboratory we have now documented the defect in more than five separate investigations of small mesenteric arteries of the STZ rat carried out over a similar number of years (for reviews see [33, 34]). This contrasts with another study of small mesenteric arteries [35] which has reported an *enhancement* of ACh relaxation after similar period of diabetes, but the degree of glycaemia induced was much less severe and the relaxation to ACh in control rats much less than that recorded in our laboratory. Recently we have shown that pregnancy confers some degree of protection against the abnormality of relaxation to ACh, as pregnant STZ diabetic rats show more pronounced relaxation to ACh when compared with virgin diabetic females [36]; this may relate to stimulation by oestrogens of ACh-induced relaxation [37]. We have also followed the offspring of these animals, which are not overtly diabetic but are insulin-resistant. At 100 days of age, these animals have a marked defect in ACh-induced relaxation [38], thus lending some support to the hypothesis that elements of diabetes and cardiovascular dysfunction could have *in utero* origins [39].

12.3 FLOW-MEDIATED, ENDOTHELIUM-DEPENDENT, DILATION IN DIABETES

Flow-mediated relaxation provides an alternative means by which to assess endothelial function. Theoretically, shear stress may be a more physiologically relevant stimulus to NO synthesis than ACh because, due to intense plasma acetylcholinesterase activity, endogenous ACh concentrations at the vascular wall are likely to be minimal, although concentrations could be locally raised at the basolateral endothelial cell membrane. Technically, assessment of flow-mediated relaxation is more challenging, both *in vivo* and *in vitro*. Flow-mediated dilation may be assessed in isolated small arteries by mounting on a perfusion myograph, pressurizing to physiological pressure and perfusing at increasing flow rates while recording artery diameter and maintaining the pressure by servo-control [40]. Using this technique, we have recorded a modest increment in flow-mediated relaxation in mesenteric small arteries from normal animals, which was mediated by NO, but arteries from the STZ diabetic animals showed flow induced *constriction* [41] (Figure 12.3).

Jin and Bohlen [42] have adopted a novel method of investigating flow-mediated relaxation in the Zucker fatty diabetic rat

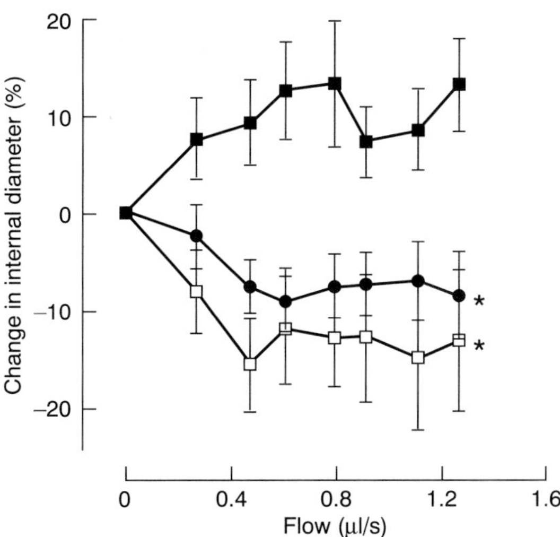

Figure 12.3 Responses to flow in small rat mesenteric arteries mounted on a pressure myograph. Arteries from control animals dilated to flow (■) and this dilation was blocked with the NOS inhibitor, L-NAME (□). Arteries from STZ diabetic rats showed constriction to flow (●). * = $p < 0.005$ compared to arteries from controls. From [4] with permission.

(NIDDM). By replacing sodium chloride with mannitol over the intestinal villi of the isolated perfused mesentery, blood flow is reduced due to inhibition of sodium-dependent metabolism; therefore flow-mediated, NO-dependent relaxation falls. Removal of sodium in the Zucker rat mesentery reduced blood flow to a lesser degree than in normoglycaemic controls, suggesting a decrement of flow mediated NO release. Lowered perineural blood flow, implicated by many in diabetic neuropathies, has been the focus of many investigations in STZ diabetic rats (for review see [32]). The administration of an NO donor leads to improvement of neuronal blood flow and NOS inhibitors exacerbate the problem. Deficiency of NO may therefore play an indirect, but important role in neuronal dysfunction.

In vivo, flow-mediated responses are now frequently investigated using high resolution Doppler ultrasound to 'visualize' conduit artery walls. The technique rests on the principle that distal hyperaemia will evoke a local increase in blood flow, through elaboration of vasoactive metabolites, and that this is transmitted proximally where flow-mediated dilation which is shear-stress-dependent, but metabolite-independent, can be recorded.

Proximal flow-mediated relaxation to distal hyperaemia was first recognized in 1933 [43] and originally thought to result from a process transmitted through the artery wall itself. A proximal increase in shear stress would now seem to be a more appropriate explanation. The relaxation to flow induced by this method, which is small (approximately 5–10% dilation) is generally determined in the brachial artery in response to hyperaemia of the hand (achieved by a cuff placed round the wrist) and is at least partially NO dependent [44]. The technique has the disadvantage that only conduit arteries may be studied and data obtained are, strictly, only relevant to conduit artery disease. Dilation may also be influenced by atheroma and by passive changes in artery compliance, and flow rates achieved by reactive hyperaemia are difficult to standard-ize and may vary if significant microvascular disease is present. Flow rates can, however, be assessed and should always be evaluated in control and patient groups.

Using this technique, but in the right com-mon femoral artery of the leg, Zenere *et al.* [45] showed a blunted response to flow in normoalbuminuric IDDM patients and com-pletely absent dilation in microalbuminuric patients. Indeed, and as in the recent inves-tigation in our laboratory of small rat arteries [41], the flow stimulus evoked constriction. GTN responses were also blunted in both groups of patients. Clarkson *et al.* [46] have shown blunted responses to flow and sub-lingual GTN in the brachial artery of 80 young adults with IDDM and reported a pro-portionately greater blunting of the flow response than of the dilation to GTN, thus suggesting the presence of an endothelial defect in association with a reduced sensitiv-ity to NO. Involvement of low density lipo-proteins (LDLs) in endothelial dysfunction was suggested by an inverse relationship between LDLs and flow-mediated responses. Brachial artery flow mediated dilatation is similarly reported to be reduced in NIDDM patients [47] but with preservation of the GTN response.

12.4 INSULIN, NO AND INSULIN RESISTANCE

Other chapters in this book deal with the topic of insulin resistance in detail; but this chapter would be incomplete without brief reference to the endothelium-dependent dila-tation which is evoked by insulin, and the consequent suggestion that poor endothelial function may contribute to insulin resis-tance.

Insulin induces vasodilation in some vas-cular beds through release of NO [48, 49] and it has been proposed that reduced glucose uptake may result from impaired blood flow responses to insulin in skeletal muscle of NIDDM subjects [50]. However, inhibition of NO synthesis by local infusion of a NOS inhibitor, while causing constriction, does not affect glucose uptake in the forearm of nor-mal subjects [49]. Moreover recent evidence has shown a clear disassociation between insulin stimulation of blood flow and glucose uptake in normal subjects [50a]. Although controversial, it is now considered unlikely that impaired dilation to insulin, resulting from endothelial dysfunction, can be the pri-mary cause of insulin resistance, although it may accentuate it.

12.5 ENDOTHELIUM-DEPENDENT CONSTRICTORS

The origin of the defect of ACh relaxation in small arteries from diabetic animals is gen-erally attributed to reduced NO availability (i.e. reduced synthesis or enhanced degrada-tion), but in some animal models of diabetes (e.g. in the larger arteries of the alloxan-treated diabetic rabbit) enhanced synthesis of constrictor prostaglandins is contributory [51]. Increased synthesis/release of endothe-lins has also been implicated in reduced peri-neural blood flow in the STZ diabetic rat, as treatment with the selective endothelin recep-tor (ETA) antagonist, BQ123, was shown to improve nerve conduction velocity and blood flow in STZ rats by 60% after two to three weeks of treatment [32].

12.6 THE DIABETIC MILIEU AND VASCULAR ENDOTHELIAL FUNCTION

Consideration of the innumerable studies of vascular endothelial function in diabetes leaves little doubt that the endothelium is dysfunctional in both NIDDM and IDDM patients. Through impairment of the dilatory NO pathway, enhanced constrictor release and increased expression of a number of pro-coagulant and pro-atherogenic molecules, the endothelium could contribute to many of the known vascular complications of the disease. The focus of many current studies is, not surprisingly, to identify the metabolic factors most responsible and, through a variety of therapeutic regimes, to attempt reversal of endothelial dysfunction. Hitherto most of the attempts at treatment have involved an animal model of diabetes; results of investigations in patients are awaited with interest.

The following paragraphs briefly cover the possible mechanisms of endothelial dysfunction and review the few studies which have attempted to improve endothelial function.

12.6.1 HYPERGLYCAEMIA

Hyperglycaemia associated with poor diabetic control may affect several metabolic pathways linked to NOS (for review see [33]). Hypergylcaemia-associated stimulation of the polyol pathway can lead to increased utilization of NADPH (the reduced form of nicotine adenine dinucleotide), an essential co-factor for constitutive NOS. A shortfall in cellular NADPH could also be deleterious to proper function of the cellular glutathione redox cycle, an important cellular antioxidant defence pathway.

Treatment of diabetic animals with aldose reductase inhibitors has produced equivocal results; conduit artery endothelial function improves with treatment in the STZ rat [52] and in the alloxan-treated diabetic rabbit [54], whereas we have found no effect on small artery function after treatment of STZ rats with the aldose reductase inhibitor, ponalrestat [54]. Glucose also stimulates membranous protein kinase C (PKC) which has been implicated in endothelial dysfunction, as PKC inhibitors can reverse glucose induced endothelial dysfunction *in vitro* [55].

The formation of advanced glycosylation endproducts (AGEs) is perhaps the most likely origin of glucose-induced vascular dysfunction (Figure 12.4). Endothelial cells express receptors for AGEs (RAGE), binding to which leads to internalization of essentially unaltered AGE molecules [56]. AGEs can play havoc in the endothelium. AGEs increase endothelial cell permeability [56] and induce macrophage adhesion to the endothelium [57]. AGEs also quench NO [58], so reducing endothelium-dependent relaxation [59]. AGEs could therefore also blunt responses to exogenous NO and so provide an explanation for the poor relaxation to nitrovasodilators often reported in diabetic animals and man. AGEs chemically modify LDL [60] rendering the LDL molecule more susceptible to oxidation. As discussed below oxidized LDLs have potent atherogenic properties and may also directly reduce endothelial NOS activity. In addition, AGE-induced modification of the LDL (which occurs principally on the lipoprotein B component of the molecule) reduces clearance of LDLs from the circulation and so contributes to elevated plasma levels [61].

AGE formation and LDLs are reduced in diabetic subjects by the nucleophilic hydrazine compound, aminoguanidine [62], but administration of this compound and assessment of vascular function have been confined to animal studies. These, however, are promising; Bucala *et al.* [58] have found aminoguanidine improves vascular endothelial function and responses to nitroglycerine in the STZ diabetic rat, and Tilton *et al.* have reported aminoguanidine-induced reduction of vascular permeability in the same animal model [63]. The role of AGEs in enhanced vascular permeability in diabetes has recently been supported by the observation that blockade of the RAGE receptor partly reversed the early vascular hyperpermeability in diabetic rats [64].

12.6.2 OXIDATIVE STRESS, LIPIDS AND ENDOTHELIAL DYSFUNCTION

Diabetes is frequently associated with an imbalance between free radical synthesis and antioxidant capacity and so is said to be a state of *oxidative stress*. In combination with certain of the lipid abnormalities of diabetes,

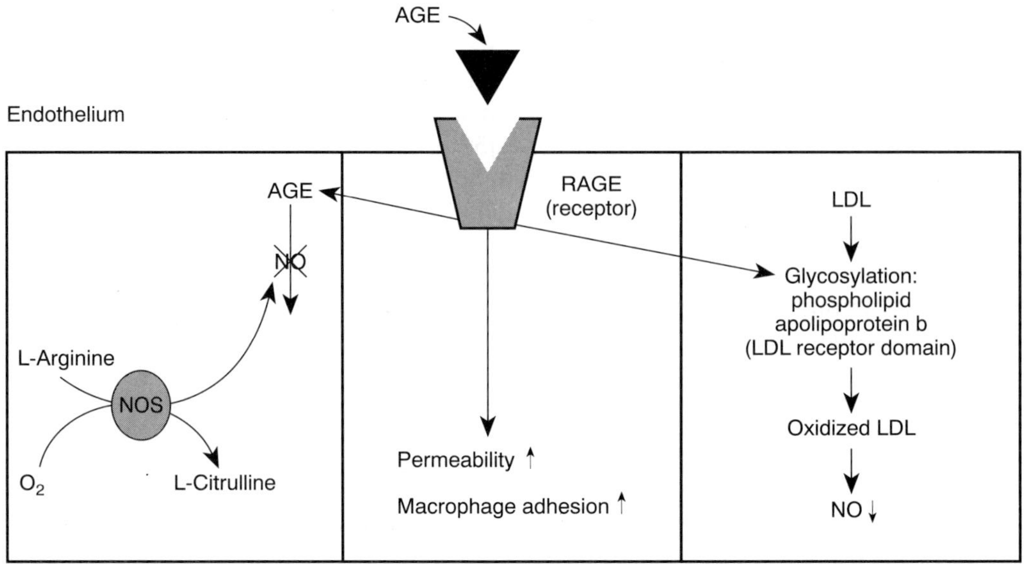

Figure 12.4 Potential mechanisms of endothelial damage induced by advanced glycosylation end-products (AGE). RAGE, receptor for AGE; LDL, low density lipoprotein; NO, nitric oxide; NOS, nitric oxide synthase.

the scene is set for the formation of lipid peroxides and the potential for interference with endothelium-dependent relaxation.

Oxidative stress may arise from elevated free radical generation, decreased levels of antioxidants and/or impaired regeneration of reduced forms of antioxidants. In diabetes increased free radical generation is likely to occur as a result of glucose induced activation of cyclooxygenase, from autoxidation of glucose or from alteration in transition metal metabolism [65]. There is some evidence that decreased antioxidant status precedes the development of diabetes in diabetic patients [66] but most investigations have been in patients or animals with established diabetes. The literature is confusing and the reader is referred to a recent detailed review [34]. Raised levels of some cellular antioxidants, e.g. superoxide dismutase, in IDDM patients may indicate an initial response to free radical challenge whereas the many reports of depletion of cellular glutathione could reflect

depletion due to chronic free radical over-production.

In animal models of uncontrolled diabetes there is substantial evidence for reduced enzymatic antioxidant status. The variability of reports in diabetic patients is likely to reflect the wide range of glycaemic control. Amongst the non-enzymatic antioxidants, platelet vitamin E was depleted in one study of NIDDM patients [67], but others have shown no change and one prospective study has suggested that low plasma vitamin E concentrations may be indicative of high risk for subsequent development of NIDDM [66]. Serum vitamin C depletion has been reported in NIDDM subjects [68] but not in poorly controlled IDDM patients [69]. There are also reports which suggest a depletion of anti-oxidant activity in the vasculature of diabetic animals [70, 71].

While free radicals are directly damaging to endothelial cells, the formation of lipid peroxides, particularly oxidized LDLs, can have further deleterious consequences. Oxidized LDLs are formed as a result of free-radical-induced oxidation of LDL within the endothelial cell. The involvement of oxidized LDL in atherogenesis is well recognized, as the molecule is taken up by the macrophage scavenger receptor and stimulates the formation of foam cells, but oxidized LDLs also reduce endothelium-dependent relaxation. In part, this may result from disruption of the G protein pathway involved in agonist-induced NO synthesis [72, 73]. Oxidized LDLs have also been shown to cause decreased expression of the endothelial NOS messenger RNA (mRNA) [74], although some recent reports do not agree [75], and to increase the synthesis of endothelin [76].

Whereas LDL concentrations in diabetic subjects are not generally raised in either IDDM or NIDDM patients, there is substantial evidence for their oxidation [34, 77] and for general lipid peroxidation [78]. LDLs in diabetic subjects are quantitatively abnormal and the LDLs consequently become more susceptible to oxidation [79]. The factors contributing to enhanced oxidation include the size of the LDL particle (LDLs are often smaller and denser [80] in diabetes) and the fact that, in patients with NIDDM, the LDLs have a high linoleic acid content [81].

The measurement of lipid peroxides is a technical minefield as lipids become rapidly oxidized if exposed to air, and most oxidized lipids are very unstable. Recently, the identification of a class of stable lipid peroxides, the isoprostanes has greatly facilitated investigations of oxidative stress. Plasma concentrations of the isoprostane, 8-epi $PGF_{2\alpha}$ are elevated in patients with NIDDM [82] and, as recently shown in our laboratory, in the plasma [83] and vasculature of the STZ diabetic rat (unpublished observations). This isoprostane also has vasoconstrictor properties in some circulations, particularly that of the heart [84] which could thus compound vascular dysfunction.

Theoretically, agents which reduce oxidative stress and/or dyslipidaemia in diabetes should reverse vascular endothelial dysfunction and reduce the risk of vasculopathy in the diabetic human and animals. Very few studies have investigated this possibility directly in diabetic subjects, although several reports are available from animal studies.

Of the few in diabetic subjects, vitamin E supplementation has been shown to reduce platelet aggregation in IDDM patients [67] and to reduce susceptibility of LDLs to oxidation [85], but no study has as yet reported effects on endothelial function in diabetic subjects. If STZ diabetic rats are fed vitamin E there is a reduction in oxidized lipids [86] and an improvement in coronary artery [87] and aorta endothelial dilator function [88]. In a recent study we have found no improvement in resistance artery endothelial function in STZ rats fed a vitamin-E-supplemented diet, despite a reversal of lipid peroxidation as assessed by measurement of isoprostanes [89]. Indeed vascular function deteriorated in the diabetic animals and, alarmingly, in the control animals fed on vitamin E (Figure 12.5). This deleterious response to Vitamin E is not an isolated observation; Trachtman *et al.* [90] have found vitamin E supplementation to reduce dramatically the survival of STZ diabetic rats and to have no affect on diabetic nephropathy.

More recently we have also shown that probucol, a mixed antioxidant and lipid-lowering drug, is as effective as vitamin E in the reversal of isoprostanes but also does not improve endothelial function [91]. Vitamin C supplementation for four months in patients with NIDDM has been shown to improve glycaemic control and to reduce plasma LDL concentrations [92]. No study has been reported of the long-term effects of vitamin C supplementation on vascular function in diabetes, but infusion of vitamin C into the forearm of NIDDM patients has shown endothelial function to improve. In STZ diabetic rats, Cotter *et al.* [93] have found an

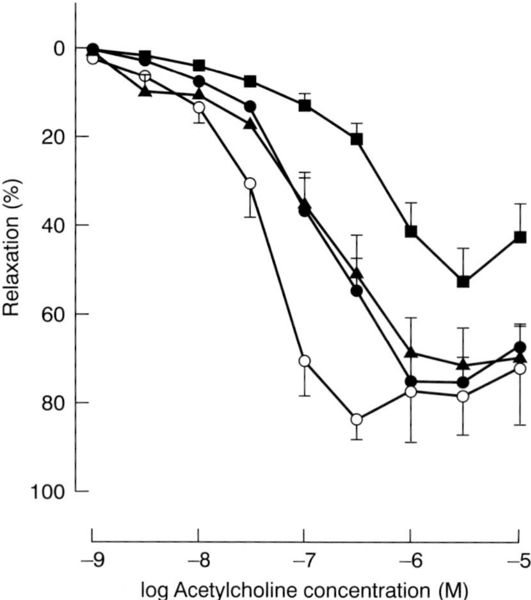

Figure 12.5 Endothelium-dependent acetycholine-induced relaxation in small mesenteric arteries from diabetic rats fed either a standard or vitamin-E-supplemented diets and from control animals fed a normal diet. Vitamin E supplementation did not reverse abnormal relaxation to acetylcholine in arteries from diabetic animals, and the higher dose led a to a further reduction of the response (STZ diabetic rats: standard diet (●), 250 mg vitamin E/kg standard diet (▲), 500 mg vitamin E /kg chow (■), and from non-diabetic rats on standard chow (○).(pEC_{50}; diabetic standard 6.70 versus control standard 7.39; $p < 0.01$; maximum relaxation; diabetic 500 mg vitamin E /kg 58.2 versus diabetic standard 84.4; $p < 0.05$). Redrawn from Palmer *et al.* [83].

increase in sciatic neural blood flow with treatment of a number of antioxidants, including vitamin C.

Other antioxidants have been used successfully to reverse endothelial dysfunction in diabetic animals. Kamata and Kobayashi [94] have suggested the involvement of the superoxide radical in endothelial dysfunction in STZ diabetic rats. These authors have shown that mRNA for the isoform of superoxide dismutase, Mn-SOD, is substantially reduced in the STZ diabetic rat and that incubation *in vitro* with SOD substantially improved endothelium-dependent relaxation. Similar *in vitro* improvement of endothelial function using SOD has been reported in the diabetic BB rat [95]. The superoxide ions rapidly destroy NO, and enhanced synthesis could contribute to reduced relaxation. Another study [96] has implicated the hydroxyl radical, as treatment of STZ rats with the hydroxyl scavenger dimethylthiourea prevented the diabetes induced impairment of the ACh response.

Lipid-lowering therapy has been shown to be effective in improving endothelial function in non-diabetic patients with atherosclerosis and/or hypercholesterolaemia [97, 98] and in hypercholestrolaemic animals [99]. No similar studies have been reported in diabetic patients but two investigations in diabetic mice have shown that the lipid-lowering drugs taurine [100] and cholestyramine [101] are effective in the reversal of endothelial function in the aorta. In our laboratory we have reversed diabetes-associated hypercholesterolaemia by treatment of the STZ diabetic rat with simvastatin and with probucol but, despite this reversal, endothelial function did not improve (unpublished observations).

In summary, there is substantial functional and biochemical evidence for endothelial dysfunction in diabetes. Potentially the most useful aspect of this knowledge for the diabetic patient is the implication that reversal of endothelial dysfunction may improve the clinical outcome of the disease, and that the therapeutic agents required are, theoretically, already available and well tolerated in diabetes. The outcome of studies in which lipid-lowering drugs, antioxidants and aminoguanidine are currently being evaluated is keenly anticipated.

ACKNOWLEDGEMENT

The author is grateful to the British Heart Foundation for financial support.

REFERENCES

1. Schmitz, O., Romer, F.K., Alberti, K.G.M.M., Hreidarsson, A.B. and Orskov, H. Angiotensin-converting enzyme in diabetes mellitus. Dependence on metabolic aberration. *Diabete Metab.*, 1983, **9,** 179–82.

2. Jensen, T., Bjerre-Knudsen, J., Feldt-Rasmussen, B. and Deckert, T. Features of endothelial dysfunction in early diabetic nephropathy. *Lancet*, 1989, **i,** 461–3.

3. Takahashi, K., Ghatei, M.A., Lam, H-C., O'Halloran, D.J. and Bloom, S.R. Elevated plasma endothelin in patients with diabetes mellitus. *Diabetologia*, 1990, **33,** 306–10.

4. Skrha, J., Vackova, I., Kvasnicka, J., Stibor, V., Stolba, P., Richter, H. and Hormann, H. Plasma free N-terminal fibronectin 30-kDa domain as a marker of endothelial dysfunction in type 1 diabetes mellitus. *Eur. J. Clin. Invest.*, 1990, **20,** 171–6.

5. Stehouwer, C.D.A., Stroes, E.S.G., Hackeng, W.H.L., Mulder, P.G.H. and Den Ottolander, G.J.H. Von Willebrand factor and development of diabetic nephropathy in IDDM. *Diabetes*, 1991, **40,** 971–6.

6. Jones, D.B., Wallace, R. and Frier, B.M. Vascular endothelial cell antibodies in diabetic patients. Association with diabetic retinopathy. *Diabetes Care*, 1992, **15,** 552–5.

7. Fasching, P., Veitl, M., Rohac, M., Streli, C., Schneider, B., Waldhausl, W. and Wagner, O.F. Elevated concentrations of circulating cell adhesion molecules and their association with microvascular complications in insulin-dependent diabetes mellitus. *J. Clin. Endocrinol. Metab.*, 1996, **81,** 4313–17.

8. Morise, T., Takeuchi, Y., Kawano, M., Koni, I. and Takeda, R. Increased plasma levels of immunoreactive endothelin and von Willebrand factor in NIDDM patients. *Diabetes Care*, 1995, **18,** 87–9.

9. Kario, K., Matsuo, T., Kobayashi, H., Matsuo, M., Sakata, T. and Miyata, T. Activation of tissue factor-induced coagulation of endothelial cell dysfunction in non-insulin dependent patients with microalbuminuria. *Arterioscler. Thromb. Vasc. Biol.*, 1995, **15,** 1114–20.

10. Chen, J.W., Gall, M.A., Deckert, M., Jensen, J.S. and Parving, H.H. Increased serum concentration of von Willebrand factor in non-insulin-dependent diabetic patients with and without diabetic nephrophathy. *BMJ*, 1995, **311,** 1405–6.

11. Garland, C.J., Plane. F., Kemp, B.K. and Cocks, T.M. Endothelium-dependent hyperpolarization: a role in control of vascular tone. *Trends Pharmacol. Sci.*, 1995, **16,** 23–30.

12. Furchgott, R.F. and Zawadski, J.V. The obligatory role of endothelial cells in the relaxation of arterial smooth muscle by acetylcholine. *Nature*, 1980, **288,** 373–376.

13. Davies, P.F. Flow-mediated endothelial mechanotransduction. *Physiol. Rev.*, 1995, **75,** 519–60.

14. Ishida, T., Peterson, T.E., Kovach, N.L. and Berk, B.C. MAP kinase activation by flow in endothelial cells. *Circulation Res.*, 1996, **79,** 310–16.

15. Corson, M.A., James, N.L., Lastta, S.E., Nerem, R.M., Berk, B.C. and Harrison, D.G. Phosphorylation of endothelial nitric oxide synthase in response to fluid shear stress. *Circulation Res.*, 1996, **79,** 984–91.

16. Khachigian, L.M., Resnick, N., Gimbrone, M.A.J. and Collins, T. Nuclear factor κβ interacts functionally with the PDFG-β chain shear stress-response element in vascular endothelial cells exposed to shear stress. *J. Clin. Invest.*, 1995, **96,** 1169–75.

17. Makimattila, S., Mantysaari, M., Groop, P.H., Summanen, P., Virkamaki, A., Schlenzka, A., Fagerudd, J. and Yki-Jarvinen, H. Hyperreactivity to nitrovasodilators in forearm vasculature is related to autonomic dysfunction in insulin-dependent diabetes mellitus. *Circulation*, 1997, **95,** 618–25.

18. Elliott, T.G., Cockroft, J.R., Groop, P-H., Earle, K., Viberti, G.C. and Ritter, J.M. Inhibition of nitric oxide synthase in forearm vasculature of insulin-dependent diabetic patients: blunted vasoconstriction in patients with microalbuminuria. *Clin. Sci.*, 1993, **85,** 687–93.

19. Johnstone, M.T., Creager, S.J., Scales, K.M., Cusco, J.A., Lee, B.K. and Creager, M.A. Impaired endothelium-dependent vasodilation in patients with insulin-dependent diabetes mellitus. *Circulation*, 1993, **88,** 2510–16.

20. Calver, A.L., Collier, J.G. and Vallance, P.J.T. Inhibition and stimulation of nitric oxide synthesis in the human forearm arterial bed

of patients with insulin-dependent diabetes. *J. Clin. Invest.*, 1992, **90**, 2546–54.

21. Makimattila, S., Virkamaki, A., Groop, P.H., Cockcroft, J., Fagerudd, J. and Yki-Jarvinen, H. Chronic hyperglycaemia impairs endothelial function and insulin sensitivity via different mechanisms in insulin-dependent diabetes mellitus. *Circulation*, 1996, **94**, 1276–82.

22. McVeigh, G.E., Brennan, G.M., Johnston, G.D., Mc Dermott, B.J., McGrath, L.T., Henry, W.R., Andrews, J.W. and Hayes, J.R. Impaired endothelium-dependent and independent vasodilation in patients with Type 2 (non-insulin-dependent) diabetes mellitus. *Diabetologia*, 1992, **35**, 771–6.

23. Williams, S.B., Cusco, J.A., Roddy, M.A., Johnstone, M.T. and Creager, M.A. Impaired nitric oxide-mediated vasodilation in patients with non-insulin dependent diabetes. *J. Am. Coll. Cardiol.*, 1996, **27**, 567–74.

24. Watts, G.F., O'Brien, S.F., Silvester and W. Millar, J.A. Impaired endothelium-dependent and independent dilation of forearm resistance arteries in men with diet treated non-insulin-dependent diabetes; role of dyslipidaemia. *Clin. Sci.*, 1996, **91**, 567–73.

25. Steinberg, H.O., Chaker, H., Leaming, R., Johnson, A., Brechtel, G. and Baron, A.D. Obesity/insulin resistance is associated with endothelial dysfunction: implications for the syndrome of insulin resistance. *J. Clin. Invest.*,1996, **97**, 2601–10.

26. Mulvany, M.J. and Halpern, W. Contractile properties of small arterial resistance vessels in spontaneously hypertensive and normotensive rats. *Circ. Res.*, 1977, **41**, 19–26.

27. McNally, P.C., Watt, P.A.C., Rimmer, T., Burden, A.C., Hearnshaw, R. and Thurston, H. Impaired contraction and endothelium dependent relaxation in isolated resistance vessels from patients with insulin dependent diabetes. *Clin. Sci.*, 1994, **87**, 31–6.

28. Cipolla, M.J., Harker, C.T. and Porter, J.M. Endothelial function and adrenergic reactivity in human type-II diabetic resistance arteries. *J. Vasc. Surg.*, 1996, **23**, 940–9.

29. Knock, G.A., McCarthy, A.L., Lowy, C. and Poston, L. Gestational diabetes is associated with abnormal maternal vascular endothelial function. *Br. J. Obstet. Gynaecol.*, 1997, **104**, 229–34.

30. Morris, S.J. and Shore, A.C. Skin blood flow responses to the iontophoresis of acetylcholine and sodium nitroprusside in man: possible mechanisms. *J. Physiol.*, 1996, **496**, 531–42.

31. Morris, S.J., Shore, A.C. and Tooke, J.E. Responses of the skin microcirculation to acetylcholine and sodium nitroprusside in patients with NIDDM. *Diabetologia*, 1995, **38**, 1337–44.

32. Cameron, N.E., and Cotter, M.A. The relationship of vascular changes to metabolic factors in diabetes mellitus and their role in development of peripheral nerve complications. *Diabetes Metab. Rev.*, 1994, **10**, 189–224.

33. Poston, L. and Taylor, P.D. Endothelium-mediated vascular function in insulin-dependent diabetes mellitus. *Clin. Sci.*, 1995, **88**, 245–55.

34. Tribe, R.M. and Poston, L. Oxidative stress and lipids in diabetes: a role in endothelium vasodilator dysfunction. *Vasc. Med.*, 1996, 1, 195–206.

35. Heygate, K.M., Davies, J., Holmes, M., James, R.F. and Thurston, H. The effect of insulin treatment and of islet transplantation on the resistance artery function in the STZ-induced diabetic rat. *Br. J. Pharmacol.*, 1996, **119**, 495–504.

36. Koukkou, E., Gerber, R.T., Lowy, C. and Poston, L. Pregnancy induced improvement in vascular function of the STZ diabetic rat persists post partum but is reversed by a high fat diet. 16th IDF Congress. Helsinki, *Diabetologia*, 1997, **40** (suppl. 1), A404.

37. Van Buren, G.A., Yang, D. and Clark, K.E. Estrogen-induced uterine vasodilation is antagonized by l-nitroarginine methyl ester, an inhibitor of nitric oxide synthesis. *Am. J. Obstet. Gynecol.*, 1992, **167**, 828–33.

38. Holemans, K., Gerber, R.T., Van Assche, F.A. and Poston, L. Adult offspring from diabetic rats show abnormal endothelium dependent relaxation and reduced heart rate. *Vasc. Res.*, 1998, **35** (suppl. 1), 6.

39. Barker D.J. Fetal nutrition and cardiovascular disease in later life. *Br. Med. Bull.*, 1997, **53**, 96–109.

40. Halpern, W., Osol, G. and Coy, G. Mechanical behaviour of pressurized *in vitro* pre-arteriolar vessels determined with a video system. *Ann. Biomed. Eng.*, 1984, **12**, 463–79.

41. Tribe, R.M., Thomas, C.R. and Poston, L. Flow-induced dilatation in isolated resistance arteries from control and streptozotocin-diabetic rats. *Diabetologia,* 1998, **41,** 34–9.

42. Jin, J.S. and Bohlen, H.G. Non-insulin dependent diabetes and hyperglycaemia impair rat intestinal flow-mediated regulation. *Am. J. Physiol.,* 1997, **272,** H728–34.

43. Schretzenmayr, A. Uber kreislaufergulatorische vorgannge and den grossen arterien bei der muskelarbeit. *Pflugers Archiv.,* 1933, **232,** 743–48.

44. Joannides, R., Hasefeli, W.E., Linder, L., Richard, V., Bakkali, E.H., Thuillez, C. and Luscher, T.F. Nitric oxide is responsible for flow dependent dilation of human peripheral conduit arteries *in vivo. Circulation,* 1995, **88,** 2511–16.

45. Zenere, B.M., Arcaro, G., Saggiani, F., Rossi. L., Muggeo, M. and Lechi, A. Noninvasive detection of functional alterations of the arterial wall in IDDM patients with and without microalbuminuria. *Diabetes Care,* 1995, **18,** 975–82.

46. Clarkson, P., Celermajer, D.S., Donald, A.E., Sampson, M., Sorensen, K.E., Adams, M., Yue, D.K., Betteridge, D.J. and Deanfield, J.E. Impaired vascular reactivity in insulin-dependent diabetes mellitus is related to disease duration and low density lipoprotein cholesterol levels. *J. Am. Coll. Cardiol.,* 1996, **28,** 573–79.

47. Goodfellow, J., Ramsey, M.W., Luddington, L.A., Jones, C.J.H., Coates, P.A., Dunstan, F., Lewis, M.J., Owens, D.R. and Henderson, A.H. Endothelium and inelastic arteries: an early marker of vascular dysfunction in non-insulin dependent diabetes. *BMJ,* 1996, *312,* 744–5.

48. Chen, Y.L. and Messina, E.J. Dilation of isolated skeletal muscle arteriole by insulin is endothelium dependent and nitric oxide mediated. *Am. J. Physiol.,* 1996, **270,** H2120–4.

49. Scherrer, U., Randin, D., Vollenweider, P., Vollenweider, L. and Nicod, P. Nitric oxide release accounts for insulin's vascular effects in humans. *J. Clin. Invest.,*1994, **94,** 2511–15.

50. Laakso, M., Edelman, S.V., Brechtel, G. and Baron, A.D. Impaired insulin-mediated skeletal blood flow in patients with NIDDM. *Diabetes,* 1992, **41,** 1076–83.

50a. Raitakari, M., Nuutila, P., Ruotsalainen, U., Laine, H., Teras, M., Iida, H., Makimattila, S., Utrainen, T., Oikonen, V., Sipila, H., Haaparanta, M., Solin, O., Wegelius, U., Knuuti, J. and Yki-Jarvinen, H. Evidence for dissociation of insulin stimulation of blood flow and glucose uptake in human skeletal muscle. *Diabetes,* 1996, **45,** 1471–7.

51. Tesfamariam, B. Selective impairment of endothelium-dependent relaxation by prostaglandin endoperoxide. *J. Hypertens.,* 1994, **12,** 41–7.

52. Cameron, N.E., and Cotter, M.A. Impaired contraction and relaxation in aorta from streptozotocin-diabetic rats: role of polyol pathway. *Diabetologia,* 1992, **35,** 1011–19.

53. Tesfamariam, B., Palacino, J.J., Weisbrod, R.M. and Cohen, R.A. Aldose reductase inhibition restores endothelial cell function in diabetic rabbit aorta. *J. Cardiovasc. Pharmacol.,* 1993, **21,** 205–11.

54. Taylor, P.D., Wickenden, A.D., Mirrlees, D.J. and Poston, L. Endothelial function in the isolated perfused mesentery and aortae of rats with streptozotocin-induced diabetes: effect of treatment with the aldose reductase inhibitor, ponalrestat. *Br. J. Pharmacol.,* 1994, **111,** 42–8.

55. Tesfamariam, B., Brown, M.L. and Cohen, R.A. Elevated glucose impairs endothelium-dependent relaxation by activating protein kinase C. *J. Clin. Invest.,*1991, **87,** 1643–8.

56. Esposito, C., Gerlach, H., Brett, J., Stern, D. and Vlassara, H. Endothelial receptor-mediated binding of glucose-modified albumin is associated with increased monolayer permeability and modulation of cell surface coagulant properties. *J. Exp. Med.,* 1989, **170,** 1387–1407.

57. Kirstein, M., Brett, J., Radoff, S., Ogawa, S., Stern, D. and Vlassara, H. Advanced protein glycosylation induces transendothelial human monocyte chemotaxis and secretion of PDGF; role in vascular disease of diabetes and aging. *Proc. Natl Acad. Sci. USA,* 1990, **87,** 9010–14.

58. Bucala, R., Tracey, K.J. and Cerami, A. Advanced glycosylation products quench nitric oxide and mediate defective endothelium-dependent vasodilation in experimental diabetes. *J. Clin. Invest.,*1991, **87,** 432–8.

59. Vlassara, H., Fuh, H., Makita, Z., Krungkrai, S., Cerami, A. and Bucala, R. Exogenous

advanced glycosylation end products induce complex vascular dysfunction in normal animals: a model for diabetic and aging complications. *Proc. Natl Acad. Sci. USA*, 1992, **89**, 12043–7.

60. Bucala, R., Makita, Z., Koshinsky, T., Cerami, A. and Vlassara, H. Lipid advanced glycosylation: pathway for lipid oxidation *in vivo*. *Proc. Natl Acad. Sci. USA*, 1993, **90**, 6434–8.

61. Bucala, R., Makita, A., Vega, G., Grundy, S., Koschinsky, T., Cerami, A. and Vlassara, H. Modification of low density lipoprotein contributes to the dyslipidaemia of diabetes and renal insufficiency. *Proc. Natl Acad. Sci. USA*, 1994, **91**, 9441–5.

62. Bucala, R. What is the effect of hyperglycaemia on atherogenesis and can it be reversed by aminoguanidine? *Diabetes Res. Clin. Pract.*, 1996, **30**, S123–30.

63. Tilton, R.G., Chang, K., Ostrow, E., Allison, W. and Williamson, J.R. Aminoguanidine reduces increased ^{131}I-albumin permeation of retinal and uveal vessels in streptozotocin-diabetic rats. *Invest. Opthalmol. Vis. Sci.*, 1990, **31**, 342.

64. Wautier, J.L., Zoukourian, C., Chappey, O., Wautier, M.P., Guillausseau, P.J., Hori, O., Stern, D. and Schmidt, A.M . Receptor-mediated endothelial cell dysfunction in diabetic vasculopathy. Soluble receptor for advanced glycosylation end products blocks hyperpermeability in diabetic rats. *J. Clin. Invest.*,1996, **97**, 238–43.

65. Wolff, S.P. Diabetes mellitus and free radicals. Free radicals, transition metals and oxidative stress in the aetiology of diabetes mellitus and complications. *Br. Med. Bull.*, 1993, **49**, 642–52.

66. Salonen, J.T., Nyyssonen, K., Tuomainen, T-P., Maenpaa, P.H., Korpela, H., Kaplan, G.A., Lynch, J., Helmrich, S.P. and Salonen, R. Increased risk of non-insulin-dependent diabetes mellitus at low plasma viamin E concentrations: a four year study in men. *BMJ*, 1995, **311**, 1124–7.

67. Kunisaki, M., Umeda, F., Inoguchi, T., Wantanabe, J. and Nawata, H. Effects of vitamin E administration in diabetes mellitus. *Diabetes Res.*, 1990, **14**, 37–42 .

68. Sinclair, A.J., Taylor, P.B., Lunec, J., Girling, A.J. and Barnett, A.H. Low plasma ascorbate levels in patients with type-2 diabetes mellitus consuming adequate dietary vitamin C. *Diabet. Med.*, 1994, **11**, 893–8.

69. Tsai, E.C., Hirsch, I.B., Brunzell, J.D. and Chait, A. Reduced plasma peroxyl radical trapping capacity and increased susceptibilty of LDL to oxidation in poorly controlled IDDM. *Diabetes*, 1994, **43**, 1010–14.

70. Dohi, T., Kawamura, K., Morita, K., Okamoto, H. and Tsujimoto, A. Alterations of the plasma selenium concentrations and the activities of tissue peroxide metabolism enzymes in streptozotocin-induced diabetic rats. *Horm. Metab. Res.*, 1988, **20**, 671–5.

71. Mooradian, A.D. The antioxidant potential of cerebral microvessels in experimental diabetes mellitus. *Brain Res.*, 1995, **671**, 164–9.

72. Jacobs, M., Plane, F. and Bruckdorfer, K.R. Native and oxidised low density lipoproteins have different inhibitory effects on endothelium-derived relaxing factor in the rabbit aorta. *Br. J. Pharmacol.*, 1990, **100**, 21–6.

73. Liao, J.K. Inhibition of Gi proteins by low density lipoproteins attenuates bradykinin stimulated release of endothelial derived nitric oxide. *J. Biol. Chem.*, 1994, **269**, 12987–92.

74. Liao, J.K., Shin, W.S., Lee, W.Y. and Clark, S.L. Oxidized low density lipoprotein decreases the expression of endothelial nitric oxide synthase. *J. Biol. Chem.*, 1995, **270**, 319–24.

75. Hirata, K., Miki, N., Kuroda, Y., Sakoda, T., Kawashima, S. and Yokoyama, M. Low concentration of oxidized low-density lipoprotein and lysophosphatidyl choline upregulate constitutive nitric oxide synthase mRNA experssion in bovine aortic endothelial cells. *Circ. Res.*, 1995, **76**, 958–62.

76. Boulanger, C.M., Tanner, F.C., Bea, M.L., Hahn, A.W., Werner, A. and Luscher, T.F. Oxidized low density lipoproteins induce mRNA expression and release of endothelin from human and porcine endothelium. *Circ. Res.*, 1992, **70**, 1191–7.

77. Bellomo, G., Maggi, E., Poli, M., Agosta, F.G., Bollati, P. and Finardi, G. Antibodies against oxidatively modified low-density lipoproteins in NIDDM. *Diabetes*, 1995, **44**, 60–6.

78. Nourooz-Zadeh, J., Tajaddini-Sarmandi, J., McCarthy, S., Betteridge, D.J. and Wolff, S.P. Elevated levels of authentic hydroperoxides in NIDDM. *Diabetes*, 1995, **44**, 1054–8.

79. Cominancini, L., Garbin, U., Pastorino, A.M., Fratta-Pasini, A., Campagnola, M., de Santis A., Davolui, A. and Lo Cascio, V. Increased susceptibility of LDL to *in vitro* oxidation in patients with insulin-dependent diabetes mellitus. *Diabetes Res.*, 1994, **36**, 173–84.

80. Stewart, M.W., Laker, M.F., Dyer, R.G., Game, F., Mitcheson, J., Winocour, P.H. and Alberti, K.G. Lipoprotein compositional abnormalities and insulin resistance in Type II diabetic patients with mild hyperlipidaemia. *Arterioscler. Thromb.*, 1993, **13**, 1046–52.

81. Dimitriadis, E., Griffin, M., Owens, D., Johnson A., Collins, P. and Tomkin, G.H. Oxidation of low-density lipoprotein in NIDDM: its relationship to fatty acid composition. *Diabetologia*, 1995, **38**, 1300–6.

82. Gopaul, N.K., Anggard, E.E., Mallet, A.I., Betteridge, D.J., Wolff, S.P. and Nourooz-Zadeh, J. Plasma 8-epi-PGF2 alpha levels are elevated in individuals with non-insulin-dependent diabetes. *FEBS Lett.*, 1995, **368**, 225–9.

83. Palmer, A.M., Thomas, C.R., Gopaul, N., Dhir, S., Anggard, E.A., Poston, L. and Tribe, R.M. Dietary antioxidant supplementation reduces lipid peroxidation but impairs vascular function in small mesenteric arteries of the streptozotocin rat. *Diabetologia*, 1998, **41**, 148–56.

84. Kromer, B.M. and Tippins, J.R. Coronary artery constriction by the isprostane 8-epi prostaglandin F2 alpha. *Br. J. Pharmacol.*, 1996, **119**, 1276–80.

85. Reaven, P.D., Herold, D.A., Barnett, J. and Edelmann, S. Effects of vitamin E on susceptibility of low-density lipoprotein and low-lipoprotein subfractions to oxidation and on protein glycation in NIDDM. *Diabetes Care*, 1995, **18**, 807–16.

86. Morel, D.W. and Chisolm, G.M. Antioxidant treatment of diabetic rats inhibits lipoprotein oxidation and cytotoxicity. *J. Lipid Res.*, 1989, **30**, 1827–34.

87. Diederich, D., Skopec, J., Diederich, A. and Dai, F.X. Endothelial dysfunction in mesenteric resistance arteries of diabetic rats: role of free radicals. *Am. J. Physiol.*, 1994, **266**, H1153–6.

88. Keegan, A., Walbank, H., Cotter, M.A. and Cameron, N.E. Chronic vitamin E treatment prevents defective endothelium-dependent relaxation in diabetic rat aorta. *Diabetologia*, 1995, **38**, 1475–8.

89. Tribe, R.M., Palmer, A.M., Thomas, C.R. and Poston, L. Effect of vitamin E and vitamin C on vascular endothelial function in the STZ diabetic rat. *J. Vasc. Res.*, 1996, **33** (suppl. 2), 23.

90. Trachtman, H., Futterweit, S., Maesaka, J., Ma, C., Valderrama, E., Fuchs, A., Tarectecan, A.A., Rao, P.S., Sturman, J.A. and Boles, T.H. Taurine ameliorates chronic streptozotocin-induced diabetic nephropathy in rats. *Am. J. Physiol.*, 1995, **269**, F429–38.

91. Palmer, A.M., Gopaul, N., Dhir, S., Thomas, C.R., Poston L. and Tribe, R.M. Endothelial dysfunction in streptozotocin rats is not reversed by probucol or simvastatin treatment. *Diabetologia*, 1998, **41**, 157–64.

92. Paolisso, G., Balbi, V., Volpe, C., Varricchio, G., Gambardella, A., Saccomanno, F., Ammendola, S., Varrichio, M. and D'Onofrio, F. Metabolic benefits deriving from chronic vitamin supplementation in aged non-insulin dependent diabetics. *J. Am. Coll. Nutr.*, 1995, **14**, 387–92.

93. Cotter, M.A., Love, A., Watt, M.J., Cameron, N.E. and Dines, K.C. Effects of natural free radical scavengers on peripheral nerve and neurovascular function in diabetic rats. *Diabetologia*, 1995, **38**, 1285–94.

94. Kamata, K. and Kobayashi, T. Changes in superoxide dismutase mRNA expression by streptozotocin-induced diabetes. *Br. J. Pharmacol.*, 1996, **119**, 583–9.

95. Pieper, G.M., Moore-Hilton, G. and Roza, A.M. Evaluation of the mechanism of endothelial dysfunction in the genetically-diabetic BB rat. *Life Sci.*, 1996, **58**, 147–52.

96. Pieper, G.M., Siebeneich, W., Roza, A.M., Jordan, M. and Adams, M.B. Chronic treatment *in vivo* with diemethylthiourea, a hydroxyl radical scavenger, prevents diabetes-induced endothelial dysfunction. *J. Cardiovasc. Pharmacol.*, 1996, **28**, 741–5.

97. Anderson, T.J., Meredith, I.T., Yeing, A.C., Frei, B., Selwyn, A.P. and Ganz, P. The effect of cholesterol lowering therapy and antioxidant therapy on endothelium-dependent coronary vasomotion. *N. Engl. J. Med.*, 1995, **332**, 488–93.

98. Goode, G.K. and Heagerty, A.M. *In vitro* responses of human peripheral small arteries

in hypercholesterolaemia and effects of therapy. *Circulation*, 1995, **91**, 2898–903.

99. Keaney J.F., Xu, A., Cunningham, D., Jackson, T., Frei, B. and Vita, J.A. Dietary probucol preserves endothelial function in cholesterol fed rabbits by limiting vascular oxidative stress and superoxide generation. *J. Clin. Invest.*, 1995, **95**, 2520–9.

100. Kamata, K., Sugiura, M., Kojima, S. and Kasuya, Y. Restoration of endothelium-dependent relaxation in both hypercholesterolaemia and diabetes by chronic taurine. *Eur. J. Pharmacol.*, 1996, **118**, 385–91.

101. Kamata, K., Suguira, M., Kojima, S. and Kasuya, Y. Preservation of endothelium-dependent relaxation in cholesterol-fed and streptozotocin-induced diabetic mice by the chronic administration of cholestryramine. *Br. J. Pharmacol.*, 1996, **118**, 385–91.

BLOOD RHEOLOGICAL CHANGES IN DIABETES

13

Alan J. Jaap and Gordon D.O. Lowe

Blood rheology is the study of factors affecting the flow properties of blood. A number of *in vitro* rheological abnormalities have been described in patients with diabetes and these are outlined below. Nonetheless, the relevance of these to the pathogenesis of diabetic angiopathy remains controversial. In this chapter, we highlight the evidence implicating a role for rheological factors in both the early functional changes and later structural changes that characterize diabetic microangiopathy.

13.1 INTRODUCTION

The prime function of blood is transport by flow, and the most important rheological property of blood is its resistance to flow, or viscosity. Plasma viscosity is about 1.6 times that of water (normal range 1.15–1.35 mPa.s at 37°C) and is largely determined by the presence of large or asymmetrical plasma proteins, especially fibrinogen, lipoproteins and immunoglobulins. The addition of erythrocytes to plasma leads to an exponential increase in viscosity with a linear increase in haematocrit. Blood is a non-Newtonian fluid, meaning that its viscosity varies with shear rate (i.e. the velocity gradient between adjacent layers in laminar flow). At high shear rates, normal blood viscosity varies from 2.5–4.5 mPa.s at 37°C. In conditions of low flow, as found in the microcirculation or in areas of flow separation in arteries, shear rate is reduced, leading to an exponential increase

in viscosity. This is due to both reduced red cell deformation and increased aggregation, each of which disturbs the streamline flow of plasma.

The deformability of the red cell determines its ability to change shape and pass through capillaries smaller than its own resting diameter of 8 μm. This is essential for oxygen delivery via the small nutritive capillaries of 3–5 μm diameter. At low shear rates, the electrostatic repulsion of red cells is overcome by the formation of cell-to-cell protein bridges, mainly consisting of fibrinogen, leading to aggregation of cells. Linear aggregates (rouleaux) of cells bind together in a side-to-side fashion, and with uptake of further cells, networks of larger aggregates are formed leading to a further increase in viscosity. This process is reversible, with disaggregation occurring as shear rates again increase, e.g. as blood flows into larger venules.

The major determinants of whole blood viscosity are therefore plasma viscosity, haematocrit, shear rate, red cell deformability and red cell aggregation.

13.2 RHEOLOGICAL CHANGES IN DIABETES

The major rheological abnormalities reported in patients with diabetes are increased plasma and whole blood viscosity [1, 2], increased red cell aggregation [2, 3] and reduced red cell deformability [3, 4]. This area has recently been reviewed in detail [5]. Some of the rheological abnormalities are interrelated, e.g. the increase in whole blood viscosity is particularly marked at low shear rates as a result of increased red cell aggregation, which is due to both increased formation and decreased dispersion of aggregates (Figure 13.1). Similar rheological changes have been described in insulin-dependent and non-insulin-dependent diabetes mellitus (IDDM and NIDDM) patients, suggesting that rheological factors are not important in determining the known differences in epidemiology and haemodynamic changes in microvascular disease in the two types of diabetes. In general, rheological abnormalities have been found to be more marked in patients with advanced microvascular complications, but are unrelated to diabetes duration [5-8].

The major factor underlying increased viscosity and red cell aggregation in patients with diabetes is an elevation in the circulating concentration of fibrinogen and globulins [5, 9]. Fibrinogen and total globulin levels are reported to be higher in patients with retinopathy, nephropathy and neuropathy in cross-sectional studies [6, 8, 10, 11]. In addition, fibrinogen and globulin levels appear to be predictive of both the development and progression of retinopathy and nephropathy in recent prospective studies in IDDM patients [10, 11]. The exact cause for increased rheologically active protein levels in patients with diabetes is uncertain, and although earlier studies suggested a link to hyperglycaemia, this was not confirmed in a large ancillary study to the Diabetes Control and Complication Trial [12]. Elevated fibrinogen levels and related rheological changes are found in a variety of other disease states where there is no associated microcirculatory damage, suggesting that other interacting factors specific to diabetes and influenced by metabolic control are necessary for the development of microvascular complications.

Serum albumin has an anti-aggregating action and it has recently been reported that this is markedly reduced by albumin glycation in patients with diabetes, further enhancing the effects of elevated fibrinogen [13].

Initial studies on red cell deformability in patients with diabetes produced conflicting results. Some suggested a reduction; others suggested no change compared with control subjects [3, 14]. This was partly due to problems in interpreting results because of the confounding effects of white blood cells. However, reduced red cell deformability has been confirmed using newer techniques which allow the red cell filtration rate to be measured independently of the sample white cell count [4, 5]. The underlying cause of reduced red cell deformability remains elusive, but may relate to a hyperglycaemia-induced increase in the microviscosity of the red cell membrane as a result of diminished ATP levels[15] or changes in the composition of membrane lipids [16]. It has been demonstrated that improved glycaemic control is associated with an increase in red cell deformability [17].

13.3 WHITE CELLS AND PLATELETS IN DIABETES

Abnormalities of the other cellular components of blood are present in patients with diabetes, and are likely to augment the effects of the rheological changes already discussed.

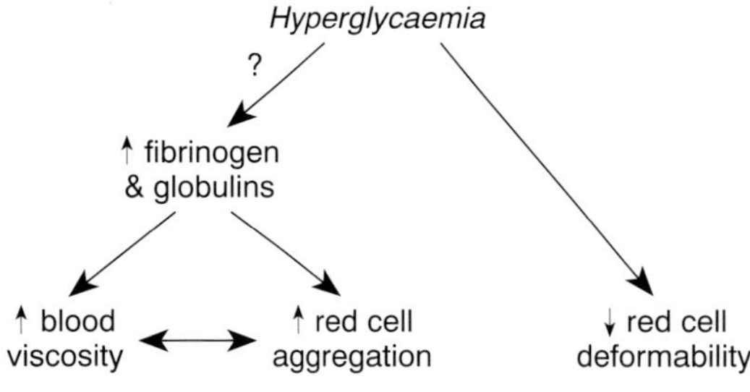

Figure 13.1 Rheological changes in diabetes.

13.3.1   WHITE CELLS

White cells are intrinsically less deformable than red cells, due to their larger volume and the presence of a nucleus. Diabetes is associated with a further reduction in white cell deformability [4], with the effects of this being compounded by the relative leucocytosis reported in patients with diabetes. In addition, there is increased adhesion of white cells to the endothelium as a result of enhanced expression of adhesion molecules, such as VCAM-1 and E-selectin [18], and the deposition of advanced glycosylation endproduct (AGE) proteins [19]. Elevated levels of soluble adhesion molecules have been found in patients with microangiopathy [20] and may relate to the degree of glycaemic control [18, 19].

13.3.2   PLATELETS

Studies in patients with diabetes have demonstrated multiple abnormalities in platelet function. Platelets from diabetic patients show evidence of increased *in vivo* activation [21, 22] and increased *in vitro* sensitivity to a variety of agonists such as ADP and collagen, resulting in increased platelet aggregation [23]. This hypersensitivity has been related to a reduction in membrane fluidity [24], similar to the situation in red cells. These abnormalities of platelet function may be more marked in patients with microvascular complications [21, 22].

13.4   RHEOLOGICAL, WHITE CELL AND PLATELET ABNORMALITIESAND THE PATHOGENESIS OF MICROANGIOPATHY

13.4.1   EARLY HAEMODYNAMIC CHANGES

Small arterioles function as resistance vessels, with the dissipation of pressure across them resulting in a high tangential force called wall shear stress. Contact of high viscosity plasma or red cell aggregates with microvascular endothelial cells results in a further increase in wall shear stress. Ditzel and Moinat [25], through direct observation of the conjunctival microcirculation, found that diabetic patients formed red cell aggregates more frequently in arterioles and that these usually disaggregated during a single cardiac systole, their disruption being required for individual red cells to flow through capillaries. Red cell changes in diabetes impede the disaggregation process, resulting in an increased peak tangential force [9]. The higher wall shear stress mediated by increased aggregation and reduced deformability of red cells may have several effects.

Firstly, there may be stimulation of endothelial cells to release vasodilator substances such as nitric oxide and prostacyclin, leading to vascular smooth muscle cell relaxation and pre-capillary vasodilation. This may possibly account for early microvascular hyperperfusion ('luxury perfusion') under resting conditions and an elevation in capillary pressure (Chapter 14). Increased tangential stress will also result in increased permeability, with greater filtration of fluid accompanied by albumin by the process of solvent drag. The final effect of increased wall shear stress may be stimulation of basement membrane synthesis.

Reduced deformability of red and white cells [4] may lead to increased endothelial contact during passage through capillaries, acting as a further stimulus to the secretion of vasodilators and repetitive endothelial damage, inducing the expression of cell adhesion molecules and increased white cell margination and migration. This latter process will occur mainly in post-capillary venules, increasing post-capillary resistance and therefore contributing to the rise in capillary pressure.

13.4.2   ESTABLISHED MICROVASCULAR DISEASE

As a result of repetitive injury, basement membrane thickening eventually leads to microvascular sclerosis and a resultant loss of flow reserve with impaired autoregulation and limited maximal vasodilation. This is compounded by reduced secretion of vaso-dilators from the denuded endothelium, also leading to exposure of the subintima and activation of the coagulation cascade and aggregation of platelets. The formation of thrombus within the microcirculation is likely to contribute to capillary non-perfusion, an early feature of retinopathy.

Although changes in blood viscosity have been described in patients with advanced microvascular disease [6, 7], findings have been inconclusive in patients with earlier microangiopathy, making it difficult to attrib-ute a primary pathological role. Also, few studies have attempted to relate measures of microvascular function with *in vitro* rheological changes. However, a negative cor-relation between transcutaneous oxygen measurements and red cell aggregation has been reported in diabetic patients with neuro-pathy [8].

As microvascular damage progresses, tis-sue hypoxia leads to the secretion of angio-genic factors and neovascularization. In this respect, it is noteworthy that cell adhesion molecules have been reported to show angio-genic activity [26]. Furthermore, the develop-ment of hypoperfusion, and therefore low shear stress, in the microcirculation may favour the development of both red cell aggregation and capillary occlusion by leuco-cytes, which may in turn promote further ischaemia. The increased tendency in patients with diabetes for both red cell aggregation under low shear conditions [3, 5] and for leucocyte capillary occlusion (due to leucocy-tosis, leucocyte activation and decreased leu-cocyte deformability [4]) may become particularly important at this stage. The potential importance of blood rheology in the progression of diabetic retinopathy has been suggested by prospective studies linking pro-gression to blood viscosity [27] and to rheo-logically-active plasma proteins [10].

Both microvascular and macrovascular complications are particularly common in diabetic patients who are hypertensive [28]. It is therefore of interest that rheological abnor-malities are greater in hypertensive compared with normotensive diabetic patients [29–31].

13.5 CONCLUSIONS

Rheological changes in diabetes are well established. They may potentially influence blood flow in both the macro- and micro-circulation, and are thus relevant to both macro- and microvascular complications. Future studies to further assess their patho-genic significance might include: (1) studies relating blood rheology to microvascular haemodynamic disturbances; (2) prospective studies of blood rheology and vascular com-plications in cohorts of diabetic patients; and (3) large randomized controlled trials of rheological interventions in patients with diabetes.

REFERENCES

1. Isogai, Y., Iida, A., Michizuki, K. and Abe, M. Hemorheological studies on the pathogenesis of diabetic microangiopathy. *Thromb. Res.*, 1976, **8**, 17–24.
2. McMillan, D.E., Utterback, N.G. and Stocki, J. Low shear rate blood viscosity in diabetes. *Biorheology*, 1980, **17**, 355–62.
3. Schmid-Schönbein, H. and Volger, E. Red cell aggregation and red cell deformability in dia-betes. *Diabetes*, 1976, **25** (supp. 2), 897–902.
4. Ernst, E., and Matrai A. Altered red and white blood cell rheology in type 2 diabetes. *Diabetes*, 1986, **35**, 1412–15.
5. MacRury, S.M. and Lowe, G.D.O. Blood rheol-ogy in diabetes mellitus. *Diabet. Med.*, 1990, **7**, 285–91.
6. Lowe, G.D.O., Ghafour, I.M., Belch, J.J.F., For-bes, C.D., Foulds, W.S. and MacCuish, A.C. Increased blood viscosity in diabetic prolifer-ative retinopathy. *Diabetes Res.*, 1986, **3**, 67–70.
7. Gordge, M.P., Merola, L. and Laibson, P.R. Blood hyperviscosity and its relationship to

progressive renal failure in patients with diabetic nephropathy. *Diabet. Med.,* 1990, **7,** 880–6.

8. Young M.J., Bennett, J.L., Liderth, S.A., Veves, A., Boulton, A.J.M. and Douglas, J.T. Rheological and microvascular parameters in diabetic peripheral neuropathy. *Clin. Sci.,* 1996, **90,** 183–7.

9. McMillan, D.E. Blood's increased transient resistance in diabetes is generated by its fibrinogen and globulin content. *Clin. Hemorheol.,* 1996, **16,** 669–76.

10. McMillan, D.E., Malone J.I. and Rand, L.I. Progression of diabetic retinopathy is linked to rheologic plasma proteins in the DCCT. *Diabetes,* 1995, **44,** 54A (abstract).

11. McMillan, D.E., Malone J.I. and Steffes M.W. Plasma fibrinogen and total globulin are elevated in albuminuria in the DCCT. *Diabetes,* 1995, **44,** 23A(abstract)..

12. McMillan, D.E. and Malone, J.I. Hemorheological effects of intensive diabetes management in the DCCT. *Clin. Hemorheol.,* 1994, **14,** 481–8.

13. Candiloros, H., Muller, S., Ziegler, O., Donner, M. and Drouin, P. Role of albumin glycation on the erythrocyte aggregation: an *in vitro* study. *Diabet. Med.,* 1996, **13,** 646–50.

14. Ritchie, D.M. Filtration of dilute erythrocyte suspension as a measure of erythrocyte deformability and its relationship to blood glucose control in diabetes mellitus. *Clin. Hemorheol.,* 1985, **5,** 257–68.

15. Rice-Evans, C. and Chapman, D. Red blood cell biomembrane structure and deformability. *Scand. J. Clin. Lab. Invest.,* 1981, **41** (suppl. 156), 99–110.

16. Otsuji, S., Baba, Y. and Kamada, T. Erythrocyte membrane microviscosity in diabetes. *Horm. Metab. Res.,* 1981, **11,** 97–102.

17. Leiper, J.M., Lowe, G.D.O., Anderson, J., Burns, P., Cohen, H.N, Manderson, W.G. *et al.* Effects of diabetic control and biosynthetic human insulin on blood rheology in established diabetics. *Diabetes Res.,* 1984, **1,** 27–30.

18. Cominacini, L., Fratta Pasini, A., Garbin, U., Davoli, A., De Santis, A., Campagnola, M. *et al.* Elevated levels of soluble E-Selectin in patients with IDDM and NIDDM: relation to metabolic control. *Diabetologia,* 1995, **38,** 1122–4.

19. Schmidt, A.M., Hori, O., Chen, J.X., Li, J.F., Crandall, J., Zhang, J. *et al.* Advanced glycation endproducts interacting with their endothelial receptor induce expression of vascular cell adhesion molecule 1 (VCAM-1) in cultured human endothelial cells and in mice. *J. Clin. Invest.,* 1995, **96,** 1395–1403.

20. Schmidt, A.M., Crandall, J., Hori, O., Cao, R. and Lakatta, E. Elevated levels of vascular cell adhesion molecule 1 (VCAM-1) in diabetic patients with microalbuminuria: a marker of vascular dysfunction and progressive vascular disease. *Br. J. Haematol.,* 1996, **92,** 747–50.

21. Fernandez-Vigo, J., Cordido, M., Fernandez Sabagul, J. and Cordido, F. Platelet function in diabetic retinopathy: levels of beta-thromboglobulin and platelet factor 4. *Metab. Paediat. Syst. Ophthalmol.,* 1992, **15,** 5–8.

22. Toth, L., Szenasi, P., Varsanyi, M.N., Szvilasi, I., Lehoczky, E., Kammerer, L. *et al.* Elevated levels of plasma and urine beta-thromboglobulin or thromboxane-B2 as markers of real platelet hyperactivation in diabetic nephropathy. *Haemostasis,* 1992, **22,** 334–9.

23. Winocour, P.D. Platelet abnormalities in diabetes mellitus. *Diabetes,* 1992, **41** (suppl. 2), 26–31.

24. Winocour, P.D., Bryszewska, M., Watala, C., Rand, M.L., Epand, R.M., Kinlough-Rathbone, R.L. *et al.* Reduced membrane fluidity in platelets from diabetic patients. *Diabetes,* 1990, **39,** 241–4.

25. Ditzel, J. and Moinat, P. Changes in serum proteins, lipoproteins and protein-bound carbohydrates in relation to pathologic alterations in the microcirculation of diabetic subjects. *J. Lab. Clin. Med.,* 1959, **54,** 843–58.

26. Koch, A.E., Halloran, M.M., Haskell, C.J., Shah, M.R. and Polverini, P.J. Angiogenesis mediated by soluble forms of E-selectin and vascular cell adhesion molecule-1. *Nature,* 1995, **376,** 517–19.

27. Barnes, A.J., Oughton, J. and Kohner, E.M. Blood rheology and the progression of diabetic retinopathy: a prospective study. *Clin. Hemorheol.,* 1987, **7,** 460 (abstract).

28. McRury, S.M., Small, M., MacCuish, A.C. and Lowe, G.D.O. Association of hypertension with blood viscosity in diabetes. *Diabet. Med.,* 1988, **5,** 830–4.

29. Rampling, M.W., Feher, M.D., Sever, P.S. and Elkeles, R.S. Haemorheological disturbances in non-insulin-dependent diabetes and the effects of concommitant hypertension. *Clin. Hemorheol.,* 1989, **9,** 101.

30. McRury, S.M., Lennie, S.E., McColl, P., Balendra, R., MacCuish, A.C. and Lowe, G.D.O. Increased red cell aggregation in diabetes mellitus: association with cardiovascular risk factors. *Diabet. Med.*, 1993, **10,** 21–6.

31. Lowe, G.D.O. Blood rheology, haemostasis and vascular disease. In *Haemostasis and Thrombosis*, (eds A.L. Bloom, C.D. Forbes, D.P. Thomas and E.G.D. Tuddenham), 3rd edn, Churchill Livingstone, Edinburgh, 1994, pp. 1169–88.

MECHANISMS UNDERLYING PATHOPHYSIOLOGICAL CHANGES IN HUMAN DIABETIC MICROANGIOPATHY

John E. Tooke

14.1 INTRODUCTION

As the previous chapters make clear, the vascular cell biochemical consequences of hyperglycaemia provide a plausible explanation for microvascular dysfunction in diabetes even if the relative importance of different pathways and the precise cellular mechanisms through which changes in microvascular performance are achieved remain unresolved. Furthermore, the central importance of the endothelial cell in the pathogenesis of microangiopathy is supported both by its anatomical credentials as the sole cell type apart from the pericytes between blood and tissue and by theoretical considerations, notably the array of relevant functions the endothelium subserves.

Knowledge of endothelial cell biology has accelerated due to the capacity to culture cells and subject them to a variety of conditions that may pertain *in vivo*. Caution is required, however, in the interpretation of findings from such studies for a number of reasons: First, endothelial cells from aorta, arteries or veins rather than the microvasculature are often used, and there is abundant evidence that microvascular endothelial responses may differ from those observed in cells derived from other larger vessels. Second, cell passage modifies cellular response to a variety of stimuli. Third, a cell culture plate poorly reproduces the intravascular environment in which cellular elements of the blood come into contact with the vessel wall, dynamic, phasic changes in pressure, flow, stretch and shear occur and intimate interactions with subjacent tissues take place.

Despite these reservations, sufficient evidence exits to implicate microvascular endothelium as the orchestrator or choreographer of a wide variety of pathophysiological phenomena observed in diabetes [1].

In this chapter, those microvascular physiological abnormalities that are characteristic of the two major types of human diabetes are scrutinized in mechanistic terms, summarizing current understanding of the cellular processes involved.

14.2 THE ORIGINS OF LUXURY PERFUSION

Early diabetes of either type is characterized by a control-related increase in resting microvascular blood flow at rest in many vascular beds. From a theoretical standpoint such a hyperaemic or 'luxury perfusion' state could result from reduced vasoconstrictor tone and/or reduced intrinsic resistance to flow possessed by the blood itself (Table 14.1). *In vitro* measurements of blood rheology support the concept of increased whole blood and plasma viscosity as well as reduced red cell deformability rather than the converse, making reduced vasoconstrictor tone the

Table 14.1 Potential causes of increased microvascular flow in diabetes

---

Reduced neurogenic tone
- sympathetic neuropathy
- secondary to raised metabolic rate

Circulating vasodilators
- insulin
- ketone bodies

Locally generated vasodilators
- neurogenic inflammation
- increased shear at endothelial surface
- vascular cell effects of hyperglycaemia
  - indirect, e.g. via kallikrein-kinin cascade
  - direct, e.g. via PKC activation

Insensitivity to vasoconstrictors
- e.g. endothelin

---

likely contender mechanism. The degree of vasoconstriction reflects the balance between vasoconstrictor and vasodilator influences and the vascular smooth muscle response to such influences. Factors influencing vascular tone may be circulating, neurally or locally derived and modified by other systemic influences. Many such factors ultimately influence the generation of endothelial cell nitric oxide (NO) and vasodilator prostanoids which have a potent influence on the intracellular calcium level of subjacent vascular smooth muscle. For example in the kidney, kallikrein synthesis (which is increased in diabetes, particularly during poor control [2]) is known to increase glomerular filtration rate (GFR). Kallikrein generates kinins (including bradykinin) from the kininogen substrate. Bradykinin binds to specific receptors and mediates its vasodilator action through the release of endothelial-derived NO, prostacyclin and endothelium-derived hyper-polarizing factor [3]. Inhibitors of kallikrein synthesis [4] or activity reduce GFR as do bradykinin receptor antagonists [5].

Hyperglycaemia may have direct effects on the endothelial cells' capacity to generate NO as well as resulting in a range of biochemical sequelae, including non-enzymatic glycation, sorbitol–*myo*-inositol changes, diacyl glycerol–protein kinase C activation and alteration in redox potential which may mirror the situation provoked by hypoxia (Chapter 10). Although protein kinase C activation results in a cascade of intracellular events resulting in increased production of reactive oxygen species including NO, the resultant oxidative stress could counter any positive effects.

What is less well appreciated is that the physical forces to which the microvascular endothelium is exposed may have a profound effect on the generation of a range of vaso-active mediators by the endothelium. Indeed, shear stress is the most potent stimulus to the release of NO [6] through increased expression of constitutive NO synthase, as well as increasing release of the vasodilator prostacyclin [7] and possibly the vasoconstrictor endothelin [8]. The cellular transduction mechanisms linking shear with NO release are imperfectly understood but involve a variety of surface receptors and the cytoskeletal machinery to provide a rapid as well as a slow gene-regulated response. It is thus conceivable that the blood rheological changes in diabetes alluded to above, rather than reducing blood flow as suggested by early workers in the field, may have their deleterious influence through stimulating luxury perfusion. In support of a rheological contribution to microangiopathy is the observation from the ancillary study of the Diabetes Control and Complications Trial that fibrinogen and total globulin levels were higher in those patients with diabetic retinopathy and nephropathy [9]. Higher levels of these plasma proteins predispose to red cell aggregation, aggregates that must be disrupted as the blood passes through arterioles to the capillaries as vessel diameter diminishes. This disaggregation process induces greater shear stress [10].

An endothelial-independent manner in which vascular tonus might be reduced in the resting state is through attenuated activity of vasoconstrictor agonists operating at the level of the vascular smooth muscle. Clearly, in the presence of peripheral neuropathy, the reduction in sympathetic nervous activity results in peripheral vasodilatation. Other organs are under lesser degrees of neurogenic control. Although culture studies have demonstrated a reduced response of vascular smooth muscle cells to vasoconstrictor agonists such as angiotensin II in a high glucose environment [11], such studies have tended to use large vessel material. Impaired vasoconstriction to endothelin 1 has been demonstrated in patients with non-insulin-dependent diabetes mellitus (NIDDM) [12]. In contrast, *in vivo* studies in man using the dorsal hand vein technique have suggested that vasoconstrictor responsiveness to noradrenaline may be enhanced rather than diminished, at least in insulin-dependent diabetes mellitus (IDDM) patients with microalbuminuria [13].

Circulating metabolites other than glucose, as well as hormones such as insulin, may also influence vasoconstrictor tone. Exposure to physiological concentrations of insulin blunted the contraction response to noradrenaline in rat mesenteric vessels via a NO-dependent mechanism [14] and human studies support the concept that, if acutely administered, insulin can act as a micro-vascular vasodilator [15]. Lactate and ketone bodies result in increased renal plasma flow, as does atrial natriuretic factor, the latter also through a NO-dependent mechanism.

14.3 THE ORIGINS OF CAPILLARY HYPERTENSION

IDDM, although not normotensive NIDDM, is characterized by control-related increases in capillary pressure [16], which, as argued in Chapter 10, implicates an increase in post- to pre-capillary resistance, or an increase in resistance at capillary level *per se* in subjects predisposed to capillary hypertension (Table 14.2). Although there is some biomicroscopical [17] and biopsy data[18] that capillary luminal diameter may be reduced in diabetes,

Table 14.2 Potential causes of capillary hypertension in insulin-dependent diabetes

Reduced pre-capillary resistance
- Mechanisms listed in Table 1

      plus

Relative increase in capillary/post-capillary resistance
- Reduced capillary number
- Reduced capillary diameter
- Increased venular tone
  - secondary to increased production of venoconstrictors, e.g. AII
  - relative deficiency of venodilators, e.g. NO
  - increased sensitivity to venoconstrictors, e.g. noradrenaline
- Increased intrinsic resistance to flow within venules secondary to red cell aggregation

particularly the arteriolar end, no systematic studies in relation to capillary pressure have been undertaken and methodological considerations make the interpretation of such results uncertain. A reduced number or density of capillaries either due to structural lack, or loss, or functional lack of recruitment, would also result in increased vascular resistance at capillary level. Such a mechanism would provide an attractive mechanism for the effects of pre-natal nutrition and development of the propensity to diabetes, hypertension and possibly nephropathy. Starting nephron number may be reduced in nephropathy-prone individuals [19] but whether or not there is any evidence of a reduction in capillary density in subjects with capillary hypertension has not been examined, although the proportion of recruitable capillaries may be reduced in subjects more prone to the development of NIDDM [20]. In hypertension in the absence of diabetes, the role of capillary rarefaction is more compelling: The offspring of two parents with high blood pressure exhibit a lower cutaneous capillary density than the offspring of two parents with low/normal blood pressure [21].

At a post-capillary level, enhanced veno-constriction could reflect the greater availability of, or enhanced response to, mediators acting on this part of the circulation. In the kidney, angiotensin II (AII) receptors are more prevalent on the efferent arteriole [22] and endothelin is known to have a greater impact on post- compared to pre-capillary resistance [23]. The angiotensin-converting enzyme (ACE) is sited on the microvascular endothelium and serum ACE levels are higher in subjects prone to diabetic nephropathy. Although this could be a generalized marker of microvascular endothelial damage, it could represent high levels of enzyme expression, perhaps genetically determined. Despite early promise, attempts to associate genetic determinants of ACE with risk of diabetic nephropathy have proved disappointing. In support of a role for ACE activity or its product AII in predisposing to accelerated microangiopathy, capillary pressure can be reduced by ACE inhibitors in patients with IDDM and incipient nephropathy [24] but not in patients without this precursor of severe complications [25].

Alternatively, if endothelin generation is not offset by a compensatory increase in vasodilator mediators such as prostacyclin, relative venoconstriction may prevail. Recent work associating reduced endothelial-dependent vasodilatation with insulin-resistant states [26] provides a mechanistic basis for greater post-capillary tone in patients with incipient or established nephropathy who tend to be more insulin resistant [27].

Another potential mediator that operates predominantly on the post-capillary segment is serotonin [28]. Sequestered in blood platelets, this chemical has complex actions including stimulating the release of NO as well as amplifying the effects of noradrenaline and angiotensin II. Relative impairment of NO release availability may again switch the balance in favour of venoconstriction.

Not only is the resistance of the post-capillary segment dependent on the cross-sectional diameter of the vascular bed at this point, but also on the flow properties of blood itself. Within the venules, low shear rates prevail favouring red cell aggregation to which diabetic blood is prone, particularly in patients predisposed to microangiopathic complications. Furthermore, white cells adhere to venular endothelium and the increased expression of adhesion molecules such as ICAM-1 mediated by increased shear [29] as well as a high glucose environment [30] may be contributory.

14.4 LIMITATION IN MAXIMAL MICROVASCULAR HYPERAEMIA

A characteristic feature of the microcirculation in diabetes is the limitation of maximum microvascular hyperaemia or limitation of microvascular vasodilatory reserve. In IDDM this phenomenon is duration-related and after initial control of diabetes is mild to moderate in the early years. In NIDDM profound reduction is observed early in diabetic life.

At a theoretical level limitation to vasodilatation could represent fixed, structural resistance or a failure of functional mechanisms designed to relax vascular smooth muscle (Table 14.3). Several lines of evidence support the concept of fixed structural resistance contributing to the reduced maximum hyperaemic response observed in IDDM. Ajjam *et al.* observed an association between reduced reactive hyperaemia and the degree of arteriolar hyalinosis in skin biopsy specimens [31]. Rayman *et al.* found a correlation between capillary basement membrane width and the hyperaemic response of the skin to a mild thermal injury[32]. As argued in Chapter 9, in this context basement membrane thickening may be a surrogate marker for more important upstream arteriolar sclerosis.

The type IV collagen present in such biopsy specimens is manufactured by the microvascular endothelium, implicating this cellular layer in the abnormality observed. In addition

Table 14.3 Potential causes of impaired maximal microvascular hyperaemia

---

Structural limitation
- Basement membrane thickening/glycation
- Arteriolar hyalinosis

Functional impairment of vascular smooth muscle relaxation
- Altered generation of local vasodilators, e.g. NO
- Quenching of NO by oxidative stress or AGE products
- Impaired vascular smooth muscle relaxation

---

to the production of vasoactive substances, increased pressure, stretch and shear results in increased production of type IV collagen as well as other extravascular matrix proteins, production that is also enhanced in high glucose environment [33]. In an elegant study, Riser *et al.* demonstrated that distension of the glomerulus resulted in the increased expression of the message for type IV collagen and laminin [34]. This alteration in extravascular matrix protein production represents the medium- to long-term gene-regulated structural adaptation to a sustained stimulus.

Whether or not the same structural adaptation occurs in NIDDM is less clear, principally because fewer systematic studies of microvascular structure have been performed in this form of the disease. The few that have been reported suggest that capillary basement membrane thickening is less marked, which is in keeping with the finding that in normotensive NIDDM capillary pressure is normal. What then is the cause of the profound reduction in microvascular vasodilatory reserve observed in NIDDM and pre-diabetic state of mildly impaired glucose tolerance?

Using laser perfusion imaging to measure cutaneous microvascular blood flow and iontophoresis to deliver endothelial-dependent and -independent mediators of vasodilatation, Morris *et al.* observed that both endothelial-dependent and -independent vasodilatation was impaired in subjects with NIDDM [35]. Similar studies in IDDM revealed impairment only of endothelial-dependent responses and only in subjects with incipient nephropathy but not those with a similar duration of disease who had avoided this complication [36]. Impaired endothelial-dependent vasodilatation was also observed in subjects with fasting hyperglycaemia, whereas non-endothelial-dependent responses were intact [37]. Further analysis revealed that the abnormality was only present in men; pre-menopausal women with fasting hyperglycaemia appearing to possess some protection. It is tempting to speculate that this protection represents the effects of oestrogen on NO synthase expression, which is lost at the menopause [38].

Evidence for impaired endothelial-dependent vasodilatation is not confined to studies of the cutaneous microvasculature. Reduced responses have been observed in the coronary circulation in the presence of diabetes and obesity [39], and flow-induced vasodilatation, which is endothelium-dependent, is reduced in conduit arteries in subjects with NIDDM [40] as well as hypercholesterolaemia [41].

The reduced endothelial-dependent vasodilatation observed in men with fasting hyperglycaemia could represent the effect of mild elevation of blood glucose or some other metabolic consequence of the insulin-resistant state and indeed correlation with calculated insulin sensitivity and overall microvascular vasodilatory reserve has been described [42]. Alternatively, endothelial dysfunction could be the primary abnormality leading to both impaired microvascular responses and the risk of NIDDM. Interestingly, other components of the insulin-resistant state or metabolic syndrome, such as hypertension [43] and dyslipidaemia [41], are also associated with impaired endothelial-dependent vasodilatory mechanisms in the absence of diabetes.

A plausible mechanism by which endothelial dysfunction could result in diabetes *per se* is through altering the capacity for glucose disposal by skeletal muscle. It has been established that insulin increases skeletal muscle blood flow through a NO-dependent mechanism [44]. Whereas insulin mediated skeletal muscle blood flow increments are blunted in the presence of obesity and NIDDM [45], the spatial correlation between blood flow and glucose uptake appears poor [46], although this could represent the gross nature of the techniques employed. In theory, insulin resistance at skeletal muscle level could represent impaired temporal and or spatial distribution of blood flow at a microvascular level, irrespective of the total flow to the muscle. An alternative hypothesis, again implicating the endothelium in the genesis of insulin resistance, is that the capillary wall may act as a key rate-limiting step in the access of insulin to the subjacent tissue [47].

Some support for the concept that endothelial dysfunction may antedate diabetes comes from the observation that plasminogen activator inhibitor-1 (PAI-1) levels are increased in proportion to insulin sensitivity in non-diabetic subjects [48]. The critical experiment demonstrating evidence of microvascular endothelial dysfunction in genetically enriched individuals at high risk of NIDDM before they develop insulin resistance or its associated metabolic derangements is yet to be performed, although a global measure of microvascular vasodilatory reserve was normal in this population [49].

14.5 CHANGES IN CAPILLARY PERMEABILITY IN DIABETES

The capillary wall comprises a single layer of endothelial cells surrounded by basement membrane produced by the endothelium. It is therefore obvious that endothelial dysfunction should be implicated in the increased microvascular permeability described in diabetes.

14.5.1 DETERMINANTS OF CAPILLARY WALL PERMEABILITY

The tubular layer of endothelial cells that comprise the capillaries may be either: (a) continuous, with cells in continuity with one another; (b) fenestrated, in which the endothelial cell cytoplasm is so thin that opposite surfaces of its membranes are very close and form circular areas called fenestrae – in the case of the renal glomerulus these fenestrae may be open directly to the basement membrane; or (c) discontinuous, with intercellular gaps communicating with holes in the basement membrane, e.g. bone marrow. Capillaries of skin, muscle, nervous tissue are continuous in type. The interendothelial cell junctional region is thought to be the major route for the passage of many molecular species. Alternative theories have postulated the existence of larger gaps or 'pores' through the vessel wall. Although transcellular 'holes' have been observed following exposure of single capillaries to high pressure [50], the anatomical basis for large pores under other conditions is scant. The concept that the traffic of vesicles invaginating from the luminal surface to engulf luminal contents and passing to the abluminal surface, or alternatively the fusion of a series of vesicles to provide a racemose channel across the endothelial cell, could act as an important means of transport for macromolecules is regaining favour. This is supported by the demonstration that inhibition of caveola movement can reduce capillary permeability [51], although transcapillary flux can still be demonstrated after vesicle formation has been experimentally arrested.

If the interendothelial cell junction is a principal route for transcapillary molecular transport, detailed knowledge of its structure and regulation are of paramount importance for the understanding of capillary permeability and its disturbance by diabetes. It has long been appreciated that the interendothelial cell gap narrows at certain points termed zonula occludens or tight junctions. In adjacent areas, the opposing cell membranes are wider apart but particularly adherent (zonular adhaerens). More detailed ultrastructural studies have revealed the presence of regularly spaced bringing structures in the interendothelial cell cleft [52] the molecular basis of which is now becoming apparent. Several molecules (vinculin, plakoglobin and catenins) are constituents of the junction, whereas cadherins and integrins are also involved. The adhesion molecule PECAM-I also plays a regulatory role, monoclonal antibodies directed against the molecule resulting in increased permeability of confluent endothelial cell layers to macromolecules [53].

In addition to the junctional complexes, the luminal surface of the capillary and the endothelial cell cleft are filled with a glycocalyx [54], a meshwork of glycoprotein onto which plasma proteins are adsorbed. The dimensions of the meshwork further contribute to the sieving properties of the capillary wall as well as acting as a charge barrier. Once beyond the endothelial cell, a molecule must traverse the basement membrane, a complex latticework of type IV collagen, laminin, fibronectin and proteoglycans. Subjected to pressure, the basement membrane acts like a compressible ultrafilter [55], becoming less permeable to large molecules as pressure rises.

14.5.2 THE MOLECULAR BASIS FOR INCREASED PERMEABILITY IN DIABETES

Remarkably little is known of the detailed molecular determinants of capillary permeability in diabetes. It is clear that disruption of the normal integrity of the interendothelial cell junctional complexes could provide a potent mechanism for permeability change and evidence is emerging for this hypothesis. For example, the prolonged incubation of

confluent monolayers of human umbilical vein endothelial cells in a high glucose medium results in reduced expression of PECAM-1 [30].

Klaentschi *et al.* have explored the impact of a high glucose environment as well as exposure to slightly raised hydrostatic pressure on the expression of PECAM-1 by dermal microvascular endothelial cells. The combination of the two conditions appears to be synergistic, resulting in significantly reduced expression of the adhesion molecule [56].

The expression of adhesion molecules may also be influenced by the interaction between advanced glycation end products (AGEs) and their cell surface receptor (RAGE) [57]. Such interaction increases endothelial cell oxidant stress, a process that is also increased by diabetes-induced auto-oxidation of glucose and the accelerated prostaglandin production that occurs in hyperglycaemia.

Junctional adhesion proteins are linked to the cytoskeletal actin myofilaments, contraction of which provides a mechanism for increasing permeability. The contractile state of the myofilaments is dependent upon intracellular calcium concentration, modulated by cyclic GMP levels, which in turn is dependent upon endothelial cell NO production [58]. As discussed above, several lines of evidence suggest that NO availability is reduced in diabetes, particularly in disease of long duration complicated by microalbuminuria, although whether this reflects reduced synthesis or excess destruction due, for example, to free radical accumulation remains to be determined. Regardless of the precise mechanism, it is clear that the loss of NO's normal modulating effect on interendothelial cell permeability could compound more direct mechanisms.

There is considerable evidence that not only is capillary basement membrane thickened in diabetes, but its chemical content and tertiary structure is also altered [59]. Loss of heparan sulphate proteoglycan results in a reduction in the charge barrier of particular relevance in the glomerulus, where basement membrane represents the key barrier component due to the discontinuous nature of the endothelial layer. Advanced glycation leads to the formation of cross-links between lysine residues of collagen molecules. Such changes may render basement membrane less compressible [60], reducing the capacity of the

Table 14.4 Potential causes of increased microvascular permeability in diabetes

---

Altered vesicular/caveola transport of macromolecules
- in response to hyperglycaemia?
- in response to capillary hypertension?

Altered expression of interendothelial cell adhesion molecules
- in response to hyperglycaemia
- in response to capillary hypertension

Altered tension on junctional adhesion molecule anchoring actin filaments
- modulated by NO availability/oxidative stress

Altered charge/physical structure of glycocalyx

Altered charge/physical structure of basement me

---

membrane to limit solute flux at high pressures. Depending on the degree of glycation, cross-linking may restrict the entry of some large molecules.

Loss of heparan sulphate proteoglycan on the endothelial cell surface may alter the adluminal charge barrier, a change regarded by some to be a key determinant of susceptibility to increased microvascular permeability/accelerated diabetic angiopathy [61]. As these proteoglycans may serve to anchor the glycocalyx, the integrity of this component of the barrier may be compromised; whether or not glycocalyx chemical structure is adversely affected by the diabetic state is unclear.

The assessment of microvascular permeability in human diabetes is compromised by the limited availability of unambiguous techniques. Early glycaemic-control-dependent increases in water and protein flux [4] could represent capillary hypertension, the presence of which has been directly verified and is related to glycaemic control [16]. Later changes in capillary filtration coefficient and capillary diffusion capacity are likely to represent changes in the intrinsic properties of the

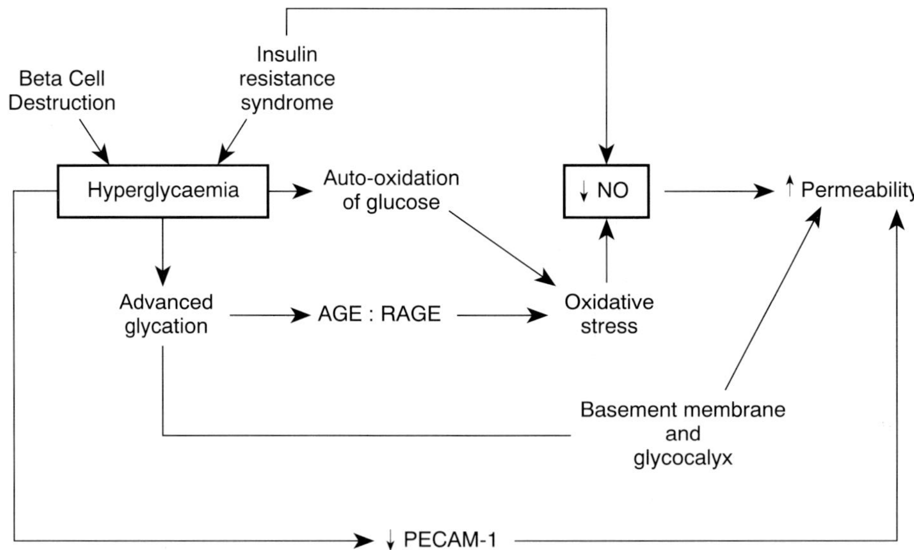

Figure 14.1 Hypothetical molecular mechanisms of increased permeability in diabetic microangiopathy.

capillary wall. In continuous capillaries, the interendothelial cell junctional complexes, about which knowledge at a molecular level is rapidly accumulating, are likely to be a key determinant of permeability in such vessels. Several molecular mechanisms associated with diabetes may now be proposed (Table 14.4) and a tentative way in which they relate outlined in Figure 14.1. Testing such hypotheses in human diabetes will be a crucial, though formidable task.

14.6 CONCLUSIONS

Metabolic and haemodynamic factors both play a role in the genesis of diabetic microangiopathy and indeed may be synergistic. Such interrelationship between physical forces and chemical environment is well accepted as far as atherosclerosis is concerned where hypertension and vessel shear rates and dyslipidaemia are indisputably involved. The endothelial cell has the capacity to respond to myriad different signals yet the subsequent transduction mechanisms are relatively limited in number. It is probably at this level that synergism occurs.

A key difficulty in grasping a clear picture of the pathogenesis of diabetic microangiopathy is that it is an evolutionary process, involving various stages and the apparently paradoxical combination of (physiologically inappropriate) over- and underperfusion. Two processes are arguably key to the evolutionary process, namely structural remodelling of the microcirculation and exhaustion of the endothelium or its replicative capacity. The concept of structural adaptation of the microcirculation in the context of hypertension is well recognized and cumulative basement membrane thickening may be considered as a similar process. Allied to the alteration in matrix dimensions is the change in their chemical structure, most notably the accumulation of AGEs. Not only may AGE proteins quench endothelial-derived NO [62], which plays the pivotal role in the regulation

of microvascular tone in health, but there is emerging evidence that AGE products and chronic hyperglycaemia may result in down-regulation of constitutive NO synthase (cNOS) yet overexpression of inducible NO synthase (iNOS) with potentially catastrophic increases in oxidative stress.

Both glucose [63] and high pressure (unpublished observation) have been shown to induce apoptosis in microvascular endothelial cells. Once the replicative capacity of the endothelium has been exhausted, permeability will be compromised as will endothelial cell cross-talk and the fine regulation of vascular tone. Exposure of the subjacent extracellular matrix may ultimately result in microthrombosis.

REFERENCES

1. Tooke, J.E. Endothelium the main actor or choreographer in the remodelling of the retinal microvasculature in diabetes? *Diabetologia*, 1996, **39**, 745–6.
2. Mayfield, R.K., Margolius, T.I.S., Levine, J.H. *et al.* Urinary kallikrein excretion in insulin-dependent diabetes mellitus and its relationship to glycaemic control. *J. Clin. Endocrinol. Metab.*, 1984, **59**, 278–86.
3. Busse, R. and Fleming, I. Molecular responses of endothelial tissue to kinins. *Diabetes*, 1996, **45** (suppl. 1), 58–513.
4. Jaffa, A.A., Rust, P.F. and Mayfield, R.K. Kinin, a mediator of diabetes induced glomerular hyperfiltration. *Diabetes,* 1995, **44**, 156–60.
5. Platts, J.K., Meadows, P. and Harvey, J.N. The relationship between urinary kallikrein and glomerular filtration rate (GFR) in Type 1 diabetes: studies with lithium. *Immunopharmacology*, 1996, **33**, 351–3.
6. Rubanyi, G.M., Romero, J.C. and Vanhoutte, P.M. Flow-induced release of endothelium-derived relaxing factor. *Am. J. Physiol.*, 1986, **255**, H783–8.
7. Frangos, J.A., Eskin, S.G., McIntire, L.V. and Ives, C.L. Flow effects on prostacyclin production by cultured human endothelial cells. *Science*, 1985, **227**, 1477–9.
8. Morita, T., Kurihara, H., Maemura, K., Yoshizumi, M. and Yazaki, Y. Disruption of cytoskeletal structures mediates shear stress-induced

endothelin-1 gene expression in cultured porcine aortic endothelial cells. *J. Clin. Invest.,* 1993, **92,** 1706–12.

9. McMillan, D.E., Malone, J.I., Rand, L.I. and Steffes, M.W. Hemorheologic plasma proteins predict future retinopathy and nephropathy in the DCCT. *Diabetologia,* 1994, **37** (Suppl. 1), A26.

10. Tooke, J.E. and Shore A.C. The regulation of microvascular function in diabetes mellitus. In *Chronic Complications of Diabetes,* eds. J.C. Pickup and G. Williams, Blackwell Oxford, 1994, pp. 34–41.

11. Williams, B., Tsai, P. and Schrier, R.W. Glucose-induced downregulation of angiotensin II and arginine vasopressin receptors in cultured rat aortic vascular smooth muscle cells. *J. Clin. Invest.,* 1992, **90,** 1992–9.

12. Nugent, A.G., McGurk, C., Hayes, J.R. and Johnston, G.D. Endothelin-1 does not cause vasoconstriction in patients with type 2 diabetes mellitus. *Diabetologia,* **38** (Suppl. 1), A48.

13. Bodmer, C.W., Patrick, A.W., How, T.V. and Williams, G. Exaggerated sensitivity to NE-induced vasoconstriction in IDDM patients with microalbuminuria. Possible etiology and diagnostic implications. *Diabetes,* 1992, **41,** 209–14.

14. Walker, A.B., Dores, J., Buckingham, R.E., Savage, M.W. and Williams, G. Impaired insulin-induced attenuation of noradrenaline-mediated vasoconstriction in insulin-resistant obese Zucker rats. *Clin. Sci.,* 1997, **93,** 235–41.

15. Tooke, J.E., Lins, P.E., Ostergren, J., Adamson, U. and Fagrell, B. The effects of intravenous insulin infusion on skin microcirculatory flow in type 1 diabetes. *Int. J. Microcirc. Clin. Exp.,* 1985, **69,** 69–83.

16. Sandeman, D.D., Shore, A.C. and Tooke, J.E. Relation of skin capillary pressure in patients with insulin-dependent diabetes mellitus to complications and metabolic control. *N. Engl. J. Med.,* 1992, **327,** 760–4.

17. Flynn, M.D., Edmonds, M.E., Tooke, J.E. and Watkins, P.J. Direct measurement of capillary blood flow in the diabetic neuropathic foot. *Diabetologia,* 1988, **31,** 652–6.

18. Rayman, G., Malik, R.A,. Metcalfe, J., Sharma, A.K. and Day, J.L. Reduced skin capillary size in the feet of insulin-dependent diabetic patients. *Diabet. Med.,* 1990, **7** (suppl. 1), 9A.

19. Sandeman, D.D. Why do some type 1 diabetic patients develop nephropathy? A possible role of birth weight. *Diabet. Med.,* 1992, **9** (Suppl. 1), 93.

20. Serné, E.H., Stehouwer, C.D.A., ter Maaten, J.C. *et al.* Insulin resistance and hypertension: role for microcirculation? *Proceedings of the Meeting of the Anglo, Danish, Dutch, Diabetes Group,* 1997, Amsterdam.

21. Noon, J.P., Walker, B.R., Webb, D.J., Shore, A.C., Holton, D.W., Edwards, H.V. and Watt, G.C.M. Impaired microvascular dilatation and capillary rarefaction in young adults with a predisposition to high blood pressure. *J. Clin. Invest.,* 1997, **99,** 1873–9.

22. Freeman, R.H. and Davis, J.O. Physiological actions of angiotensin II on the kidney. *Fed. Proc.,* 1979, **38,** 2276–9.

23. Haynes,W.G. and Webb, D.J. Endothelium-dependent modulation of responses to endothelin-I in human veins. *Clin. Sci.,* 1993, **84,** 427–33.

24. Shore, A.C., Donohoe, M., Jaap, A.J. and Tooke, J.E. The effect of increasing doses of an angiotensin converting enzyme inhibitor on capillary pressure levels in patients with insulin-dependent-diabetes mellitus and microalbuminuria. *Diabet. Med.,* 1993, **10** (suppl. 1), A18.55.

25. Shore, A.C., Sandeman, D.D. and Tooke, J.E. Nailfold capillary pressure in non-nephropathic diabetic patients of moderate disease duration the effect of angiotensin converting enzyme inhibition by enalapril. *Int. J. Microcirc. Clin. Exp.,* 1992, **11,** 445.

26. McVeigh, G.E. Hyperinsulinaemia, insulin resistance, and endothelial dysfunction. *Curr. Op. Nephrol. Hypertens.,* 1994, **3,** 365–9.

27. Yip, J., Mattock, M.B., Morocutti, A., Sethi, M., Trevisan, R. and Viberti,G.C. Insulin resistance in insulin-dependent diabetic patients with microalbuminuria. *Lancet,* 1993, **342,** 883–7.

28. Vanhoutte, P.M. Cardiovascular effects of serotonin. *J. Cardiovasc. Pharmacol.,* 1987, **10** (suppl. 3), S8–11.

29. Nagel,T., Resnick, N., Atkinson,W.J., Dewey, C.F. Jr. and Gimborne, M.A. Jr. Shear stress selectively upregulates intercellular adhesion molecule-1 expression in cultured human vascular endothelial cells. *J. Clin. Invest.,* 1994, **94,** 885–91.

30. Baumgartner-Parzer, S.M., Wagner, L., Pettermann, M., Gessl, A. and Waldhausl, W. Modulation by high glucose of adhesion molecule

expression in cultured endothelial cells. *Diabetologia*, 1995, **38**, 1367–70.

31. Ajjam, Z.S., Barton, S., Corbett, M., Owens, D. and Marks, R. Quantitative evaluation of the dermal vasculature of diabetics. *Q. J. Med.*, 1985, **54**, 229–39.

32. Rayman, G., Malik, R.A., Sharma, A.K. and Day, J.L. Microvascular response to tissue injury and capillary ultrastructure in the foot skin of Type I diabetic patients. *Clin. Sci.*, 1995, **89**, 467–74.

33. Cagliero, E., Maiello, M., Boeri, D., Roy, S. and Lorenzi, M. Increased expression of basement membrane components in human endothelial cells cultured in high glucose. *J. Clin. Invest.*, 1988, **82**, 735–8.

34. Riser, B.L., Cortes, P., Zhao, X., Bernstein, J., Dumler, F., Narins, R.G., Hassett, C.C., Sastry, K.S.S., Atherton, J. and Holcomb, M.A. Intraglomerular pressure and mesangial stretching stimulate extracellular matrix formation in the rat. *J. Clin. Invest.*, 1992, **90**, 1932–43.

35. Morris, S.J., Shore, A.C. and Tooke, J.E. Response of the skin microcirculation to acetylcholine and sodium nitroprusside in patients with NIDDM. *Diabetologia*, 1995, **38**, 1337–44.

36. Shore, A.C., Morris, S.J. and Tooke, J.E. Impaired skin microvascular endothelial cell responses in IDDM patients with microalbuminuria. *Diabet. Med.*, 1997, **14**, (Suppl. 1), A54.

37. Morris, S.J., Jaap, A.J., Shore, A.C. and Tooke, J.E. Responses of the skin microcirculation to acetylcholine and sodium nitroprusside in subjects with fasting hyperglycaemia. *J. Physiol.*, 1996, **491**, P, 14P.

38. Hishikawa, K., Nakaki, T., Marumo, T. *et al.* Up-regulation of nitric oxide synthase by estradiol in human aortic endothelial cells. *FEBS Lett.*, 1995, 360, **3**, 291–3.

39. Nitenberg, A., Valensi, P., Sachs, R., Dali, M., Aptecar, E. and Attali, J.R. Impairment of coronary vascular reserve and AcH-induced coronary vasodilation in diabetic patients with angiopgraphically normal left ventricular systolic function. *Diabetes*, 1993, **42**, 1017–25.

40. Goodfellow, J., Ramsey, M.W., Luddington, L.A., Jones, C.J.H., Coates, P.A., Dunstan, F., Lewis, M.J., Owens, D.R. and Henderson, A.H. Endothelium and inelastic arteries an early marker of vascular dysfunction in non-insulin dependent diabetes. *BMJ*, 1996, **312**, 744–6.

41. Chowienczyk, P.J., Watts,G.F., Cockcroft, J.R. and Ritter, J.M. Impaired endothelium-dependent vasodilation of forearm resistance vessels in hypercholesterolaemia. *Lancet,* 1992, **340**, 1430–2.

42. Jaap, A.J., Shore, A.C. and Tooke, J.E. Relationship of insulin resistance to microvascular dysfunction in subjects with fasting hyperglycaemia. *Diabetologia,* 1997, **40**, 238–43.

43. Vallance, P., Calver, A. and Collier, J. The vascular endothelium in diabetes and hypertension. *J. Hypertens.*, 1992, **10** (suppl. 1), S25–9.

44. Steinberg, H.O., Brechtel,G., Johnson, A., Fineberg, N. and Baron, A.D. Insulin-mediated skeletal muscle vasodilation is nitric oxide dependent. *J. Clin. Invest.*, 1994, **94**, 1172–9.

45. Laakso, M., Edelman, S.V., Brechtel, G. and Baron, A.D. Impaired insulin-mediated skeletal muscle blood flow in patients with NIDDM. *Diabetes*, 1992, **41**, 1076–83.

46. Utriainen, T., Makimattila, S., Virkamaki, A., Bergholm, R. and Yki-Jarvinen, H. Dissociation between insulin sensitivity of glucose uptake and endothelial function in normal subjects. *Diabetologia*, 1996, **39**, 1477–82.

47. Yang, Y.J., Hope, I.D., Ader, M. and Bergman, R.N. Insulin transport across capillaries is rate limiting for insulin action in dogs. *J. Clin. Invest.*, 1989, **84**, 1620–8.

48. Juhan-Vague, I., Vague, P., Alessi, M.C., Backer, C., Valadier, J., Aillard, M.F. and Atlan, C. Relationship between plasma insulin triglyceride body mass index and plasmingen activator inhibitor 1. *Diabete Metab.*, 1987, **13**, 331–6.

49. Lee, B.C., Humphreys, J.M., Shore, A.C., Tooke, J.E. and Hattersley, A.T. Maximum microvascular hyperaemia in offspring of 2 NIDDM parents. *British Diabetic Association, Medical and Scientific Section Spring Meeting,* March 1998, pp. 26–27.

50. Neal, C.R. and Michel, C.C. Transcellular openings through endothelium of frog mesenteric microvessels following perfusion with A23187 and exposure to high transmural pressure. *J. Physiol. (Lond.)*, 1993, **467**, 39P.

51. Schnitzer, J.E., Allard, J. and Oh, P. NEM inhibits transcytosis, endocytosis and capillary permeability: implication of caveolae fusion in endothelia. *Am. J. Physiol.*, 1995, **37**, H48–55.

52. Schulze, C. and Fortu, A. The interendothelial junction in myocardial capillaries: evidence for the existence of regularly spaced, cleft spanning structures. *J. Cell. Sci.*, 1992, **101**, 647–55.

53. Ferrero, E., Ferrero, M.E., Pardi, R. and Zocchi, M.R. The platelet endothelial adhesion molecule-1 (PECAM 1) contributes to endothelial barrier function. *FEBS Lett.*, 1995, **374**, 323–6.
54. Curry, F.E. and Michel, C.C. A fiber matrix model of capillary permeability. *Microvasc. Res.*, 1980, **20**, 96–9.
55. Robinson, G.B. and Walton, H.A. Glomerular basement membrane as a compressible ultrafilter. *Microvasc. Res.*, 1989, **38**, 36–48.
56. Klaentschi, K., Shore, A. and Tooke, J.E. Effect of pressure and glucose on PECAM expression by microvascular endothelial cell. *British Diabetic Association, Medical and Scientific Section Spring Meeting,* March 1998, pp. 26– 27.
57. Wautier, J.L., Schmidt, A.M., Zoukourian, C., Chappey, O., Wautier, M., Hori, O., Stern, D. and Lariboisiere, C. Diabetic erythocytes bearing cell surface advanced glycation endproducts interact with the receptor for advanced glycation endproducts to induce oxidant stress in endothelium and increase vascular permeability. *Circulation*, 1994, **90**, I-576, 3105.
58. van Hinsbergh, V.W.M. Endothelial permeability for macromolecules: mechanistic aspects of pathophysiological modulation. *Arterioscler. Thromb. Vasc. Biol.*, 1997, **17**, 1018–23.
59. Williamson, J.R. and Kilo, C. Current status of capillary basement-membrane disease in diabetes mellitus. *Diabetes*, 1977, **26**, 65–73.
60. Klaentschi, K., Brown, J.A. and Tooke, J.E. Crosslinking of Matrigel basement membrane results in a decreased permeability to both glycated and non-glycated albumin. *Diabet. Med.*, 1996, **13** (suppl. 7), 19.
61. Deckert, T., Feldt-Rasmussen, B., Borch-Johnsen, K., Jensen,T. and Kofoed Enevoldsen, A. Albuminuria reflects widespread vascular damage: The Steno hypothesis. *Diabetologia*, 1989, **32**, 219–26.
62. Bucala, R., Tracey, K.J. and Cerami, A. Advanced glycosylation products nitric oxide and mediate defective endothelium-dependent vasodilation in experimental diabetes. *J. Clin. Invest.*, 1991, **87**, 432–8.
63. Baumgartner-Parzer, S.M., Wagner, L., Pettermann, M., Grillari, J., Gessl, A. and Waudhausl, W. High-glucose-triggered apoptosis in cultured endothelial cells. *Diabetes*, 1995, **44**, 1323–7.

PART FOUR

ORGAN-SPECIFIC VASCULAR CHANGES

Eva M. Kohner and Rakesh Chibber

15.1 INTRODUCTION

Of the microvascular complications of diabetes retinopathy is probably the most interesting one, because the retinal circulation can be observed *in vivo* repeatedly without interfering with its function. While colour photographs show us the larger vessels, injection of fluorescein allows for visualization of capillaries, and the study of functional changes such as leakage. Because of this clear visibility of the retina we know the evolution of the lesions and the natural history of the disease. Unfortunately we still do not know all the pathogenic mechanisms which lead to this sight-threatening disease, nor do we know the interaction of the various pathogenic mechanisms.

With improvement in technology during the last 10 years, considerable advances have been made in understanding of what happens both on the physiological and biochemical level in diabetic retinopathy. This chapter gives an overview of our knowledge to date.

15.2 THE EVOLUTION OF DIABETIC RETINOPATHY

The earliest changes of diabetic retinopathy are only recognized by careful histological examination. They include basement membrane thickening, loss of pericytes and occlusion of capillaries. These changes are followed by the clinically recognized lesions of microaneurysms and haemorrhages. Later, increased permeability is recognized associated with the formation of hard exudates. Other early abnormalities are dilatation of both major arteries and veins. These are all features of non-proliferative or background retinopathy (Figure 15.1 a, 15.1b). This condition is not associated with visual impairment unless there is excessive permeability involving the foveal area, resulting in macular oedema.

Occlusion of capillaries is a continuous process and eventually involves venules and arterioles, so that large areas of the retina are not perfused. This pre-proliferative retinopathy is recognized by abnormalities of the veins such as beading, loop formation and reduplication, by intra-retinal microvascular abnormalities (IRMA) (dilated capillaries in areas of capillary non-perfusion), multiple cotton wool spots, and clusters of haemorrhages (Figure 15.2). The avascular, ischaemic retina is responsible for the liberation of vasoactive factors, resulting in new vessel and fibrous tissue formation (Figures 15.3, 15.4). While the evolution of the early lesions is specific for diabetes, neovascularization is not; it is the consequence of large areas of ischaemic retina. Proliferative retinopathy is a feature of many diseases resulting in ischaemia, including vein occlusion, sickle cell disease and vasculitis.

The late complications of proliferative retinopathy, resulting in advanced diabetic eye disease, are the result of vascular proliferation which always involves both new vessels and accompanying fibrous tissue.

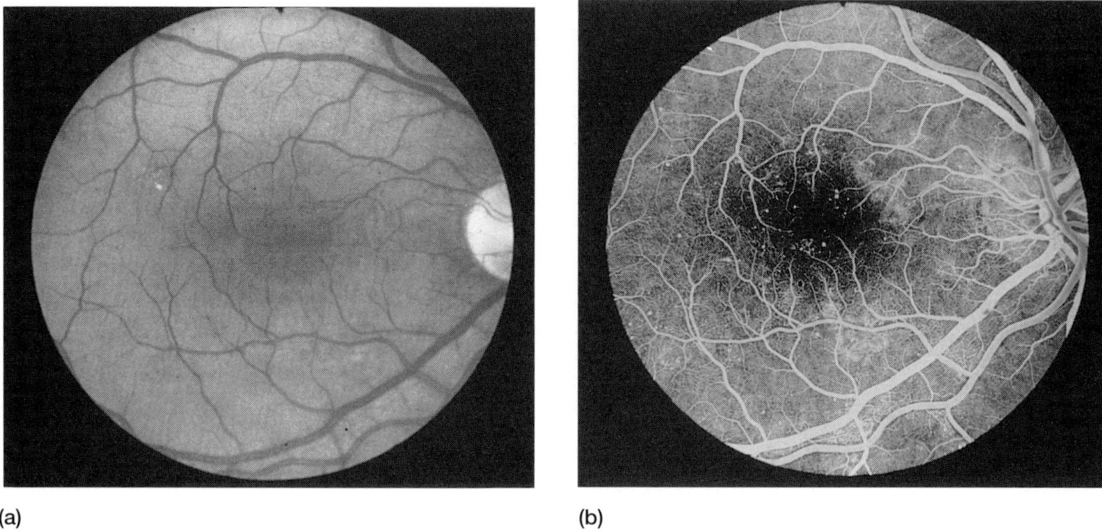

(a)

(b)

Figure 15.1 Photographs showing retinopathy. (a) From a colour photograph of right macular region showing mild background retinopathy with microaneurysms and haemorrhages and a few hard exudates. (b) Fluorescein angiogram of area shown in (a). Note many more microaneurysms are seen, and small areas of non-perfusion in perifoveal area. Also note leakage in area of hard exudates.

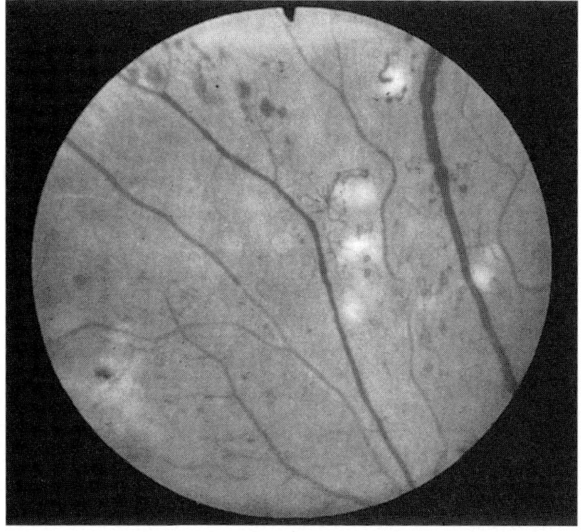

Figure 15.2 From a colour photograph showing left superior area with pre-proliferative retinopathy. There are marked venous abnormalities, IRMA and multiple cotton wool spots. There are also blot haemorrhages.

These are not discussed further in this chapter, which focuses primarily on the early changes specific to diabetic retinopathy.

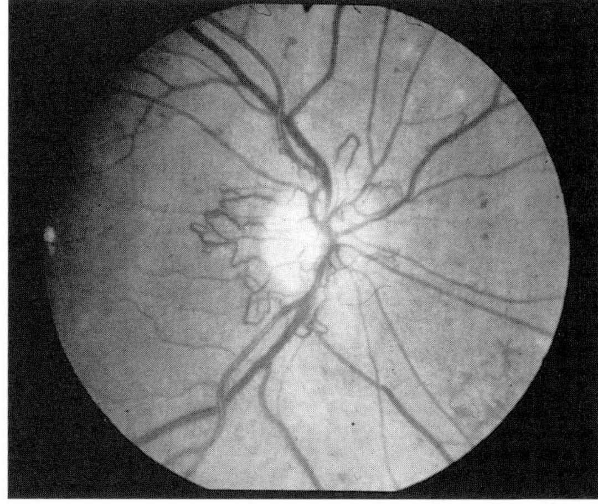

Figure 15.3 Proliferative retinopathy with new vessels arising from the optic disc.

15.3 PATHOGENIC MECHANISMS IN DIABETIC RETINOPATHY

The underlying abnormality in diabetes is high blood glucose with its accompanying metabolic changes. Engerman *et al.* [1] have

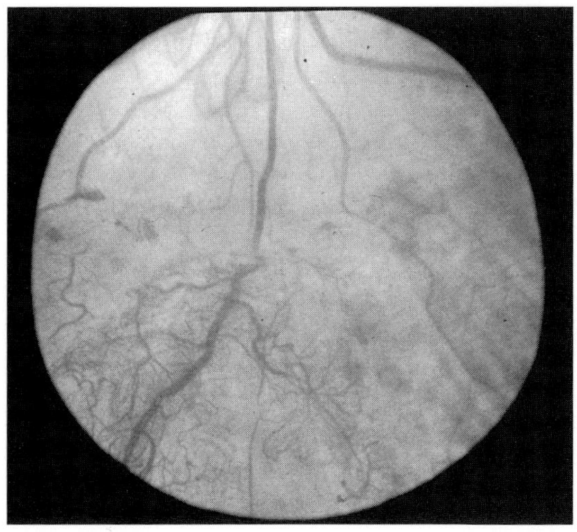

Figure 15.4 New vessels arising from the retinal periphery .

shown that in experimental diabetes in dogs strict control of the blood glucose could prevent the formation of microaneurysms and acellular capillaries. In human type 1 diabetes, the Diabetes Control and Complications Study [2, 3] has shown that intensive insulin treatment could delay the onset of retinopathy and slow the progression of background retinopathy already present. However, in this study it was not clear whether the control of blood glucose or the accompanying metabolic abnormalities were primarily responsible. Similarly the work by Okhubo *et al.* in Japan [4] in type 2 diabetes suffers from the same criticism. It was work by Engerman and Kern which showed that elevation of hexose sugar alone without the accompanying diabetic metabolic changes resulted in the early abnormalities of diabetic retinopathy [5]. It is therefore reasonable to assume that the major cause of diabetic retinopathy is elevation of blood glucose.

High blood glucose has marked haemodynamic effects, and important toxic effects on the capillary wall. These are shown in Figure 15.5.

15.3.1   HAEMODYNAMIC CHANGES

High blood glucose results in increase in retinal blood flow. The high glucose also influences vascular autoregulation. This is particularly important in the retina, since the retina has no functioning autonomic nerves, and therefore relies on autoregulation for the control of blood flow.

That retinal blood flow may be increased and cause at least some features of retinopathy was proposed by L'Esperance [6] who suggested that the preference for the perifoveal area involvement in early retinopathy was due to the specific vascular pattern in the macular area allowing for increased blood flow.

Early changes

The changes in early diabetes are controversial. Grunwald *et al.* [7] found increased blood flow due primarily to increased vessel diameters in patients with type 1 diabetes and less than four years diabetes duration. These workers used the laser Doppler velocimeter for measurement of red cell velocity and measured vessel diameters from retinal photographs in order to measure volume flow. Using video fluorescein angiography, Bursell *et al.* [8] found increased transit time and reduced flow. The reasons for this are several. Bursell used fluorescein, which actually measures plasma flow rather than total blood flow, and the layers near the vessel wall flow more slowly than the red cells. The vessel diameters were measured in pixels by Bursell, and this could be inaccurate because of the relatively poor resolution of digitized images. Also he measured mean transit time and estimated blood flow. Finally, the measurements were made not at the time of diagnosis but after the diabetes was controlled.

Animal studies performed at the Joslin Clinic suggest that retinal blood flow is reduced in diabetic rats, and this could be

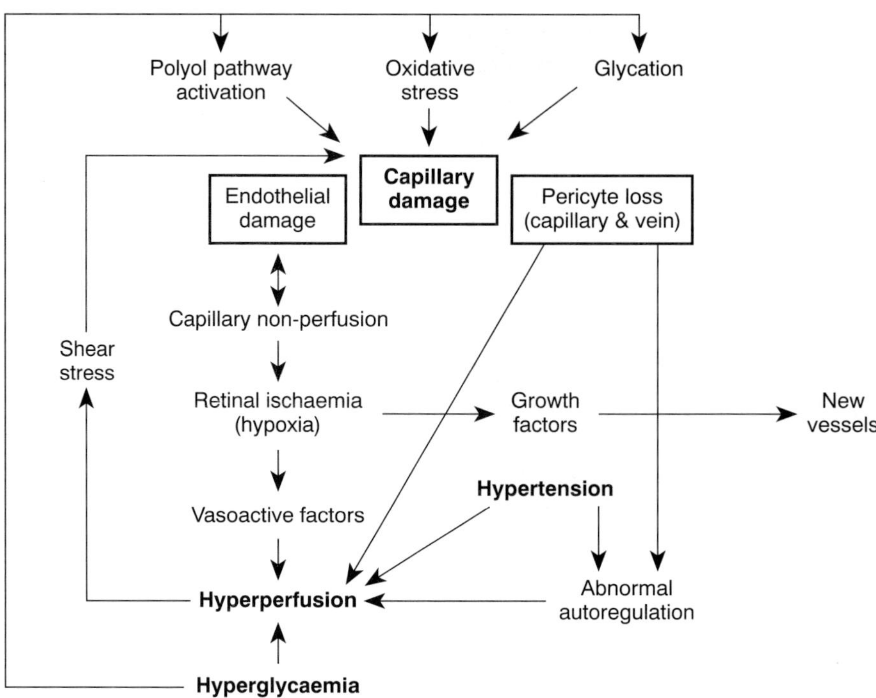

Figure 15.5 Schematic representation of the role of different pathogenic mechanisms in the development of diabetic retinopathy. Hyperperfusion is made worse by reduced endothelin production and pericyte loss. Capillary occlusion is caused by the damage to the vascular wall, including apoptosis, increased coagulation and abnormal white cells with abnormal adhesion properties. Hyperglycaemia stimulates protein kinase C production which together with hypoxia and growth factors result in proliferative retinopathy.

normalized by a number of procedures [9–11]. However, it must be emphasized that rats differ significantly from humans. The diabetic rat is one of only a few species in which growth hormone (GH) is reduced when diabetes is induced. GH increases retinal blood flow (unpublished observation). In uncontrolled human diabetes GH is elevated. GH increases red cell mass and plasma volume, which in turn increases cardiac output, contributing to increased blood flow [12]. Also, diabetic rats have considerably higher blood glucose and are probably dehydrated, a condition which will result in reduced plasma volume.

Effect of retinopathy and blood glucose control on retinal blood flow

Grunwald found increased retinal blood flow in early diabetic retinopathy [13]. The Hammersmith workers also used laser Doppler velocimetry [14] and in patients without retinopathy, they found that blood flow was similar to non-diabetic controls. However, with increasing severity of retinopathy the blood flow increased, being highest in those who had proliferative retinopathy. Following successful pan-retinal photocoagulation, there was significant reduction of blood flow in these patients. In pregnant diabetic subjects, Chen *et al.* [15] found blood flow increased in those in whom retinopathy deteriorated or who developed retinopathy for the first time during pregnancy. Using the pulsatility of blood flow, Feke *et al.* noted increase of flow with increasing retinopathy [16].

That blood glucose control is of importance in determining retinal blood flow was also shown by Grunwald in two studies. In the first study, poorly controlled diabetic subjects had their blood flow measured before and two hours after starting intravenous insulin infusion and resulting in the normalization of blood glucose. They found that blood flow decreased by about 20% [17]. In the second study, patients were examined before and after five days of intensified insulin treatment. The patients in whom blood flow did not decrease during these five days were the ones in whom retinopathy deterioration was noted six months after starting intensified insulin treatment.

Abnormal autoregulation

As mentioned above, autoregulation is of particular importance in the control of retinal vascular regulation. There are several studies which indicate that this regulation is abnormal in diabetes, and that diabetic vessels fail to adjust effectively to changes in blood pressure and alterations in the metabolic environment.

In the strict physiological sense autoregulation means the ability to keep blood flow constant during changes in perfusion pressure [18]. The normal reaction to an increase in blood pressure is vascular constriction. If blood glucose is high, this vasoconstriction is impaired and blood flow is increased. In experimental hypertension achieved by tyramine infusion, Rassam *et al.* [19] found that in normal subjects there was no increase in blood flow until the mean pressure increased by about 40% above normal. This is also the limit of autoregulation for the cerebral circulation. In diabetic subjects, when their blood glucose was under 10 mmol/l, autoregulation

had already broken down at 30% rise in mean arterial pressure. In the same diabetic subjects when the blood glucose was high, autoregulation was absent at 15% rise in mean arterial pressure and flow increased by over 70% at higher levels.

Guyton expanded the concept of autoregulation by defining it as the ability of the blood vessels to adjust flow according to the needs of the tissue or organ [20]. In the retina, the most vasoactive substance is oxygen. While breathing 100% oxygen, normal subjects reduced their retinal blood flow by 63%. In diabetic subjects this was considerably reduced, more markedly so in those with more severe retinopathy. However, following effective photocoagulation this reduction was restored towards the non-retinopathic level [21]. Rassam *et al.* [22] found that in hypertensive diabetic subjects there was considerable reduction in oxygen reactivity, more so when the blood glucose was high. Controlling blood pressure without controlling blood glucose had little effect but, when both blood glucose and blood pressure were controlled, autoregulation returned towards that of the normotensive diabetic subjects with blood glucose under 10 mmol/l. Studies by Grunwald have also shown that, when blood glucose is controlled, blood flow is reduced but at the same time the response to oxygen breathing is improved [17].

Causes and effects of increased blood flow

During hyperglycaemia, retinal metabolism is increased and this is thought to be the main reason for increased retinal blood flow. It has also been shown that when blood glucose is high much of the glucose is metabolized to lactic acid, a substance which dilates retinal vessels [23]. Blood flow is also increased during hypoglycaemia [24], to enable retinal functioning to continue, since the retina depends on glucose. Later in the disease when there are large areas of capillary, non-perfusion blood flow in the remaining vessels is increased, possibly in response to retinal hypoxia. Furthermore, blood flow through new vessels is also high, as there are no contractile elements in their wall.

The result of the increased blood flow is an increase in wall shear stress. Shear stress is the viscous drag that exists between the laminae of blood flow nearest to the vessel wall and the vessel wall itself. Shear stress is directly related to blood viscosity and blood flow, and inversely related to the radius of the vessel cubed. Increased shear stress may damage the vessel wall in several ways. It promotes a haemostatic response [25], extravascular matrix production [26] and increased cell turnover and proliferation by stimulating DNA [27, 28]. It also decreases the production of endothelin, a potent vasoconstrictor, and increases production of certain vasodilators [29–30], worsening hyperperfusion. Thus both hyperglycaemia as well as hypoglycaemia have a deleterious effect on the retinal vessels.

15.3.2   DIRECT EFFECT OF HYPERGLYCAEMIA ON RETINAL VASCULAR CELLS

The observation that pericytes are preferentially lost in diabetic retinopathy and the finding that capillary occlusion is associated with loss of endothelial cells within the capillaries led to a number of hypotheses accounting for these findings.

Sorbitol accumulation

This hypothesis was based on the observation that glucose is metabolized to sorbitol by the enzyme aldose reductase under conditions of hyperglycaemia [31]. Under normal glucose conditions the enzyme activity is low because of the low affinity of the enzyme for glucose. As cell membranes are impermeable to sorbitol, its increased production in diabetes will lead to excessive intracellular accumulation in vascular, neuronal and other tissues resulting

in osmotic damage [32]. Elevated polyol levels have been reported in diabetic and galactosaemic human and animal tissues [33].

Evidence for the involvement of the polyol pathway in diabetic retinopathy was provided by Akagi *et al.* [34], demonstrating the presence of aldose reductase in pericytes but not in endothelial cells. However, other workers have either failed to detect aldose reductase in retinal microvessels [35] or have localized the enzyme in both pericytes and endothelial cells [36]. In some animal studies, inhibitors of aldose reductase have been reported to greatly retard the development of retinopathy-like changes, including pericyte loss, microaneurysms and capillary acellularity [37, 38]. In contrast, in other animal studies inhibitors of aldose reductase have failed to prevent the onset and progression of retinopathy-like changes despite inhibiting the polyol accumulation by 90–96% in the retina [39]. The aldose reductase inhibitor, Tolrestat, was ineffective in preventing glucose-induced toxicity in cultured vascular cells [40]. Finally, the clinical trial using aldose reductase inhibitor did not show significant difference between patients treated with the active drug and placebo [41].

Non-enzymatic glycation

The basis of the glycation hypothesis is that glucose can react covalently with amino groups of proteins (Maillard reaction) to form a Schiff base, which then undergoes further rearrangements and oxidative reactions to form irreversible advanced glycation endproducts (AGEs). This reaction is determined by the rate of turnover of proteins and the degree and duration of hyperglycaemia [42, 43]. In diabetes, AGE products accumulate in tissues, on vascular wall collagen, basement membranes and the circulation of diabetic patients.

Experimental evidence supports a causal relationship between accelerated accumulation of AGEs in diabetes and the development of chronic diabetic complications. There seems to be a good correlation between the extent to which AGE accumulates on patient's dermal collagen and the degree of diabetic retinopathy [44]. Excessive accumulation of AGEs could contribute to microvascular damage in diabetes by two pathways: directly or indirectly through interaction with cell surface receptors. The direct damage could result from cross-linking, polymerization, decreased solubility and sensitivity to proteolytic enzyme degradation of connective tissue [45]. AGE-modified proteins can also inactivate nitric oxide (NO), trap plasma macromolecules and low density lipoprotein (LDL) [46]. The formation of AGE cross-links on the extracellular matrix proteins can increase vessel wall rigidity [47].

AGE-modified proteins bind specifically to specific receptors on the cell surface of endothelial cells, macrophages, mesanglial cells and other diverse cell types [48, 49]. Two of these membrane-bound receptors, a 50–60 kDa protein, identical to a component of the olgiosaccharyltransferase-48 complex (OST-48) [50] and a 90 kDa protein, identical to 80 K-H, a protein kinase C substrate [51], have now been well characterized. AGE-receptor interaction results in receptor-mediated endocytosis, changes in cellular proliferation, chemotaxis, cell activation, endothelial cell permeability, coagulant functions [52] and altered expression of endothelial-derived relaxing activity [53]. The interaction can also promote cytokine release and upregulate the synthesis of a variety of products, including extracellular matrix components, cytokines, insulin-like growth factor-1 and vascular endothelial growth factor (VEGF) [54–57]. Western blot analyses have also localized the p60 component of the AGE receptor on retinal capillary pericytes and endothelial cells *in vitro* and *in vivo* [58]. Interaction of AGE with AGE receptor has been reported as toxic to cultured bovine retinal capillary pericytes but mitogenic to endothelial cells [58, 59]. In support of these *in vitro* studies, the work of Hammes *et al.* [60] has demonstrated: (i) the presence of AGE products in retinal capillaries of diabetic rats and (ii) significant reduction in the number of diabetes-induced formation of acellular capillaries and pericyte loss when the formation of AGE is inhibited with aminoguanidine. Recently, Stitt *et al.* [61] have reported that AGE, which accumulates in the retinal capillaries of diabetic rats, co-localizes with cellular AGE receptors resulting in increased accumulation in pericytes and formation of acellular capillaries.

Another receptor termed RAGE (receptor for AGEs) is a member of the immunoglobulin superfamily and has been found to be expressed on endothelial cells, smooth muscle cells and mononuclear phagocytes [62]. The binding of AGE-modified proteins with RAGE has been shown to mediate monocyte migration and activation [62], induce oxidative stress on endothelial cells [63] and increase the expression of the vascular adhesion molecule-1 (VCAM-1) [64]. Soluble RAGE, the extracellular domain of the membrane-anchored receptor, has been shown to prevent vascular hyperpermeability in diabetic rats [65].

Oxidative stress

An imbalance between the production of free radicals and cellular antioxidant defence mechanisms plays an important role in many disease processes, including diabetes mellitus. Possible sources of oxidative stress and damage to proteins in diabetes include free radicals generated by autooxidation reaction of sugars and sugar adducts to proteins and by autooxidation of unsaturated lipids in plasma and membrane proteins. Reactive oxygen species (ROS) arising from processes such as non-enzymatic glycation, the polyol pathway and pseudo-hypoxia [66–68] can break down cell membranes, denature proteins, damage DNA and break down glucose to toxic hydrogen peroxide and oxo-aldehydes. Recently, Kaneto *et al.* [69] demonstrated that reducing sugars can trigger the production of ROS through the glycation reaction and induce apoptosis of pancreatic β-cells.

Changes in glucose transport activity and glucose-induced apoptosis

Mandarino *et al.* [70] have proposed the idea that despite pericytes being exposed to hyperglycaemia they may be lost in diabetes through possible glucose starvation. This is an interesting hypothesis which is based on the author's observation that high concentrations of glucose downregulate glucose transport activity and glucose transporter 1 (GLUT 1) content in retinal capillary pericytes but not endothelial cells. This glucose starvation may lead to apoptosis of pericytes as demonstrated by Li *et al.* [71]. Pericytes which are chronically exposed to high glucose respond to an abrupt lowering of glucose by undergoing apoptosis or programmed cell death. Similar fluctuation of glucose had no effect on endothelial cells and this may be relevant in diabetes where marked variations in glucose are known to take place [72]. Baumgartner-Parzer *et al.* [73] have demonstrated that glucose at high concentration can promote apoptosis of endothelial cells. These studies are particularly interesting because apoptosis of pericytes and endothelial cells has been observed in human and in experimentally induced diabetes [74]. These studies suggest that there is an equal amount of endothelial and pericyte loss at least in the diabetic rat. The imbalance between pericyte and endothelial cell number could then be due to proliferation of endothelial cells which is induced by a number of mechanisms, such as increased shear stress and non-enzymatic glycation.

15.3.3 CAPILLARY OCCLUSION

The abnormalities discussed in the previous sections explain some of the vascular changes, but do not explain fully the occlusion of capillaries and the increased permeability seen in diabetes. Although Lorenzi believes that capillaries are not occluded but destroyed by the increased apoptosis, there is no adequate proof for this. There is evidence for increased haemostasis in diabetes, and increased activity of platelets [75–78], but these are at least in part due to the endothelial damage and to increased shear stress. More recently, abnormalities of the white cells have been suggested.

Capillary occlusion by leucocytes

There is now strong experimental evidence supporting the concept that leucocytes may be involved in the pathogenesis of diabetic retinopathy. Because the diameter of leucocytes exceeds that of the average capillary [79], they are subject to considerable amount of deformation as they pass through the capillary network. Leucocytes show increased adhesion to vascular endothelium in diabetes [80–81] and can release oxygen-derived free radicals and/or proteolytic enzymes [82–83]. Activated leucocytes can increase blood flow resistance [84] and glucose can increase the production of superoxide radical from stimulated leucocytes removed from diabetic cats. The report by Schroder *et al.* [85] further points to a causal relationship between capillary occlusion by leucocytes and the development of diabetic retinopathy. Working with control and diabetic rats, the authors observed diabetes-induced capillary occlusion by leucocytes leading to areas of endothelial cell damage capillary loss and neovascularization in the retina. More recently, Fukushima *et al.* [86] have presented evidence of a relationship between capillary occlusion by leucocytes and retinal capillary drop-out in diabetic patients. Recent data [87] suggest that increased activity of the Golgi glycosylating enzyme, core 2 GlcNAc-T, may be responsible for increased adhesion of leucocytes to vascular endothelium in diabetes.

15.3.4 VASCULAR PROLIFERATION

Once there are large areas of capillary nonperfusion, new vessels will grow. In diabetes this involves both hypoxic activation of protein kinase C (PKC) and growth factors, which may also contribute to the increased permeability seen in diabetes.

Protein kinase C

For many years now King's research group at the Joslin Diabetes Centre have examined the potential involvement of protein PKC in diabetes-induced vascular dysfunction [88]. PKC is ubiquitously distributed in cells, and enzyme activities in the membrane pool (the active fraction) have been shown to be elevated in many vascular tissues which are affected in diabetes, such as retina, aorta, heart and renal glomeruli [89–91]. In conjunction with this PKC translocation from the cytosolic pool to the membrane fraction there is a corresponding increase in total diacylglycerol (DAG) content of the tissues [92]. This supports the concept that DAG, generated by *de novo* synthesis or through the phosphotidylcholine breakdown pathways [92], activates PKC. In diabetes, the activation of the DAG/PKC pathway is not transitory but is persistent, as demonstrated by Xia *et al.* [92]. These authors demonstrated that PKC and DAG levels continue to be elevated in vascular tissues of diabetic dogs even after five years of diabetes. Another important finding in this study [92] was that once the activation of DAG/PKC had occurred its reversal to baseline level was only achieved after many weeks of normal blood glucose levels. These observations further strengthen the potential role of PKC in diabetic complications.

There is now increasing evidence supporting the hypothesis that PKC plays an important role in a wide range of vascular functions which are altered in diabetes, including vascular permeability, contractility, coagulation, blood flow, angiogenesis and the synthesis and turnover of basement membrane components [93]. PKC can also regulate gene expression of many other proteins in the vasculature, including intracellular adhesion molecules, proteins involved in smooth muscle contraction, and cytokines such as transforming growth factor β [94, 95]. Activation of PKC can alter endothelial cell barrier function causing increased permeability to albumin and other macromolecules [96], possibly through the development of intercellular gaps in the endothelial cell monolayer with reorganization of vinculin and F-actin filaments [97].

Using a specific inhibitor of PKC-β_1 and PKC-β_2, Ishii *et al.* [98] have recently provided further evidence for the direct involvement of PKC-β_2 in the pathogenesis of diabetic vascular complications. Oral administration of the inhibitor (LY333531) was found to correct diabetes-induced changes in the glomerular filtration rate, albumin excretion rate and retinal circulation in diabetic rats [98]. It is important to emphasize that, although the inhibitor is specific for PKC-β_2, this enzyme is also expressed in other tissues, particularly in the central nervous system (CNS) and the endocrine tissues such as pancreatic islets and pituitary gland [99]. Results from long-term toxicity studies will help in the future clinical application of the novel PKC inhibitors.

In a recent study, Xia *et al.* [100] were able to demonstrate that vascular endothelial growth factor (VEGF) may act through the activation of the PKC-γ and PKC pathway, involving mainly the PKC-β isoform in endothelial cells. These results are particularly interesting since VEGF, which is a potent endothelial cell mitogen, is now considered a major player in hypoxia-stimulated retinal neovascularization in diabetes [101]. The results suggest that specific inhibitors of PKC-

β_2 activity may prove useful in preventing proliferative eye disease and VEGF-induced vascular permeability changes in diabetes.

Growth factors

In 1953 Poulsen reported a patient with diabetic retinopathy in whom post-partum haemorrhage followed by hypopituitarism resulted in improvement of the retinopathy [102] This finding resulted in pituitary ablation for the treatment of proliferative diabetic retinopathy, and this was found to be effective in eliminating or at least improving the new vessels, provided abolition of GH secretion was complete [103, 104]. GH was implicated not only because this hormone is elevated in diabetic patients [105, 106], but also because the other known pituitary hormones were replaced. GH acts through insulin-like growth factor-1 (IGF-1). IGF-1 is low in most insulin-dependent diabetic subjects, but is elevated in the rapidly progressive forms of retinopathy [107] and is elevated in patients as new vessels develop [108]. IGF-1 is produced by the retinal endothelial cells. Both endothelial cells and pericytes express receptors for IGF-1, which are structurally similar to those localized on other cell types [109]. In a recent excellent experimental study, Smith *et al.* have shown that in the ROP mouse model proliferation can be reduced by one-third using a somatostatin analogue, and proliferative lesions are reduced in transgenic GH deficient mice [110]. These studies confirm a role for these hormones in the development of proliferative retinopathy.

Of the other growth factors, the one most closely linked with retinal neovascularization is VEGF [111–114], which is also induced by hypoxia, PKC and AGEs. Other growth factors which may be of importance include basic and acidic fibroblast growth factor (bFGF and aFGF), transforming growth factor β (TGFβ) and platelet-derived growth factor (PDGF) [115].

This chapter shows that there are many factors which interact in the formation of the lesions of diabetic retinopathy. Near-normalization of blood glucose will improve the prognosis for diabetic eye disease, but the metabolic abnormalities of diabetes are many and it is unlikely that this alone will prevent all visual loss. The hope and expectation is that a better understanding of the pathogenic mechanisms involved in the development of retinopathy will lead to new preventive and therapeutic strategies.

REFERENCES

1. Engerman, R., Bloodworth, J.M.B. Jr, Nelson, S. *et al.* Relationship of microvascular disease in diabetes to metabolic control. *Diabetes,* 1977, **26,** 760–9.
2. The Diabetes Control and Complications Trial Research Group. The effect of intensive treatment of diabetes on the development and progression of long term complications in insulin dependent diabetes mellitus. *N. Engl. J. Med.,* 1993, **329,** 977–86.
3. The Diabetes Control and Complications Trial Research Group. The effect of intensive diabetes treatment on the progression of retinopathy in insulin dependent diabetes mellitus: the diabetes control and complications trial. *Arch. Ophthalmol.,* 1995, **113,** 36–51.
4. Ohkubo, Y., Kishikawa, H., Araki, E., Miyata, T., Motoyoshi, S. *et al.* Intensive insulin therapy prevents progression of diabetic microvascular complications in Japanese patients with non-insulin dependent diabetes mellitus. *Diabetes Res. Clin. Pract.,* 1995, **28,** 103–17.
5. Engerman, R.L., Kern, T.S., Engerman, R.L. and Kern, T.S. Progression of incipient diabetic retinopathy during good glycemic control. *Diabetes,* 1987, **36,** 808– 12.
6. L'Esperance, F.A. The pathologic haemodynamics of diabetic retinopahy: a theory. *Am. J. Ophthalmol.,* 1971, **71,** 251–260.
7. Grunwald, J.E., DuPont, J. and Riva, C.E. Retinal haemodynamics in patients with early diabetes mellitus. *Br. J. Ophthalmol.,* 1996, **80,** 327–31.
8. Bursell, S.E., Clermont, A.C., Kinsley, B.T., Simpson, D.C., Aiello, L.M. and Wolpert, H.A. Retinal blood flow changes in patients with insulin dependent diabetes mellitus and no diabetic retinopatny: a video fluorescein

angiography study. *Invest. Ophthalmol. Vis. Sci.*, 1996, **37,** 886–97.

9. Takagi, C., Bursell, S.E. Clermont, A.C., Takagi, H., Jirousek, M.R. and King, G.L. Mimicking abnormal retinal haemodynamics in diabetes by enhancing DAG/PKC levels in the retina of non-diabetic rats. *Diabetes,* 1994, **43,** 1372.

10. Takagi, C., King, G.L., Clermont, A.C., Cummins, D.R., Takagi, H. and Bursell, S.E. Reversal of abnormal retinal haemodynamics in diabetic rats by acabose, an α-glucosidase inhibitor. *Curr. Eye Res.,* 1995, **14,** 741–9.

11. Kunisaki, M., Bursell, E.E., Clermont, A.C., Ishii, H., Ballas, L.M., Jirousek, M.R. *et al.* Vitamin E treatment prevents diabetes induced abnormality in retinal blood flow via the diacyl-glycerol-protein kinase C pathway. *Am. J. Physiol.,* 1995, **269,** E239–46.

12. Christ, E., Cummings, M.H., Westwood, N.B., Sawyer, B.M., Pearson, T.C. *et al.* The role of growth hormone in regulating erythropoesis, red cell mass and plasma volume in adults with growth hormone deficiency. *J. Clin. Endocrinol. Metab.,* 1997, **8,** 2985–90.

13. Grunwald, J.E., Riva, C.E., Sinclair, S.H., Brucker, A.J. and Petrig, B.L. Laser Doppler velocimetry study of the retinal circulation in diabetes mellitus. *Arch. Ophthalmol.,* 1986, **104,** 991–6.

14. Patel, V., Rassam, S.M.B., Newson, R.S.B., Wiek, J. and Kohner, E.M. Retinal blood flow in diabetic retinolpathy. *BMJ,* 1992, **305,** 678–84.

15. Chen, H.C., Patel, V., Newsome, R.S.B., Cassar, J., Mather, H. and Kohner, E.M. Retinal blood flow changes during pregnancy in women with diabetes. *Invest. Ophthalmol. Vis. Sci.,* 1994, **35,** 3199–208.

16. Feke, G., Tagawa, H., Yoshida, A., Goger, D.G., Weiter, J.J., Busney, S.M. and McMeel, J.W. Retinal circulatory changes related to retinopathy: progression in insulin dependent diabetes mellitus. *Ophthalmology,* 1985, **92,** 1517–22.

17. Grunwald, J.E., Riva, C.E., Martin, D.B., Quint, A.R. and Epstein, P.A. Effect of an insulin induced decrease in blood glucose on the human diabetic retinal circulation *Ophthalmology,* 1987, **94,** 1614–20.

18. Johnson, P.C. Origin localisation and haemostatic significance of autoregulation in the intestine. *Circ. Res.,* 1964, **15** (suppl.) 225–32.

19. Rassam, S.M.B., Patel, V. and Kohner, E.M. The effect of experimental hypertension on retinal autoregulation in humans: a mechanism for progression of diabetic retinopathy. *Exp. Physiol.,* 1995, **80,** 53–68.

20. Guyton, A.C. and Coleman, T.G. Long term regulation of the circulation In *Physiological Basis of Circulatory Transport,* (eds E.B. Reeve and A.C. Guyton), Saunders, Philadelphia, 1967, pp. 179–202.

21. Grunwald, J.E., Riva, C.E., Brucker, A.J., Sinclair, S.H. and Petrig, B.L. Altered retinal vascular response to 100% oxygen breathing in diabetes mellitus. *Ophthalmology,* 1984, **91,** 1447–52.

22. Patel, V., Rassam, S.M.B., Chen, H.C. and Kohner, E.M. Oxygen reactivity in diabetes mellitus: effect of hypertension and hyperglycaemia. *Clin. Sci.,* 1994, **86,** 689–95.

23. Keen, H. and Chlouverakis, C. Metabolic factors in diabetic retinopathy. In *Biochemistry of the Retina,* (ed. E. Graymore) Blackwell, London, 1965, pp. 138–47.

24. Caldwell, G., Davies, E.G., Sullivan, P.M., Morris, A.H. and Kohner, E.M. A laser Doppler velocimetry study of the effect of hypoglycaemia on retinal blood flow in the minipig. *Diabetologia,* 1990, **33,** 262–5.

25. Iba, T., Shin, T. Sonoda, T., Rosales, O. and Sumpio, B.E. Stimulation of endothelial secretion of tissue type plasminogen activator by repetitive stretch. *J. Surg. Res.,* 1991, **50,** 457–60.

26. Parving, H.H., Viberti, G.C., Keen, H., Christiansen, J.S. and Lassen, N.A. Haemodynamic factors in the in the genesis of diabetic microangiopathy. *Metabolism,* 1983, **32,** 943–9.

27. Ando, J., Nomura, H. and Kamiya, A. The effect of fluid shear stress on the migration and proliferation of cultured endothelial cells. *Microvasc. Res.,* 1987, **33,** 62–70.

28. Davies, P.S., Remuzzi, A., Gordon, A.J., Dewey, D.F. and Gimborne, M.A. Turbulent fluid shear stress induces vascular endothelial turnover *in vitro. Proc. Natl Acad. Sci. USA,* 1986, **83,** 2114–17.

29. Davis, P.F. and Tripathi, S.C. Mechanical stress mechanism and the cell: an endothelial paradigm. *Circ. Res.,* 1993, **72,** 239–43.

30. Kuchan, M.J. and Frangos, J.A. Shear stress regulates endothelin-1 release via protein kinase C and cGMP in cultured endothelial cells. *Am. J. Physiol.,* 1993, **264,** H150–6.

31. Gabbay, K.H. The sorbitol pathway and the complications of diabetes. *N. Engl. J. Med.*, 1973, **288**, 831–6.

32. Kinoshita, J.H. Cataracts in galactosemia. *Invest. Ophthalmol.*, 1985, **4**, 786–99.

33. Dvornik, D., Simard-Dequesne, N., Krami, M., Gabbay, K.H., Kinoshita, J.H, Verma, S.D. and Merola, L.O. Polyol accumulation in diabetic and galactosemic rats. *Science*, 1973, **182**, 1146–8.

34. Akagi, Y., Terubayashi, H., Millen, J. *et al.* Aldose reductase localisation in human retinal mural cells. *Invest. Ophthalmol. Vis. Sci.*, 1983, **24**, 1516–19.

35. Kern, T.S. and Engerman, R.L. Distribution of aldose reductase in ocular tissues. *Exp. Eye. Res.*, 1981, **33**, 175–82.

36. Kennedy, A., Frank, R.N. and Verma, S.D. Aldose reductase activity in retinal and cerebral microvessels. *Invest. Ophthalmol. Vis. Sci.*, 1983, **24**, 1250–8.

37. Kador, P.F., Akagi, Y., Takahashi, Y., Ikebe, H., Wyman, M. and Kinoshita, J.H. Prevention of retinal vessel changes associated with diabetic retinopathy in galactose-fed dogs by aldose reductase inhibitors. *Arch. Ophthalmol.*, 1990, **108**, 1301–9.

38. Robison, W.G. Jr, Nagata, M., Laver, N., Hohman, T.C. and Kinoshita, J.H. Diabetic-like retinopathy in rats prevented with an aldose reductase inhibitor. *Invest. Ophthalmol. Vis. Sci.*, 1989, **30**, 2285–92.

39. Engerman, R.L. Pathogenesis of diabetic retinopathy. *Diabetes*, 1989, **38**, 1203–6.

40. Chibber, R., Molinatti, P.A., Wong, J.S.K., Mirlees, D. and Kohner, E.M. The effect of aminoguanidine and tolrestat on glucose toxicity in bovine retinal capillary pericytes. *Diabetes*, 1984, **43**, 758–63.

41. Sorbinil Retinopathy Trial Research Group. A randomised trial of sorbinil, an aldose reductase inhibitor, in diabetic retinopathy. *Arch. Ophthalmol.*, 1990, **108**, 1234–44.

42. Makita, Z., Radoff, S., Rayfield, E.J., Yang, Z., Scolnik, E., Friedman, C.A., Cerami, A. and Vlassara, H. Advanced glycosylation endproducts in patients with diabetic nephropathy. *N. Engl. J. Med.*, 1991, **325**, 836–42.

43. Monnier, V.M., Kohn, R.R. and Cerami, A. Accelerated age-related browning of human collagen in diabetes mellitus. *Proc. Natl Acad. Sci. USA*, 1984, **81**, 583–7.

44. Beisswinger, P.J., Makita, Z., Curphey, T.J., Moore, L.L., Jean, S., Brink-Johnsen, T., Bucala, R. and Vlassara, H. Formation of immunochemical advanced glycosylation end products precedes and correlates with early manifestation of renal and retinal disease in diabetes. *Diabetes*, 1995, **44**, 824–9.

45. Brownlee, M., Cerami, A. and Vlassara, H. Advanced glycosylation end products in tissue and the biochemical basis of diabetic complications. *N. Engl. J. Med.*, 1988, **318**, 1315–21.

46. Vlassara, H. Receptor-mediated interactions of advanced glycosylation end products with cellular components within diabetic tissues. *Diabetes*, 1992, **41** (suppl. 2), 52–6.

47. Brownlee, M., Cerami, A. and Vlassara, H. Advanced products of nonenzymatic glycosylation and the pathogenesis of diabetic vascular disease. *Diabetes Metab. Rev.*, 1988, **4**, 437–51.

48. Vlassara, H. Recent progress on the biologic and clinical significance of advanced glycosylation end products. *J. Lab. Clin. Med.*, 1994, **124**, 19–30.

49. Brownlee, M. Glycation and diabetic complications. *Diabetes*, 1994, **43**, 836–41.

50. Siberstein, S., Kelleher, G. and Gilmore. The 48-kDa subunit of the mammalian oligosaccharyltransferase complex is homologous to the essential yeast protein WBP1. *J. Biol. Chem.*, 1992, **267**, 23658–63.

51. Sakei, K., Hirai, M., Minoshima, S., Kudoh, J., Fukuyama, R. and Shimzu, Y. Purification of two distinct proteins of approximate Mr 80000 from human epithelial cells and identification as proper substrates for protein kinase C. *Genomics*, 1989, **5**, 309–15.

52. Esposito, C., Gerlach, H., Brett, J., Stern, D. and Vlassara, H. Endothelial receptor binding of glucose-modified albumin is associated with increased monolayer permeability and modulation of cell surface coagulant properties. *J. Exp. Med.*, 1989, **170**, 1387–1407.

53. Vlassara, H., Brownlee, M. and Cerami, A. High affinity-receptor-mediated uptake and degradation of glucose-modified proteins: a potential mechanism for the removal of senescent macromolecules. *Proc. Natl Acad. Sci. USA*, 1985, **82**, 5588–92.

54. Doi, T., Vlassara, H., Kirstein, M., Yamada, Y., Striker, G.E. and Striker, L.J. Receptor-specific increase in extracellular matrix production in

mouse mesangial cells by advanced glycosylation endproducts is mediated by PDGF. *Proc. Natl Acad. Sci. USA,* 1991, **89,** 11823–7.

55. Kirstein, M., Aston, C., Hintz, R. and Vlassara, H. Receptor-specific induction of insulin-like growth factor 1 (IGF-1) in human monocytes by advanced glycosylation endproducts-modified proteins. *J. Clin. Invest.,* 1992, **90,** 439–46.

56. Vlassara, H., Brownlee, M., Monogue, K., Dinarello, C.A. and Pasagian, A. Cachectin/TNF and IL-1 induced by glucose-modified proteins: role in normal tissue remodelling. *Science,* 1988, **240,** 1546–8.

57. Shigeta, H., Nakano, K., Nakamura, K., Hirata, C., Kitagawa, Nakamura, N. and Kondo. AGEs promote diabetic retinopathy by the production of vascular endothelial growth factor. *Diabetes,* 1997, **46** (suppl.), 10A.

58. Chibber, R., Molinatti, P.A., Rosatto, N., Lamborne, B. and Kohner, E.M. Toxic action of advanced glycation end products on cultured retinal capillary pericytes and endothelial cells: relevance to diabetic retinopathy. *Diabetologia,* 1997, **40,** 156–64.

59. Yamagishi, S., Hsu, C., Taniguchi, M., Harada, S., Yamamoto, Y., Ohsawa, K.S., Kobayashi, K.I. and Yamamoto, H. Receptor-mediated toxicity to pericytes of advanced glycation end products: a possible mechanism of pericyte loss in diabetic microangiopathy. *Biochem. Biophys. Res. Commun.,* 1995, **213,** 681–7.

60. Hammes, H.P., Martin, S., Federlin, K., Geison, K. and Brownlee, M. Aminoguanidine treatment inhibits the development of experimental diabetic retinopathy. *Proc. Natl Acad. Sci. USA,* 1991, **88,** 11556–8.

61. Stitt, A.W., Li, Y.M., Gardiner, T.A., Buccala, R., Archer, D.B. and Vlassara, H. Advanced glycation end products (AGEs) co-localise with AGE-receptors in the retinal vasculature of diabetic and of AGE-infused rats. *Am. J. Pathol.,* 1997, **150,** 523–531.

62. Schmidt, A.M., Yan, S.D., Brett, J., Mora, R., Nowygrod, R. and Stern, D.M. Regulation of human mononuclear phagocyte migration by cell surface-binding proteins for advanced glycation end products. *J. Clin. Invest.,* 1993, **91,** 2155–68.

63. Yan, S.D., Schmidt, A.M., Anderson, G.M., Zhang, J., Brett, J., Zou, Y.S., Pinsky, D. and Stern, D. Enhanced cellular oxidant stress by the interaction of advanced glycation end products with their receptor binding proteins. *J. Biol. Chem.,* 1994, **269,** 9889–97.

64. Schmidt, A.M., Hori, O., Chen, J., Brett, J. and Stern, D. AGE interaction with their endothelial receptor induces expression of VCAM-1: a potential mechanism for accelerated vaculopathy of diabetes. *J. Clin. Invest.,* 1995, **96,** 1375–1403.

65. Wautier, J.L., Zoukourian, C., Chappey, O., Wauter, M.L., Guilausseau, P.J., Cao, R., Hori, O., Stern, D. and Schmidt, A.M. Receptor-mediated endothelial cell dysfunction in diabetic vasculopathy. *J. Clin. Invest.,* 1996, **97,** 238–43.

66. Mullarkey, C.J., Edlestein, D. and Brownlee, M. Free radicals generation by early glycation products: a mechanism for accelerated atherogenesis in diabetes. *Biochem. Biophys. Res. Commun.,* 1990, **173,** 932–9.

67. Williamson, J.R., Chang, K., Frangos, M., Hasan, K.S. *et al.* Hyperglycemic pseudohypoxia and diabetic complications. *Diabetes,* 1993, **42,** 801–13.

68. Nagasaka, Y., Fujii, S. and Kaneko, T. Effect of high glucose and sorbitol pathway on lipid peroxidation of erythrocytes. *Horm. Metab. Res.,* 1989, **21,** 275–6.

69. Kaneto, H., Fujii, J., Myint, T., Miyazawa, N., Islam, K.N., Kawasaki, Y., Suzuki, K. *et al.* Reducing sugars trigger oxidative modification and apoptosis in pancreatic B-cells by provoking oxidative stress through the glycation reaction. *Biochem. J.,* 1996, **320,** 855–63.

70. Mandarino, L.J., Finlayson, J. and Hassell, J.R. High glucose downregulates glucose transport activity in retinal capillary pericytes but not endothelial cells. *Invest. Ophthalmol. Vis. Sci.,* 1994, **35,** 964–72.

71. Li, W., Liu, X., Yanoff, M., Cohen, S. and Ye, X. Cultured retinal capillary pericytes die by apoptosis after an abrupt fluctuation from high to low glucose levels: a comparative study with retinal capillary endothelial cells. *Diabetologia,* 1996, **39,** 537–47.

72. Van Balleogooie, E., Hooymans, J.M., Timmerman, Z. *et al.* Rapid deterioration of diabetic retinopathy during treatment with continuous subcuteneous insulin infusion. *Diabetes Care,* 1984, **7,** 236–42.

73. Baumgartner-Parzer, S., Wagner, L., Pettermann, M., Grillari, J., Gessl, A. and Waldhausl, W. High glucose triggered apoptosis in

cultured endothelial cells. *Diabetes*, 1995, **44,** 1323–7.

74. Mizutani, M., Kern, T.S. and Lorenzi, M. Accelerated death of retinal microvascular cells in human and experimental diabetic retinopathy. *J. Clin. Invest.*, 1996, **97,** 2883–90.

75. Colwell, J.A. Platelets, endothelium and diabetic vascular disease. *Diabete Metab.*, 1988, **14,** 512–18.

76. Kuijper, P.H.M., Gallardo, T.H.I., Van der Linden, J.A.M., Lammers, J.W.J., Sixma, J.J. *et al.* Platelet-dependent primary hemostasis promotes selectin- and integrin-mediated neutrophil adhesion to damaged endothelium under flow conditions. *Blood*, 1996, **87,** 3271–81.

77. Tschoepe, D., Driesch, E., Schwippert, B., Nieuwenhuis, H.K. and Gries, F.A. Exposure of adhesion molecules on activated platelets in patients with newly diagnosed IDDM is not normalised by near-normoglycemia. *Diabetes*, 1995, **44,** 890–894.

78. Colwell, J.A., Winocour, P.D. and Halushka, P.V. Do platelets have anything to do with microvascular disease? *Diabetes*, 1993, **32,** 14–18.

79. Schmidt-Schonbein, G.W., Shih, Y.Y. and Chien, S. Morphometry of human leukocytes. *Blood*, 1980, **56,** 866–75.

80. Setiadi, H., Wautier, J.L., Courillon-Mallet, A., Passa, P. and Caen, J. Increased adhesion to fibronectin and MO-1 expression by diabetic monocytes. *J. Immunol.*, 1987, **138,** 3230–34.

81. Harris, A.G., Skalak, T.C., and Hatchell, D.L. Leucocyte capillary plugging and network resistance are increased in skeletal muscles of rats with streptozotocin-induced hyperglycaemia. *Int. J. Microcirc. Clin. Exp.*, 1994, **14,** 159–66.

82. Fantorle, J.C. and Ward, P.A. Role of oxygen-derived free radicals and metabolites in leukocyte-dependent inflammatory reactions. *Am. J. Pathol.*, 1982, **107,** 397–418.

83. Nathan, C.F., Murray, H.W. and Cohn, Z.A. The macrophage as an effector cell. *N. Engl. J. Med.*, 1980, **303,** 622–6.

84. Harris, A.G. and Skalak, T.C. Effects of leukocyte activation on capillary hemodynamics in skeletal muscle. *Am. J. Physiol.*, 1993, **264,** H909–16.

85. Schroder, S., Palinski, W. and Schmidt-Schonbein, G.W. Activated monocytes and granulocytes, capillary nonperfusion, and neovascularisation in diabetic retinopathy. *Am. J. Pathol.*, 1991, **139,** 81–100.

86. Fukushima, I., Mcleod, D.S., Merges, C. and Lutty, G. Relationship of neutrophils to capillary dropout and adhesion molecules in the diabetic retina. *Invest. Ophthalmol. Vis. Sci.*, 1997, **38,** S769 (abstract).

87. Chibber, R., Belgore, F., Coppini, D., Christ, E., Sonksen, P.H. and Kohner, E.M. Raised activity of glycosylating enzyme, core 2 GlcNAc-T in leukocytes from diabetic patients: a novel mechanism for the pathogenesis of diabetic retinopathy. *Diabet. Med.*, 1997, **14** (suppl. 1), S10 (abstract).

88. King, G.L., Shiba, T., Oliver, J., Inoguchi, T. and Bursell, S. Cellular and molecular abnormalities in the vascular endothelium of diabetes mellitus. *Annu. Rev. Med.*, 1994, **45,** 179–88.

89. Siba, T., Inoguchi, T., Sportman, J.R., Heath, W.F., Bursel, S. and King, G.L. Correlation of diacylglycerol level and protein kinase C activity in rat retina to retinal circulation. *Am. J. Physiol.*, 1993, **265,** E783–93.

90. Inoguchi, T., Battan, R., Handler, E., Sportman, J.R., Heath, W. and King, G.L. Preferential elevation of protein kinase C isoform βII and diacylglycerol in the aorta and heart of diabetic rats: differential reversibility glycemic control by islet transplantation. *Proc. Natl Acad. Sci. USA*, 1992, **89,** 11059–63.

91. Tanaka,Y., Kashiwagi, A., Ogawa, T., Abe, N., Asashina, T., Ikebuchi, M., Takagi, Y. and Shigeta, Y. Effect of verampil on cardiac protein kinase C activity in rats. *Eur. J. Pharamacol.*, 1991, **200,** 353–6.

92. Xia, P., Inoguchi, T., Kern, T.S., Engerman, R.L., Oates, P.J. and King, G.L. Characterisation of the mechanism for the chronic activation of diacylglycerol protein kinase F pathway in diabetes and hypergalactosemia. *Diabetes*, 1994, **43,** 1122–9.

93. King, G.L. The role of protein kinase C activation in the development of vascular disease in diabetes. *Curr. Opin. Endocrinol. Diabetes*, 1996, **3,** 285–90.

94. Nagpala, P.G., Malik, A.B., Vuong, P.T. and Lum, H. Protein kinase Cβ1 overexpression augments phorbol ester-induced increase in endothelial permeability. *J. Cell. Physiol.*, 1996, **166,** 249–55.

95. Weiss, R.H., Yabes, A.P. and Sinaee, R. TGFβ and phorbol esters inhibit mitogenesis utilising protein kinase C dependent pathways. *Kidney Int.*, 1995, **48**, 738–44.

96. Nagpala, P., Malik, A.B., Vuong, T. and Lum, H. Protein kinase C β_1 overexpression augments phorbol ester-induced increase in endothelial permeability. *J. Cell. Physiol.*, 1996, **166**, 249–55.

97. Schilwa, M., Nakamura, T., Porter, K.R. and Ursular, E. A tumour promoter induces rapid and coordinated reorganisation of actin and vinculin in cultured cells. *J. Cell. Biol.*, 1994, **99**, 1045–59.

98. Ishii, H., Jirousek, M.R., Koya, D., Takagi, C., Xia, P., Clermont, A. *et al.* Amelioration of vascular dysfunctions in diabetic rats by an oral PKC β inhibitor. *Science,* 1997, **272**, 728–31.

99. Nishizuka, Y. The molecular hetrogeniety of protein kinase C and its implications for cellular regulation. *Nature*, 1988, **334**, 661–5.

100. Xia, P., Aiello, L.P., Ishii, H., Jiang, Z.Y., Park, D.J., Robinson, G.S., Takagi, H., Newsome, W.P., Jirosek, M.R. and King, G.L. Characterisation of vascular endothelial growth factor's effect on the activation of protein kinase C, its isoforms, and endothelial cell growth. *J. Clin. Invest.*, 1996, **98**, 2018–26.

101. Ferrara, N., Houck, K.A., Kakeman, L.B. and Leung, D.W. Molecular and biological properties of the vascular endothelial growth factor family of proteins *Endocrinol. Rev.,* 1992, **13**, 18–32.

102. Poulsen, J.E. Recovery from retinopathy in a case of diabetes with Simmond's disease. *Diabetes*, 1953, **2**, 7–12.

103. Wright, A.D., Kohner, E.M., Oakley, N.W., Hartog, M., Joplin, G.F. and Fraser, T.M. Serum GH levels and response of diabetic retinopathy to pituitary ablation. *Lancet,* 1969, **ii**, 343–8.

104. Lundbaek, K., Malmros, R., Anderson, H., Rasmussen, J.H., Bruntse, E., Madsen, P. and Jensen, V.A. Hypophysectomy for diabetic angiopathy: A controlled clinical trial. In *Symposium on the Treatment of Diabetic Retinopathy,* (eds M.F. Goldberg and S.T. Fine), Department of Health Education and Welfare, Washington, 1969, pp. 291–311.

105. Passa, P., Gauville, C. and Canivet, J. Influence of muscular excerise on plasma level of growth hormone in diabetics with and without retinopathy. *Lancet,* 1974, **ii**, 72–4.

106. Sundkvist, G., Almer, L. and Pandolfi, M. Growth hormone and endothelial function during excerise in diabetics with and without retinopathy. *Acta Med. Scand.,* 1984, **215**, 55–61.

107. Merimee, T.J., Zapf, J. and Froesch, E.R. Insulin like growth factors: studies in diabetics with and without retinopathy. *N. Engl. J. Med.,* 1983, **309**, 257–60.

108. Hyer, S.L., Sharp, P.S., Brooks, R.A., Burrin, J.M. and Kohner, E.M. A two- year follow-up study of serum insulin-like growth factor-1 in diabetics with retinopathy. *Metabolism,* 1989, **38**, 586–9.

109. Jialal, I., Crettaz, M., Hachiya, H.L., Kahn, C.R., Moses, A.C., Buzney, S.M. and King, G.L. Characterisation of receptors for insulin and the insulin-like growth factors on micro- and macrovascular tissues. *Endocrinology,* 1984, **117**, 1222–29.

110. Smith, L., Kopchick, J.K., Chen, W., Knapp, J., Kinose, F., Daley, D. *et al.* Essential role of growth hormone in ischemia-induced retinal neovascularisation. *Science,* 1997, **276**, 1706–9.

111. Shweiki, D., Itin, D., Soffer, D. and Keshet, E. Vascular endothelial growth factor induced by hypoxia may mediate hypoxia-initiated angiogenesis. *Nature,* 1992, **359**, 843–5.

112. Aiello, L.P., Avery, R.L., Arrigg, P.G., Keyt, H.D., Jampel, S.T. *et al.* Vascular endothelial growth factor in ocular fluid of patients with diabetic retinopathy and other retinal disorders. *N. Engl. J. Med.,* 1994, **331**, 1480–7.

113. Miller, J.W., Adamis, A.P., Shima, P.A., D'Amore, P.A., Moulton, R.S., O'Reilly, S. *et al.* Vascular endothelial growth factor/vascular permeability factor is temporally and spatially correlated with ocular angiogenesis in a primate model. *Am. J. Pathol.,* 1994, **145**, 574–84.

114. Leung, D.W., Cachianes, G., Kuang, W.J., Goeddel, D.V. and Ferrara, N. Vascular endothelial growth factor is a secreted angiogenic mitogen. *Science,* 1989, **246**, 1306–9.

115. Forrester, J.V., Shaifiee, A., Schroder, S., Knott, R. and Mcintosh, L. The role of growth factors in proliferative diabetic retinopathy. *Eye,* 1993, **7**, 276–87.

Allan Kofoed-Enevoldsen

16.1 INTRODUCTION

From 1930 to 1982 the incidence of diabetic nephropathy declined by almost 50%, resulting in a concomitant impressive reduction in relative mortality among insulin-dependent diabetes mellitus (IDDM) patients [1–3]. This was not a gradual process; the major reduction was found among patients with onset of diabetes between 1940 and 1960.

The 1980s and 1990s may become recognized for the *second* major drop in morbidity and mortality from diabetic nephropathy, at least in parts of the world where appropriate resources for treatment and control are available. Encouraging reports of the beneficial effects of improved blood glucose control and antihypertensive treatment on the development and progression of diabetic nephropathy may justify this optimistic view.

Nevertheless, at the present time, it seems that the development of diabetic nephropathy remains a menace for 30–40% of patients with IDDM. Non-insulin-dependent diabetes mellitus (NIDDM) patients face considerable additional vascular morbidity that may be viewed as a greater threat, but they still represent some 50% of the diabetic population developing end-stage renal disease.

The past decade has seen the generation of a vast amount of data concerning the pathophysiology and molecular biology of diabetic nephropathy, and some discoveries have led to trials of novel therapeutic modalities. This chapter summarizes the current, albeit somewhat fragmented, knowledge of the key aspects of the pathogenesis of diabetic nephropathy with emphasis on glomerular pathology.

16.2 THE NATURE OF DIABETIC RENAL DISEASE

Overt diabetic nephropathy is present when urinary albumin excretion exceeds 300 mg/24 h (200 µg/min). Due to the considerable day-to-day variation in urinary albumin excretion, the clinical diagnosis requires a positive sample in two out of three urine samples collected within six months. The annual incidence of overt diabetic nephropathy in relation to duration of diabetes follows a bell shaped curve with a peak after 15–20 years of diabetes duration (Figure 16.1). Patients with overt diabetic nephropathy either already exhibit, or carry an increased risk of developing, widespread angiopathy including arterial hypertension, coronary heart disease, peripheral vascular diseases and proliferative diabetic retinopathy. Overt diabetic nephropathy carries a poor prognosis with a median life expectancy of seven years from its onset [4], although current therapy may have resulted in an improved rate of survival [5].

Microalbuminuria, i.e. elevated urinary albumin excretion within the range of 30–300 mg/24 h, precedes the development of overt diabetic nephropathy. It is also referred to as incipient diabetic nephropathy and rarely develops before five years of diabetes duration. The presence of widespread angiopathy is already evident at this early stage of diabetic nephropathy [6]. The cumulative incidence of microalbuminuria slightly exceeds

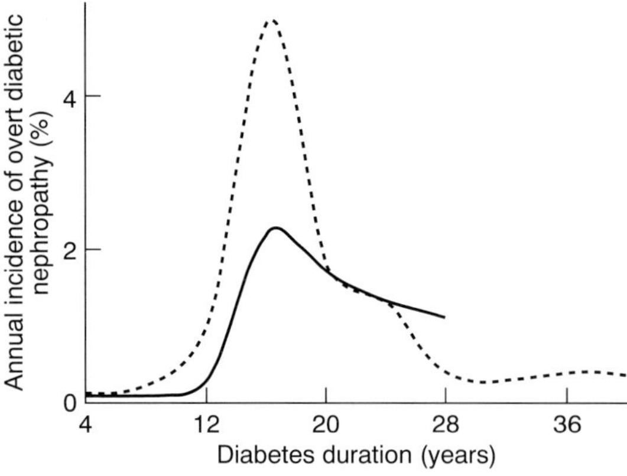

Figure 16.1 The declining incidence of diabetic nephropathy. The annual incidence of diabetic nephropathy in two cohorts of IDDM patients is shown. (- - -) Patients with onset of diabetes from 1933–42; (–) those with onset of diabetes from 1953–62. Note also that in addition to the differences in the peak incidence, both curves demonstrate the reduction in annual incidence of diabetic nephropathy appearing after 20 years of diabetes duration. Data from Kofoed-Enevoldsen *et al.* (1987).

that of overt diabetic nephropathy, but the risk of progression to overt diabetic nephropathy within 10 years may be as high as 80% [7]. This risk is highly modifiable by therapeutic intervention, primarily improved blood glucose control and antihypertensive treatment.

The course of the glomerular filtration rate from the onset of diabetes to the eventual development of end-stage renal failure has led to the definition of two pre-microalbuminuria stages of diabetic renal involvement, both characterized by glomerular hyperfiltration [8]. The consensus is, however, that the definition of diabetic nephropathy must be based on urinary albumin excretion, not the glomerular filtration rate [9].

16.3 MORPHOLOGICAL CHANGES

Kimmelstiel and Wilson [10] reported that '. . . *in a certain group of cases this change* [broad-ening of the glomerular intercapillary connective tissue] *may so dominate the histological picture as to give characteristic appearance'* and they noted that at least seven of their eight cases had diabetes. Since then, the unravelling of the pathogenesis of diabetic nephropathy has been focused upon glomerular pathology.

Advanced glomerular lesions are evenly distributed between the juxtamedullary and cortical zones. Thickening of the glomerular basement membrane is found in most diabetic patients whether or not urinary albumin excretion is elevated. However, the width of the glomerular basement membrane increases with the development of microalbuminuria until, in overt diabetic nephropathy, the width is doubled compared with healthy non-diabetic controls [11].

Higher specificity for the development of diabetic nephropathy is found in the increased mesangial matrix volume fraction. It remains within the normal range (10% of total glomerular volume) in patients with normal urinary albumin excretion, but is significantly increased in patients with micro-albuminuria (to 15% of total glomerular volume), but still exhibits substantial overlap with the normal range. Mesangial volume fraction then increases further (to 25%) in overt diabetic nephropathy, exceeding the normal range [11].

Local segmental 'fluffy intrinsic structures' of the peripheral glomerular basement membrane, which may be sites of protein leakage, have been described by Østerby and Nyberg [12].

The area of the glomerular peripheral filtration surface correlates with glomerular filtration rate. Hyperfiltrating newly diagnosed diabetic patients have large filtration surface areas, whereas a reduction in the filtration surface area is associated with the decrease in glomerular filtration rate with the progression of diabetic nephropathy. This reduction in the global filtration surface results primarily from glomerular closure, i.e. loss of functioning nephrons. Filtration surface per open glomerulus remains intact as compensatory enlargement of total glomerular volume accompanies the mesangial expansion [12a–14].

16.4 GENETIC DETERMINANTS

Evidence for a genetic component in the pathogenesis of diabetic nephropathy is found in the shape of the annual incidence curve (Figure 16.1); its decline after 20 years of diabetes duration suggests the presence of a non-susceptible sub-population. That diabetic nephropathy indeed coincides among siblings with diabetes has been confirmed in three major studies. The most recent [15] found a 70% cumulative 25-year risk of developing diabetic nephropathy among diabetic siblings of probands with overt diabetic nephropathy, compared with 25% for siblings of probands with normo- or microalbuminuria. The likely explanation, according to the investigators, for this remarkable difference is genetic, possibly of dominant autosomal origin, rather than environmental.

Several candidate genes (as discussed below) have been proposed and positive associations have been reported in early studies. Frequently, however, secondary confirmation of such association has failed, and so far no genes with a major effect have been clearly identified and confirmed. Linkage studies, using affected sibling or relative pairs, thus allowing whole genome screening, are ongoing.

As outlined by Krolewski *et al.* [16], a genetic predisposition, certainly acting in concert with environmental factors such as blood glucose control, may serve either to initiate the onset of microalbuminuria (an interactive effect) or to determine the risk of progression from microalbuminuria to overt diabetic nephropathy (an additive effect). Inasmuch as diabetic nephropathy is an organ-specific manifestation of a more generalized angiopathy which is manifest already at the stage of microalbuminuria, it follows that the transformation from normoalbuminuria to microalbuminuria is of primary pathogenetic importance. In this respect the interactive gene effects are of major interest.

16.5 HAEMODYNAMIC CHANGES

The case presented by Berkman and Rifkin [17], where unilateral renal arterial stenosis may have protected against development of nodular sclerosis, is frequently brought up as the experiment of nature which confirms the detrimental effect of glomerular hyperperfusion and hypertension in diabetes. The observation remains intriguing, although the case of a 64-year-old obese man who died in 1940 with hypertension, peripheral vascular disease, liver cirrhosis and proteinuria only two years after the diagnosis of NIDDM is hardly representative of today's young newly diagnosed IDDM patient.

Nevertheless, although neither hyperfiltration alone [18] nor long-term IDDM with elevated glomerular filtration rate [19] necessarily induce the morphological and clinical hallmarks of diabetic nephropathy, glomerular haemodynamics almost certainly influence the disease process.

Renal haemodynamics are markedly disturbed from the onset of diabetes, as discussed elsewhere in this book. With respect to the glomerulus, a significant increase (>40%) in glomerular filtration rate, and to a minor extent renal plasma flow, is associated with metabolic derangement including hyperglycaemia, ketosis, elevated glucagon and growth hormone [20].

The glomerular filtration rate is determined by renal plasma flow, transglomerular hydraulic pressure, oncotic pressure and the ultrafiltration coefficient. In the diabetic glomerulus the renal plasma flow may be increased by reduction in intrarenal vascular resistance, the ultrafiltration coefficient increased by enlargement of the filtration surface and the capillary pressure elevated by relative dilation of the afferent glomerular arteriole compared with the efferent arteriole. For technical reasons, no direct measurements of glomerular capillary pressure are available in man but animal experiments suggest that glomerular capillary pressure is indeed increased in diabetes [21].

Factors that may contribute to diabetic glomerular hyperfiltration thus include: (1) metabolic factors: hyperglycaemia, glucagon, insulin-like growth factor 1 (IGF-1), ketones; (2) vasoactive factors: prostaglandins, atrial natriuretic peptide, nitric oxide, the renin-angiotensin-aldosterone system, kinins; (3) structural factors: increased filtration surface. As diabetic nephropathy develops the number of functioning glomeruli is reduced [19] so that a normal glomerular filtration rate at this stage may still result from single nephron hyperfiltration.

Increased glomerular haemodynamic stress leads, in animal models, to albuminuria and a focal segmental glomerulosclerosis [22, 23] which may, however, not be comparable with the development of diabetic nephropathy in man [24]. Evidence from clinic-based studies with a focus on elevated glomerular filtration rate as the proposed risk marker has been conflicting. A strong case for the pathogenetic importance of haemodynamics comes from the eight-year prospective study of 64 IDDM adolescents by Rudberg *et al.* [25] who found that elevated glomerular filtration rate (>125 ml/min) was a most significant determinatant for progression from normoalbuminuria to incipient or overt diabetic nephropathy. Loss of glomerular capillary autoregulation in patients with overt diabetic nephropathy will add to glomerular haemodynamic stress [26].

Progression of diabetic nephropathy may be retarded by antihypertensive therapy [26a, 27]. This beneficial effect relates in part to blood pressure lowering rather than the choice of drug, as shown by Elving *et al.* [28]. In a two-year randomized study of 29 IDDM patients with overt diabetic nephropathy (11 of whom had hypertension), they found no difference in the efficacy of an angiotensin-converting enzyme (ACE) inhibitor (captopril) compared with a β-blocking agent (atenolol) in postponing progressive renal dysfunction.

Thus haemodynamic stress apparently contributes to the development of diabetic nephropathy. One possible mechanism could be through direct impairment of endothelial and mesangial cell metabolism and matrix synthesis (section 16.7).

16.5.1   RENIN–ANGIOTENSIN SYSTEM

There has been considerable interest in the use of ACE inhibitors in the prevention and treatment of diabetic nephropathy and the role of the renin–angiotensin system in the development of diabetic nephropathy has been the subject of several studies.

Although Miller *et al.* [28a] found circulating renin activity to be increased after 12h of hyperglycaemia, the general impression is that plasma renin activity and circulating angiotensin II remain unchanged or suppressed in patients with newly diagnosed IDDM (except in the presence of dehydration) as with the development of diabetic nephropathy [29, 30]. The interpretation of these findings is, however, hampered by a possible increase in the response to angiotensin II and by local glomerular angiotensin II production (review in [31]). Serum angiotensin converting enzyme activity is increased in patients with diabetic nephropathy [32, 33].

In addition to the direct haemodynamic effects, angiotensin II has growth factor properties and will, for example, stimulate transforming growth factor β (TGF-β) expression with possible consequences for extracellular matrix synthesis, as discussed below. The significance of the high circulating levels of the renin precursor prorenin found in IDDM patients with diabetic nephropathy [34] remains unknown.

The genetics of the renin–angiotensin system has been extensively investigated. The DD genotype of the ACE 'insertion/deletion' (I/D) polymorphism was originally found to confer excess risk of developing myocardial infarction in the non-diabetic population. The initial study in a diabetic population suggested that the II genotype was related to a reduced risk of development of diabetic nephropathy [35]. Subsequent studies have not confirmed this finding and the current evidence is that the I/D polymorphism is not related to the development of diabetic nephropathy *per se* but remains a significant cardiovascular risk factor in diabetic patients [36]. The polymorphism may however relate to the rate of progression of diabetic nephropathy [37].

Nor have initially promising polymorphisms in the angiotensinogen gene and the angiotensin-II type 1 receptor withstood confirmatory tests in secondary populations [38, 39].

16.5.2 HYPERTENSION

There is evidence that a familial predisposition to the development of arterial hypertension may be involved in the development of diabetic nephropathy [40]. A crucial debate has centred around whether the blood pressure *per se*, or some underlying genetic derangement, confers the risk.

In a three-year study of 24 h ambulatory blood pressure in 44 IDDM patients, no initial differences in blood pressure were found between the six patients who progressed from normo- to microalbuminuria. A rise in blood pressure, however, followed closely the development of microalbuminuria [41]. In this, as in other studies, e.g. [42], it was demonstrated that those who developed microalbuminuria already had elevated urinary albumin excretion (yet still within the normal range) at entry to the study. This is evidence that the process of diabetic nephropathy had been initiated at this early stage when blood pressure was not elevated. Thus when microalbuminuria is considered a stage rather than predictor of diabetic nephropathy, the development of hypertension is a concomitant expression of the disease process, not its initiator.

The prevalence of hypertension in a Danish cohort of normoalbuminuric IDDM patients was strikingly similar to the prevalence in the general population [43]. This indicates that the phenotype 'essential hypertension' may not predispose to the development of diabetic nephropathy.

Angiotensinogen gene polymorphisms (methionine/threonine substitutions at position 235 or 174) may be involved in the pathogenesis of arterial hypertension in non-diabetic people as well as in IDDM patients with nephropathy. However, the polymorphisms do not seem to be associated with the presence of diabetic nephropathy *per se* [38].

The arguments above serve to illustrate that, to the extent that a familial history of hypertension does predispose to development of diabetic nephropathy, it does not mediate this effect directly through an elevation of the arterial pressure.

16.6 GLOMERULAR SIZE AND CHARGE SELECTIVITY

Glomerular macromolecular permeability is selective for size and charge, and proteinuria in diabetic nephropathy reflect defects in both types of selectivity. The major glomerular filtration barrier consists of the fenestrated capillary endothelium, the glomerular basement membrane and the epithelial cells. The selectivity of the filtration barrier depends on the integrated function of these three layers.

Impairment of glomerular size selectivity is not found until advanced diabetic nephropathy, characterized by urinary albumin excretion exceeding 300 mg/24 h and reduced glomerular filtration rate. At this late stage, dextran clearance measurements have demonstrated a loss of size selectivity that may be explained by 5–10% of the glomerular filtrate passing through non-size-selective shunts. The remaining major part of the glomerular filtration barrier shows normal or even more restrictive size selectivity. This mechanism of proteinuria appears to be operating in a wide range of glomerular diseases [44–47]. The structural and biochemical origin of the shunt has not been identified, although the 'fluffy intrinsic structures' of the peripheral glomerular basement membrane mentioned above are possible candidates [12].

In contrast, glomerular charge selectivity is markedly impaired from the onset of microalbuminuria [46]. This loss of charge selectivity may explain the onset of microalbuminuria, and suggests a specific molecular derangement within the glomerular basement membrane, i.e. loss of heparan sulphate (see below). Reduced glomerular charge selectivity in IDDM patients with microalbuminuria may be restored by strict metabolic control [48].

16.7 DERANGEMENT OF THE EXTRACELLULAR MATRIX

The glomerular extracellular matrix includes the glomerular basement membrane and the mesangial matrix. These structures not only offer physical support for the embedded cellular components, but are deeply involved in regulation of cell growth and filtration barrier permeability. Major macromolecular constituents of the extracellular matrices are collagen type IV, laminin and heparan sulphate proteoglycan (Figure 16.2). Impairment of extracellular matrix metabolism is intimately involved in the pathogenesis of diabetic nephropathy.

The amino acid and carbohydrate composition of the expanded glomerular basement membrane in diabetic nephropathy does not differ significantly from normal [49], indicating an overabundance of the normal constituents in the expanded matrix. At the macromolecular level, however, a selective decrease is found in the content of heparan sulphate in glomerular basement membranes from diabetic patients [50–52]. This finding can be reproduced in experimental diabetes, as well as *in vitro* models. With the progression of diabetic nephropathy and the appearance of late nodular sclerosis, a decrease in glomerular basement membrane content of collagen IV and laminin is observed, although still exceeded by the decrease in heparan sulphate content.

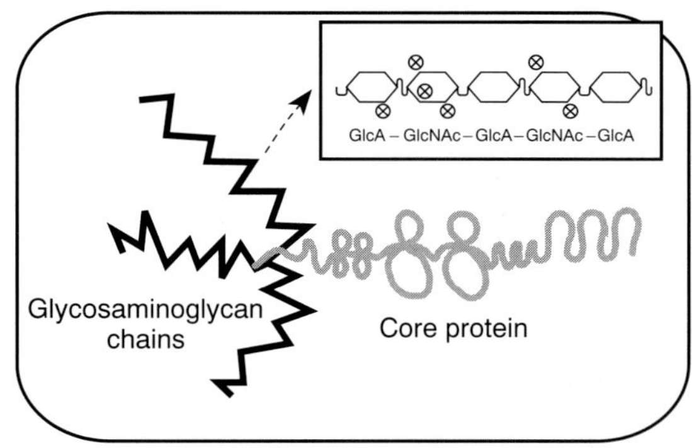

Figure 16.2 The basement membrane heparan sulphate proteoglycan is composed of a 400 kDa core protein with three 50–100 kDa glycosaminoglycan chains attached. The insert illustrates the repeated disaccharide structure of D-glucuronic acid (GlcA) and N-acetylglucosamine (GlcNAc) of the heparan sulphate glycosaminoglycan chain. Sulphation (⊗) of the glycosaminoglycan chain has major impact on the biological function of heparan sulphate. The pattern of sulphation is highly polymorphic but also very structured. Diabetes seems to impair heparan sulphate proteoglycan biosynthesis either by inducing a relative reduction in core protein synthesis, or by direct inhibition of the glycosaminoglycan sulphation through inhibition of the enzyme N-deacetylase. Both will result in failure of the several important functions of heparan sulphate: glomerular permeability, endothelial and vascular smooth muscle cell growth, lipid metabolism and anticoagulant properties.

The change in the composition of the extracellular matrix results from increased synthesis (mRNA expression) of collagen IV (α1 and α2) and laminin in combination with a relative or absolute decrease in the synthesis of glomerular basement membrane heparan sulphate proteoglycan [53–55]. In addition, appearance of collagen III in the mesangial matrix [55a], and of chondroitin sulphate in the rat glomerular basement membrane [56] indicates the major impact of diabetes on extracellular matrix metabolism. The mechanisms by which diabetes influences glomerular extracellular matrix metabolism are possibly several. Mechanical stress, e.g. cyclic stretching of mesangial cells, induces vascular endothelial permeability factor (VEPF) and TGF-β expression by mesangial and endothelial cells with concomitant alteration of matrix synthesis [57]. Metabolic factors including polyol pathway activation and reactive non-enzymatic glycation products may, through induction of protein kinase C, activity induce TGF-β expression and other factors potentially influencing the regulation and balancing of extracellular matrix synthesis (further discussed below).

Heparan sulphate proteoglycan has a central role in maintaining glomerular filtration barrier function including charge selectivity. Enzymatic removal of glomerular basement membrane heparan sulphate or exposure to monoclonal antibody directed against the heparan sulphate glycosaminoglycan chain induce increased permeability for albumin and loss of charge selectivity [58, 59]. In a study of 16 IDDM patients, Vernier *et al.* [60] found evidence for an inverse correlation between the level of urinary albumin excretion and the number of anionic sites (i.e. heparan sulphate) in the lamina rara externa of the glomerular basement membrane within the range from normo- to macroalbuminuria. These findings have, however, been questioned by Goode *et al.* [61]. They also found a (non-significant) reduction in glomerular basement membrane anionic charge density

in a smaller and mixed IDDM/NIDDM population with no normo- and microalbuminuric subjects included.

16.7.1 HEPARAN SULPHATE PROTEOGLYCAN (STENO HYPOTHESIS)

The Steno hypothesis suggests that loss of extracellular matrix heparan sulphate represents a common cause of the late diabetic vascular lesions [62]. It is based on the known role of heparan sulphate in the regulation of glomerular basement membrane charge selectivity, vascular endothelial and smooth muscle cell growth, lipid metabolism and anticoagulant properties. The hypothesis thereby provides an explanation for the combined appearance of albuminuria and premature atherosclerosis and it offers a possible target for the development of novel therapeutic strategies.

The mechanism underlying the diabetes-induced impairment of heparan sulphate metabolism is likely to include inhibition of a key enzyme in heparan sulphate biosynthesis, the glucosaminyl *N*-deacetylase, as the activity of this enzyme is closely linked to blood glucose control and, in experimental diabetes, to certain yet undefined genetic factors [63, 64] Also, cultured skin fibroblasts from patients with diabetic nephropathy have shown reduced synthesis of heparan sulphate, indicating a constitutively possible genetic defect in the regulation of the extracellular matrix biosynthesis [65]. A polymorphism in the glomerular basement membrane heparan sulphate core-protein gene that seems to protect against the development of diabetic nephropathy has been identified, but with a very low prevalence in the normo-albuminuric IDDM population [66].

Ongoing studies directed at specific pharmacological intervention towards the impairment of heparan sulphate metabolism have provided encouraging results. *In vitro*, heparin stimulates heparan sulphate biosynthesis and in experimental diabetes it has been shown to prevent the development of diabetes induced albuminuria and basement membrane thickening [67]. In IDDM patients with elevated urinary albumin excretion, 1–3 months of low-dose heparin treatment lead to a significant decrease in albuminuria [55a, 68].

16.8 CELLULAR AND MOLECULAR MECHANISMS

16.8.1 Na^+/H^+ EXCHANGER AND SODIUM-LITHIUM COUNTERTRANSPORT ACTIVITY

The Na^+/H^+ exchanger is involved in intracellular pH regulation, cell proliferation and renal sodium reabsorption. It is activated by growth factors, possibly through protein kinase C activation. Sodium-lithium countertransport on the other hand probably has no physiological function, but is thought to reflect Na^+/H^+ exchanger activity. Increased activity of these systems is a recognized risk factor for development of essential hypertension and possibly also for the development of diabetic nephropathy.

Increased leucocyte and cultured skin fibroblast Na^+/H^+ exchanger activity has been found in patients with diabetic nephropathy [69–71]. In cultured lymphoblasts, glucose seems to increase Na^+/H^+ antiport activity in cells from patients with diabetic nephropathy compared with normoalbuminuric diabetic patients [72]. The increased activity is due to an increase in the turnover per Na^+/H^+ exchanger site rather than an increase in the amount of the exchanger [73].

It is not known whether the increased exchanger activity itself contributes to the development of diabetic nephropathy, e.g. by intracellular alkalinization, or whether it is a secondary phenomenon. An interesting hypothesis has been proposed by Siffert and Düssing [74] that a general increased activation of pertussis-toxin-sensitive G proteins could explain the findings.

Several studies have emphasized the finding of increased sodium-lithium countertransport activity in diabetic nephropathy [40]. It may reflect Na^+/H^+ exchanger activity but its exact nature has not been established. Some of the controversies in the reported results may have been caused by methodological flaws, and guidelines for future measurements have been published [75].

The prognostic significance of an elevated Na^+/H^+ exchanger or sodium-lithium countertransport activity is unknown as prospective data are not available. Normotensive NIDDM patients with seven years of diabetes duration, left ventricular hypertrophy and elevated sodium-lithium countertransport may have normal urinary albumin excretion [76].

16.8.2 POLYOL PATHWAY AND PSEUDOHYPOXIA

The low affinity conversion of glucose to sorbitol and further to fructose (catalysed by the enzymes aldose reductase and sorbitol dehydrogenase) is activated when intracellular glucose is elevated. The process leads to declining intracellular reduced glutathione levels with possible diminished protection against peroxidative damage, and to a reduction in the cytosol $NAD^+/NADH$ ratio. The reduction in the $NAD^+/NADH$ ratio has been termed hyperglycaemic pseudohypoxia because hypoxic conditions also change the redox state of the $NAD^+/NADH$ couple. A detailed discussion of the widespread consequences of this pseudohypoxia can be found in Chapter 10.

An important metabolic consequence linked to the altered $NAD^+/NADH$ ratio, and which has been demonstrated to be likely to take place within the kidney, is increased diacylglycerol synthesis leading to protein kinase C activation [77, 78]. This in turn may increase the synthesis of vasodilatatory prostaglandins, increase free radical formation, increase nitric oxide production and eventually modify extracellular matrix metabolism [79].

Inhibitors of the aldose reductase enzyme, and thus of the increased activation of the polyol pathway, have been demonstrated to reduce early (2–4 weeks) raised glomerular prostaglandin synthesis, glomerular filtration rate and urinary albumin excretion [80]. However, they did not correct diabetes-induced undersulphation of basement membrane heparan sulphate after 4–5 weeks of streptozotocin (STZ) diabetes [81] or urinary albumin excretion after 32 weeks [82]. In normoalbuminuric IDDM patients with elevated glomerular filtration rate six months of aldose reductase inhibition reduced glomerular filtration rate by 5–10% without changing urinary albumin excretion [83].

The biological significance of the recently found association between a dinucleotide repeat polymorphic marker in the 5'-region of the human aldose reductase gene and the presence of diabetic nephropathy [84] remains to be determined.

16.8.3   NON-ENZYMATIC GLYCATION

Elevated levels of circulating advanced glycation endproducts (AGEs) have been found in patients with diabetic nephropathy, but so far only in patients with reduced glomerular filtration rate [85] where accumulation of circulating AGE products may add to the overall increase in cardiovascular morbidity. Evidence from experimental diabetes, however, suggests that reactive glycation products may contribute more directly to the development of diabetic nephropathy. The basics of non-enzymatic glycation is covered in Chapter 12.

Through interaction with their specific receptor on endothelial and mesangial cells, AGEs may interfere with glomerular matrix metabolism. In mouse mesangial cells, AGEs induce increased collagen IV mRNA transcription rate, as well as increasing laminin and heparan sulphate core protein and TGF-β1 mRNA [86, 87]. Long-term (eight week) culture of rat mesangial cells on glycated and cross-linked matrix lead to a reduction in charge and sulphation of newly synthesized proteoglycans, and also to a reduction in collagen synthesis [88]. Note that in these studies, AGEs did not induce the dyscoordinated matrix metabolism discussed above (section 16.7). 'Pre-AGE' Amadori glycation products also stimulate murine mesangial cell collagen IV synthesis *in vitro*, and the administration of antibody directed against Amadori adducts reduces diabetes-induced albuminuria and mesangial expansion in diabetic mice [89, 90].

Increased formation of free radicals [91] and impairment of the binding of the endothelial extracellular superoxide dismutase to cell surface heparan sulphate [92] are additional potentially hazardous effects of non-enzymatic glycation. Several studies have examined the effect of the AGE formation inhibitor aminoguanidine on experimental diabetic glomerulopathy. Nyengaard *et al.* [93] found in long-term (seven-month) diabetic rats aminoguanidine treatment inhibited the formation of AGEs and reduced albuminuria to some extent, whereas morphological hallmarks of diabetic nephropathy, such as increased mesangial volume and glomerular basement membrane width, were unaltered. Postulated inherited differences in the ability to detoxify AGE intermediates as an explanation of the varying inter-individual risk of developing diabetic nephropathy [94] awaits experimental confirmation.

16.8.4   PROTEIN KINASE C

Increased glomerular protein kinase C activity has been found in short-term (1–2 weeks) diabetic rats [77], and 15 mmol/l glucose induced a maximal increase in protein kinase C activity in cultured rat vascular smooth muscle cells [95]. The increased protein kinase C activity seems related to a glucose-induced increase in diacylglycerol production [77] which in turn may be due to an increase in cytosolic $NADH/NAD^+$ ratio (see above).

Protein kinase C activity may influence extracellular matrix metabolism [96] and angiotensin-II-mediated TGF-β expression [97]. Also, the glucose-induced increase in vascular smooth muscle cell and leucocyte Na^+/H^+ exchanger activity is dependent on increased protein kinase C activity [98, 99]. Protein kinase C is also involved in controlling mesangial cell contractility [100] and may thus take part in several of the pathogenetic processes possibly involved in the development of diabetic nephropathy.

Diabetes-induced changes in glomerular haemodynamics and increase in urinary albumin excretion in diabetic rats have been attenuated by a specific inhibitor of protein kinase C [101]. This has reinforced the interest in the role of protein kinase C in the development of diabetic nephropathy.

16.8.5   TGF-β

TGF-β is a potent regulator of extracellular matrix metabolism, and its expression is highly influenced in a diabetic environment. Urinary TGF-β excretion may be elevated in normoalbuminuric young IDDM patients [102]. Increased TGF-β immunostaining correlating with the severity of diabetic nephropathy has been found in one study [103]. In another study, glomerular TGF-β mRNA correlated with haemoglobin A1c and collagen-staining intensity, and not with the presence or absence of albuminuria/nephropathy [104].

In experimental diabetes, increased glomerular TGF-β mRNA expression and immunostaining is an early event, found within 24 h

of the induction of diabetes [105]. TGF-β expression can be induced by mechanical stretching, or by some of the factors already considered for their role in the pathogenesis of diabetic nephropathy: high glucose, angiotensin II, AGE receptor stimulation, IGF-1, protein kinase C activation [57, 97, 106].

TGF-β affects glomerular mesangial, endothelial and epithelial cells, stimulating the synthesis of extracellular matrix components: collagen (I, III, IV, VI), laminin, fibronectin and chondroitin sulphate [107–110]. However, the synthesis of basement membrane heparan sulphate proteoglycan may remain unstimulated [108], resulting in the relative loss of heparan sulphate discussed above (section 16.5).

Treatment with a neutralizing anti-TGF-β antibody attenuates experimental diabetes-induced glomerular hypertrophy and increase in TGF-β, collagen IV(α1) and fibronectin mRNA expression [111]. Also ACE inhibitors as well as angiotensin II receptor antagonists may modulate TGF-β mediated effects, including the autostimulated TGF-β-mediated increase in TGF-β expression (reviewed in [112]). Thus increased glomerular TGF-β expression is an attractive candidate as the possible common mediator of the multiple diabetes induced glomerular stress factors.

16.8.6   NITRIC OXIDE

Induction of nitric oxide (NO) synthesis may play a role in the increased glomerular filtration rate in experimental diabetes [113, 114]. It has been suggested that some of the favourable effects of the AGE formation inhibitor aminoguanidine results from its capability to inhibit stimulation of the inducible NO synthase [115]. Mesangial-inducible NO synthase on the other hand is downregulated by TGF-β which, as discussed above, is likely to be overexpressed in diabetes. At the present time, the possible relevance of increased glomerular NO synthesis to the development of diabetic nephropathy remains uncertain.

16.8.7   GROWTH HORMONE AND IGF-1

In experimental diabetes, renal and glomerular enlargement in the early days is associated with increased binding of IGF-1, probably mediated by increased expression of IGF binding proteins. If initiated from the day of onset of experimental diabetes, growth hormone suppressing treatment with octreotide attenuates increased urinary albumin excretion and kidney weight [116]. No obvious role in the development of long-term renal complications has been established, and the role of possible intervention in the GH/IGF-1 axis may only turn out to be of interest in experimental diabetes.

16.8.8   INSULIN RESISTANCE

The possible role of insulin resistance in the pathogenesis of generalized diabetic angiopathy is discussed in more detail in Chapter 8. That insulin resistance could be involved in the development of diabetic nephropathy is inferred from the reduced insulin sensitivity in non-diabetic and IDDM patients with elevated sodium-lithium countertransport [117, 118], and the evidence of insulin resistance in first-degree relatives of IDDM and NIDDM patients with incipient or overt diabetic nephropathy [119, 120]. Low birth weight, a risk factor for development of insulin resistance, seems to be only a weak predictor, if anything, of development of diabetic nephropathy as evident from a case-control study of 184 IDDM patients with diabetic nephropathy [121]. A putative link between increased protein kinase A activation, the likely consequence of insulin resistance, and impairment of heparan sulphate biosynthesis

by downregulation of *N*-deacetylase activity awaits further confirmation [122].

16.9   DIABETIC NEPHROPATHY IN NIDDM VERSUS IDDM

The occurrence of diabetic nephropathy in NIDDM patients is influenced by their much more prevalent competing causes of morbidity and mortality. Elevated urinary albumin excretion, on the other hand, was found in 25% of 68 newly diagnosed NIDDM patients [123]. The Pima Indians have a high risk of developing NIDDM at a young age; they develop a diabetic nephropathy which functionally, morphologically and with regard to prognosis for survival and the development of endstage renal failure, is almost identical to that of IDDM [124, 125].

In newly onset NIDDM, as in IDDM, glomerular filtration rate, renal plasma flow and renal volume are increased, although to a somewhat lesser extent [126–128]. Glomerular morphological changes (basement membrane thickness and mesangial volume fraction) may appear less pronounced in NIDDM patients with proteinuria compared with IDDM patients at similar level of urinary albumin excretion [129]; however, the IDDM patients in that study had lower glomerular filtration rate and longer known diabetes duration.

It seems that the rate of progression of overt diabetic nephropathy in NIDDM, as in IDDM, is accelerated by elevated blood pressure [130]. An interesting observation in relation to the debate about the importance of blood pressure is that in Pima Indians developing NIDDM, increased prediabetic blood pressure may be associated with an increased risk of developing diabetic nephropathy [131].

Current knowledge gives no reason to doubt that similar central mechanisms are operating in the pathogenesis of diabetic nephropathy in NIDDM and IDDM. However, the common concurrence of hypertension, renovascular disease and other features of the insulin-resistance syndrome may modify the rate and mode of expression.

REFERENCES

1. Borch-Johnsen, K., Kreiner, S. and Deckert, T. Mortality of type 1 (insulin-dependent) diabetes mellitus in Denmark. *Diabetologia*, 1986, **29**, 767–72.
2. Krolewski, A.S., Warram, J.H., Christlieb, A.R., Busick, E.J. and Kahn, C.R. The changing natural history of nephropathy in type 1 diabetes. *Am. J. Med.*, 1985, **78**, 785–94.
3. Kofoed-Enovoldsen, A., Borch-Johnsen, K., Kreiner, S., Nerup, J. and Deckert, T. Declining incidence of persistent proteinuria in Type 1 diabetic patients in Denmark. *Diabetes*, 1987, **2**, 205–9.
4. Andersen, A.R., Christiansen, J.S., Andersen, J.K., Kreiner, S. and Deckert, T. Diabetic nephropathy in type 1 (insulin-dependent) diabetes, an epidemiological study. *Diabetologia*, 1983, **25**, 496–501.
5. Parving, H.H. and Hommel, E. Prognosis in diabetic nephropathy. *Br. Med. J.*, 1989, **299**, 230–3.
6. Jensen, T. Albuminuria – a marker of renal and generalized vascular disease in insulin-dependent diabetes mellitus. *Dan. Med. Bull.*, 1991, **38**, 134–44.
7. Mogensen, C.E. and Christensen, C.K. Predicting diabetic nephropathy in insulin-dependent patients. *N. Engl. J. Med.*, 1984, **311**, 89–93.
8. Mogensen, C.E., Christensen, C.K. and Vittinghus, E. The stages in diabetic renal disease. *Diabetes*, 1983, **32** (suppl 2), 64–78.
9. Mogensen, C.E. *The Kidney and Hypertension in Diabetes Mellitus*, 3rd edn. Kluwer, Boston, Dordrecht and London, 1997, pp. 11–23.
10. Kimmelstiel, P. and Wilson, C. Intercapillary lesions in the glomeruli of the kidney. *Am. J. Pathol.*, 1936, **12**, 83–97.
11. Østerby, R. Glomerular structural changes in type 1 (insulin-dependent) diabetes mellitus – causes, consequences, and prevention. *Diabetologia*, 1992, **35**, 803–12.
12. Østerby, R and Nyberg, G. New vessel formation in the renal corpuscles in advanced diabetic glomerulopathy. *J. Diab. Compl.*, 1987, **1**, 122–7.
12a. Hirose, K., Tsuchida, H., Østerby, R. and Gundersen, H.J.G. A strong correlation between glomerular filtration rate and filtration surface in diabetic kidney hyperfunction. *Lab. Invest.*, 1980, **43**, 434–7.
13. Ellis, E.N., Steffes, M.W., Goetz, F.C., Sutherland, D.E.R. and Mauer, S.M. Glomerular filtration surface in type 1 diabetes mellitus. *Kidney Int.*, 1986, **29**, 889–94.
14. Østerby, R., Parving, H.H., Nyberg, G., Homme, E., Jorgensen, H.E., Lokkegaard, H. and Svalander, C. A strong correlation between glomerular filtration rate and filtration surface in diabetic nephropathy. *Diabetologia*, 1988, **31**, 265–70.
15. Quinn, M., Angelico, M.C., Warram, J.H. and Krolewski, A.S. Familial factors determine the development of diabetic nephropathy in patients with IDDM. *Diabetologia*, 1996, **39**, 940–5.
16. Krolewski, A.S., Doria, A., Magre, J., Warram, J.H. and Housman, D. Molecular genetic approaches to the identification of genes involved in the development of nephropathy in insulin-dependent diabetes mellitus. *J. Am. Soc. Nephrol.*, 1992, **3**, S9–S17.
17. Berkman, J. and Rifkin, H. Unilateral nodular diabetic glomerulosclerosis (Kimmelstiel–Wilson) – report of a case. *Metabolism*, 1973, **22**, 715– 22.
18. Nyberg, G., Andersson, C., Persson, H. and Østerby, R. Twenty years of hyperfiltration without diabetic-type glomerulosclerosis. *Am. J. Kidney. Dis.*, 1989, **13**, 345–7.
19. Mauer, S.M., Steffes, M.W., Ellis, E.N., Sutherland, D.E.R., Brown, D.M. and Goetz, F.C. Structural–functional relationships in diabetic nephropathy. *J. Clin. Invest.*, 1984, **74**, 1143–55.
20. Christiansen, J.S., Gammelgaard, J., Tronier, B., Svendsen, P.A. and Parving, H.H. Kidney function and size in diabetics before and during initial insulin treatment. *Kidney Int.*, 1982, **21**, 683–8.
21. Hostetter, T.H., Troy, J.L. and Brenner, B.M. Glomerular hemodynamics in experimental diabetes. *Kidney Int.*, 1981, **19**, 410.
22. Zatz, R., Meyer, T.W., Rennke, H.G. and Brenner, B.M. Predominance of hemodynamic

rather than metabolic factors in the pathogenesis of diabetic glomerulopathy. *Proc. Natl Acad. Sci. U.S.A.*, 1985, **82**, 5963–7.

23. Zatz, R., Dunn, B.R., Meyer, T.W., Anderson, S., Rennke, H.G. and Brenner, B.M. Prevention of diabetic glomerulopathy by pharmacological amelioration of glomerular capillary hypertension. *J. Clin. Invest.*, 1986, **77**, 1925–30.

24. Fioretto, P., Steffes, M.W., Brown, D.M. and Mauer, S.M. An overview of renal pathology in insulin-dependent diabetes mellitus in relationship to altered glomerular hemodynamics. *Am. J. Kidney. Dis.*, 1992, **20**, 549–58.

25. Rudberg, S., Persson, B. and Dahlquist, G. Increased glomerular filtration rate as a predictor of diabetic nephropathy. *Kidney Int.*, 1992, **41**, 822–8.

26. Parving, H.H., Kastrup, H., Smidt, U.M., Andersen, A.R., Feldt-Rasmussen, B. and Sandahl Christiansen, J. Impaired autoregulation of glomerular filtration rate in type 1 (insulin-dependent) diabetic patients with nephropathy. *Diabetologia*, 1984, **27**, 547–52.

26a. Parving, H.H., Andersen, A.R., Smidt, U.M. and Svendsen, P.A. Early aggressive antihypertensive treatment reduces rate of decline in kidney function in diabetic nephropathy. *Lancet*, 1983, 1175–80.

27. Mogensen, C.E. Long-term antihypertensive treatment inhibiting progression of diabetic nephropathy. *Br. Med. J.*, 1982, **285**, 685–8.

28. Elving, L.D., Wetzels, J.F.M., van Lier, H.J.J., de Nobel, E. and Berden, J.H.M. Captopril and atenolol are equally effective in retarding progression of diabtic nephropathy. *Diabetologia*, 1994, **37**, 604–9.

28a. Miller, J.A., Floras, J.S., Zinman, B. and Skorecki, K.L. Effect of hyperglycaemia on arterial pressure, plasma renin activity and renal function in early diabetes. *Clin. Sci.*, 1996, **90**, 189–95.

29. Christiansen, J.S., Giese, J., Damkjaer, M. and Parving, H.H. The renin-angiotensin system and kidney function during initial insulin treatment in diabetic man. *Scand. J. Clin. Lab. Invest.*, 1988, **48**, 451–6.

30. Norgaard, K. Hypertension in insulin-dependent diabetes. *Dan. Med. Bull.*, 1996, **43**, 21–38.

31. Hostetter, T.H. Diabetic nephropathy – metabolic versus hemodynamic considerations. *Diabetes Care*, 1992, **15**, 1205–15.

32. van Dyk, J., Erman, A., Erman, F., Chen-Gal, B., Sulkes, J. and Boner, G. Increased serum angiotensin converting enzyme activity in type 1 insulin-dependent diabetes mellitus, its relation to metabolic control and diabetic complications. *Eur. J. Clin. Invest.*, 1994, **24**, 463–67.

33. Hallab, M., Bled, F., Ebran, J.M., Suraniti, S., Girault, A., Fressinaud, P.H. and Marre, M. Elevated serum angiotensin I converting activity in type I, insulin-dependent diabetic subjects with persistent microalbuminuria. *Acta Diabetologia*, 1992, **29**, 82–5.

34. Wilson, D.M. and Luetscher, J.A. Plasma prorenin activity and complications in children with insulin dependent diabetes mellitus. *N. Engl. J. Med.*, 1990, **323**, 1101–16.

35. Marre, M., Bernadet, P., Gallois, Y., Savagner, F., Guyene, T.T., Hallab, M., Cambien, F., Passa, P.H. and Alhenc-Gelas, F. Relationships between angiotensin I converting enzyme gene polymorphism, plasma levels, and diabetic retinal and renal complications. *Diabetes*, 1994, **43**, 384–8.

36. Tarnow, L., Cambien, F., Rossing, P., Nielsen, F.S., Hansen, B.V., Lecerf, L., Poirier, O., Danilov, S., Boelskifte, S., Borch-Johnsen, K. and Parving, H.H. Insertion/deletion polymorphism in the angiotensin-I-converting enzyme gene is associated with coronary heart disease in IDDM patients with diabetic nephropathy. *Diabetologia*, 1995, **38**, 798–803.

37. Parving, H.H., Jacobsen, P., Tarnow, L., Rossing, P., Lecerf, L., Poirier, O. and Cambien, F. Effect of deletion polymorphism of angiotensin converting enzyme gene on progression of diabetic nephropathy during inhibition of angiotensin converting enzyme, observational follow up study. *Br. Med. J.*, 1996, **313**, 591–4.

38. Tarnow, L., Cambien, F., Rossing, P., Nielsen, F.S., Hansen, B.V., Ricard. S., Poirier, O. and Parving, H.H. Angiotensinogen gene polymorphisms in IDDM patients with diabetic nephropathy. *Diabetes*, 1996, **45**, 367–9.

39. Tarnow, L., Cambien, F., Rossing, P., Nielsen, F.S., Hansen, B.V., Ricard, S., Poirer, O. and Parving, H.H. Angiotensin-II type 1 receptor gene polymorphism and diabetic microangiopathy. *Nephrol. Dial. Transpl.*, 1996, **11**, 1019–23.

40. Trevisan, R. and Viberti, G.C. Genetic factors in the development of diabetic nephropathy. *J. Lab. Clin. Med.*, 1995, **126**, 342–9.

41. Poulsen, L., Hansen, K.W. and Mogensen, C.E.Ambulatory blood pressure in the transition from normo- to microalbuminuria. *Diabetes*, 1994, **43**, 1248–53.

42. Mathiesen, E.R., Rønn, B., Jensen, T., Storm, B. and Deckert, T. The relationship between blood pressure and urinary albumin excretion in the development of microalbuminuria. *Diabetes*, 1990, **39**, 245–9.

43. Norgaard, K., Feldt-Rasmussen, B., Borch-Johnsen, K., Sælan, H. and Deckert, T. Prevalence of hypertension in type 1 (insulin-dependent) diabetes mellitus. *Diabetologia*, 1990, **33**, 407–10.

44. Deen, W.M., Bridges, C.R., Brenner, B.M. and Myers, B.D.Heteroporous model of glomerular size selectivity, application to normal and nephrotic humans. *Am. J. Physiol.*, 1985, **249**, F374–89.

45. Myers, B.D., Winetz, J.A., Chui, F. and Michaels, A.S. Mechanisms of proteinuria in diabetic nephropathy. A study of glomerular barrier function. *Kidney Int.*, 1982, **21**, 633–41.

46. Deckert, T., Kofoed-Enevoldsen, A., Vidal, P., Nørgaard, K., Andreasen, H.B. and Feldt-Rasmussen, B. Size- and charge selectivity of glomerular filtration in IDDM patients with and without albuminuria. *Diabetologia*, 1993, **36**, 244–51.

47. Kofoed-Enevoldsen, A. Heparan sulphate in the pathogenesis of diabetic nephropathy. *Diabetes Metab. Rev.*, 1995, **11**, 137–60.

48. Bangstad, H.J., Kofoed-Enevoldsen, A., Dahl-Jørgensen K. and Hanssen, K.F. Glomerular charge selectivity and the influence of improved blood glucose control. *Diabetologia*, 1992, **35**, 1165–9.

49. Wahl, P., Deppermann, D. and Hasslacher, C. Biochemistry of glomerular basement membrane of the normal and diabetic human. *Kidney. Int.*, 1982, **21**, 744–9.

50. Shimomura, H. and Spiro, R.G. Studies on macromolecular components of human glomerular basement membrane and alterations in diabetes. *Diabetes*, 1987, **36**, 374–81.

51. Nerlich, A. and Schleicher, E. Immunohistochemical localization of extracellular matrix components in human diabetic glomerular lesions. *Am. J. Pathol.*, 1991, **139**, 889–99.

52. Tamsma, J.T., van den Born, J., Bruijn, J.A., Assmann, K.J.M., Weening, J.J., Berden, J.H.M., Wieslander, J., Schrama, E., Hermans, J., Veerkamp, J.H., Lemkes, H.H.P.J. and van der Woude, F.J. Expression of glomerular extracellular matrix components in human diabetic nephropathy – decrease of heparan sulphate in the glomerular basement membrane. *Diabetologia*, 1994, **37**, 313–20.

53. Ledbetter, S., Copeland, E.J., Noonan, D., Vogeli and Hassell. J. Altered steady-state mRNA levels of basement membrane proteins in diabetic mouse kidneys and thromboxane synthease inhibition. *Diabetes*, 1990, **39**, 196–203.

54. Fukui, M., Nakamura, T., Ebihara, I., Shirato, I., Tomino, Y. and Koide, H. ECM gene expression and its modulation by insulin in diabetic rats. *Diabetes*, 1992, **41**, 1520–7.

55. Couchman, J.R., Beavan, L.A. and McCarthy, K.J. Glomerular matrix – synthesis turnover and role in mesangial expansion. *Kidney Int.*, 1994, **45**, 328–35

55a. Tamsma, J.T., van der Woude, F.J. and Lemkes, H.H. Effect of sulphated glycosaminoglycans on albuminuria in patients with overt diabetic (type 1) nephropathy. *Nephrol. Dial. Transpl.*, 1996, **11**, 182–5.

56. McCarthy, K.J., Abrahamson, D.R., Bynum, K., St John, P.L. and Couchman, J.R. Basement membrane-specific chondroitin sulfate proteoglycan is abnormally associated with the glomerular capillary basement membrane of diabetic rats. *J. Histochem. Cytochem.*, 1994, **42**, 473–84.

57. Riser, B.L., Cortes, P., Zhao, X., Bernstein, J., Dumler, F., Narins, R.G,, Hassett, C.C., Sury-Sastry, K.S., Atherton, J. and Holcomb, M.A. Intraglomerular pressure and mesangial stretching stimulate extracellular matrix formation in the rat. *J. Clin. Invest.*, 1992, **90**, 1932–43.

58. Rosenzweig, L.J. and Kanwar, Y. Removal of sulfated (heparan sulfate) or nonsulfated (hyaluronic acid) glycosaminoglycans results in increased permeability of the glomerular basement membrane to ^{125}I-bovine serum albumin. *Lab. Invest.*, 1982, **47**, 177–84.

59. van den Born, J., van den Heuvel, L.P.W.J., Bakker, M.A.H., Veerkamp, J.H., Assmann, K.J.M. and Berden, J.H.M. A monoclonal antibody against GBM heparan sulfate

induces an acute selective proteinuria in rats. *Kidney Int.*, 1992, **41**, 115–23.

60. Vernier, R.L., Steffes, M.W., Sisson-Ross, S. and Mauer, S.M. Heparan sulfate proteoglycan in the glomerular basement membrane in type 1 diabetes mellitus. *Kidney Int.*, 1992, **41**, 1070–80.

61. Goode, N.P., Shires, M., Crellin, D.M., Aparicio. S.R. and Davison, A.M. Alterations of glomerular basement membrane charge and structure in diabetic nephropathy. *Diabetologia*, 1995, **38**, 1455.

62. Deckert, T., Feldt-Rasmussen, B., Borch-Johnsen, K., Jensen, T. and Kofoed-Enevoldsen, A. Albuminuria reflects widespread vascular damage. *Diabetologia*, 1989, **32**, 219–26.

63. Kofoed-Enevoldsen, A., Noonan, D. and Deckert, T. Diabetes induced inhibition of glucosaminyl *N*-deacetylase – effect of short-term blood glucose control. *Diabetologia*, 1993, **36**, 310–15.

64. Kofoed-Enevoldsen, A., Kotinis, A. and Deckert, T. Poor metabolic control decreases *N*-deacetylase activity type-1 diabetic-patients. *Diabetologia*, 1994, **37** (suppl 1),A3 (abstract).

65. Deckert, T., Horowitz, I.M., Kofoed-Enevoldsen, A., Kjellén, L., Deckert, M., Lykkelund, C. and Burchart, F. Possible genetic defects in regulation of glycosaminoglycans in patients with diabetic nephropathy. *Diabetes*, 1991, **40**, 764–70.

66. Hansen, P.M., Jensenm, J.S., Pociot, F. and Deckert, T. Possible association between genetic variation in the perlecan gene and urinary albumin excretion. *Diabetologia*, 1995, **38** (suppl 1), A229 (abstract).

67. Gambaro, G., Cavazzana, A.O., Luzi, P., Piccolo, A., Borsatti, A., Crepaldi, G., Marchi, E., Venturini, A.P. and Baggio, B. Glycosaminoglycans prevent morphological renal alterations and albuminuria in diabetic rats. *Kidney Int.*, 1992, **42**, 285–91.

68. Myrup, B., Hansen, P.M., Jensen, T., Kofoed-Enevoldsen, A., Feldt-Rasmussen, B., Gram, J., Kluft, C., Jespersen, J. and Deckert, T. Effect of low-dose heparin on urinary albumin excretion in insulin-dependent diabetes mellitus. *Lancet*, 1995, **345**, 421–2.

69. Ng, L.L., Simmons, D., Frighi, V., Garrido, M.C., Bomford, J. and Hockaday, T.D.R. Leucocyte Na^+/H^+ antiport activity in type 1 (insulin-dependent) diabetic patients with diabetic nephropathy. *Diabetologia*, 1990, **33**, 371–7.

70. Davies, J.E., Ng, L.L, Kofoed-Enevoldsen, A., Li, L.K., Earle, K.A., Trevisan, R. and Viberti, G.C. Intracellular pH and Na^+/H^+ antiport activity of cultured fibroblasts in diabetic nephropathy. *Kidney Int.*, 1992, **42**, 1184–90.

71. Trevisan, R., Li, L.K., Messent, J., Tariq, T., Earle. K., Walker, J.D. and Viberti G.C. Na^+/H^+ antiport activity and cell growth in cultured skin fibroblasts of IDDM patients with nephropathy. *Diabetes*, 1992, **41**, 1239–46.

72. Davies, J.E., Siczkowski, M,, Sweeney, F.P., Quinn, P.A., Krolewski, B., Krolewski, A.S. and Ng, L.L. Glucose-induced changes in turnover of Na^+/H^+ exchanger of immortalized lymphoblasts from type 1 diabetic patients with nephropathy. *Diabetes*, 1995, **44**, 382–8.

73. Siczkowski, M., Davies J.E., Sweeney, F.P., Kofoed-Enevoldsen, A. and Ng, L. Na^+/H^+ exchanger isoform-1 abundance in skin fibroblasts of type I diabetic patients with nephropathy. *Metabolism*, 1995, **44**, 791–5.

74. Siffert, W. and Düsing, R. Na^+/H^+ exchange in hypertension and in diabetes mellitus – facts and hypotheses. *Basic Res. Cardiol.*, 1996, **91**, 179–90.

75. Canessa, M., Zerbini,G. and Laffel, L.M.B. Sodium activation kinetics of red blood cell Na^+/Li^+ countertransport in diabetes, methodology and controversy. *J. Am. Soc. Nephrol.*, 1992, **3**, 41–9.

76. Sampson, M.J., Denver, E., Foyle, W.J., Dawson, D., Pinkney, J. and Yudkin, J.S. Association between left ventricular hypertrophy and erythrocyte sodium-lithium exchange in normotensive subjects with and without NIDDM. *Diabetologia*, 1995, **38**, 454–60.

77. Craven, P.A. and DeRubertis, F.R. Protein kinase C is activated in glomeruli from streptozotocin diabetic rats. *J. Clin. Invest.*, 1989, **83**, 1667–75.

78. Tilton, R.G., Baier, L.D., Harlow, J.E., Smith, S.R., Ostrow, E. and Williamson, J.R. Diabetes-induced glomerular dysfunction, links to a more reduced cytosolic ratio of $NADH/NAD^+$. *Kidney Int.*, 1992, **41**, 778–88.

79. Williamson, J.R., Chang, K., Frangos, M., Hasan, K.S., Ido, Y., Kawamura, T., Nyengaard, J.R., van den Enden, M., Kilo, C. and Tilton, R.G. Hyperglycemic pseudohypoxia

and diabetic complications. *Diabetes*, 1993, **42,** 801–813.

80. Chang, W.P., Dimitriadis, E., Allen, T., Dunlop, M.E., Cooper, M. and Larkins. The effect of aldose reductase inhibitors on glomerular prostaglandin production and urinary albumin excretion in experimental diabetes mellitus. *Diabetologia*, 1991, **34,** 225–31.

81. Cohen, M.P., Klepser, H. and Wu, V.Y. Undersulfatation of glomerular basement membrane heparan sulfate in experimental diabetes and lack of correction with aldose reductase inhibition. *Diabetes*, 1988, **37,** 1324–27.

82. Soulis-Liparota, T., Cooper, M.E., Dunlop, M. and Jerums, G. The relative roles of advanced glycation oxidation and aldose reductase inhibition in the development of experimental diabetic nephropathy. *Diabetologia*, 1995, **38,** 387–94.

83. Pedersen, M.M., Christensen, J.S. and Mogensen, C.E. Reduction of glomerular hyperfiltration in normoalbuminuric IDDM patients 6 mo of aldose reductase inhibition. *Diabetes*, 1991, **40,** 527–31.

84. Heesom, A.E.E., Hibberd, M.L., Millward, A. and Demaine, A.G. Polymorphism in the 5′-end of the aldose reductase gene is strongly associated with the development of diabetic nephropathy in type I diabetes. *Diabetes*, 1997, **46,** 287–91.

85. Makita, Z., Radoff, S., Rayfield, E.J., Yang, Z.Y., Skolnik, E., Delaney, V., Friedman, E.A., Cerami, A. and Vlassara, H. Advanced glycosylation end products in patients with diabetic nephropathy. *N. Engl. J. Med.*, 1991, **325,** 836–42.

86. Doi, T., Vlassara, H., Kirstein, M., Yamada, Y., Striker, G.E. and Striker, L.J. Receptor-specific increase in extracellular matrix production in mouse mesangial cells by advanced glysosylation end products is mediated via platelet-derived growth factor. *Proc. Natl Acad. Sci. U.S.A.*, 1992, **89,** 2873–7.

87. Yang, C.W., Vlassara, H., Peten, E.P., He, C.J., Striker, G.E. and Striker, L.J. Advanced glycosylation endproducts upregulate gene expression found in diabetic glomerular disease. *Proc. Natl Acad. Sci. U.S.A.*, 1994, **90,** 9436–40.

88. Silbiger, S., Crowley, S., Shan, Z., Brownlee, M., Satriano, J. and Schlondorff, D. Non-enzymatic glycation of mesangial matrix and prolonged exposure of mesangial matrix to elevated glucose reduced collagen synthesis and proteoglycan charge. *Kidney Int.*, 1993, **43,** 853–64.

89. Cohen, M.P. and Ziyadeh, F.N. Amadori glucose adducts modulate mesangial cell growth and collagen expression. *Kidney Int.*, 1994, **45,** 475–84.

90. Cohen, M.P., Hud, E. and Wu, V.Y. Amelioration of diabetic nephropathy by treatment with monoclonal antibodies against glycated albumin. *Kidney Int.*, 1994, **45,** 1673–9.

91. Sakurai, T. and Tsuchiya, S. Superoxide production from nonenzymatically glycated proteins. *FEBS Lett.*, 1988, **236,** 406–10.

92. Adachi, T., Ohta, H., Hirano, K., Hyashi, K. and Marklund, S.L. Non-enzymatic glycation of human extracellular superoxide dismutase. *Biochem. J.*, 1991, **279,** 263–7.

93. Nyengaard, J.R., Chang, K., Berhorst, S., Reiser, K.M., Williamson, J.R. and Tilton, R.G. Discordant effects of guanidines on renal structure and function and on regional vascular dysfunction and collagen changes in diabetic rats. *Diabetes*, 1997, **46,** 94–106.

94. Brownlee, M. Glycation and diabetic complications. *Diabetes*, 1994, **43,** 836–41.

95. Williams, B. and Schrier, R.W. Characterization of glucose-induced *in situ* protein kinase C activity in cultured vascular smooth muscle cells. *Diabetes*, 1992, **41,** 1464–72.

96. Studer, R.K., Craven, P.A. and DeRubertis, F.R. Role for protein kinase C in mediation of increased fibronectin accumulation by mesangial cells grown in high-glucose medium. *Diabetes*, 1993, **42,** 118–26.

97. Gibbons, G.H., Pratt, R.E. and Dzau, V.J. Vascular smooth muscle cell hypertophy vs hyperplasia. Autocrine transforming growth factor-β1 expression determines growth response to angiotensin II. *J. Clin. Invest.*, 1992, **90,** 456–61.

98. Williams, B. and Howard, R.L. Glucose-induced changes in Na$^+$/H$^+$ antiport activity and gene expression in cultured vascular smooth muscle cells. Role of protein kinase C. *J. Clin. Invest.*, 1994, **93,** 2623–31.

99. Ng, L.L., Simmons, D., Frighi, V., Garrido, M.C. and Bomford, J. Effect of protein kinase C modulators on the leucocyte Na$^+$/H$^+$ antiport in type 1 (insulin-dependent) diabetic subjects with albuminuria. *Diabetologia*, 1990, **33,** 278–4.

100. DeRubertis, F.R. and Craven, P.A. Activation of protein kinase C in glomerular cells in diabetes. *Diabetes,* 1994, **43,** 1–8.

101. Ishii, H., Jirousek, M.R., Koya, D., Takagi, C., Xia, P., Clermont, A., Bursell, S.E., Kern, T.S., Ballas, L.M., Heath, W.F., Stramm, L.E., Feener, E.P. and King, G.L. Amelioration of vascular dysfunctions in diabetic rats by an oral PKC beta inhibitor. *Science,* 1996, **272,** 728–31.

102. Korpinen, E., Teppo, A.M., Groop, P.H., Fagerudd, J., Åkerblom, H.K. and Vaarala, O. Elevated levels of urinary transforming growth factor-fl1 in young IDDM patients. *Diabetologia,* 1996, **39** (suppl 1), A293 (abstract).

103. Yamamoto, T., Nakamura, T., Noble, N.A., Rouslathi, E. and Border, W.A. Expression of transforming growth factor β is elevated in human and experimental diabetic nephropathy. *Proc. Natl Acad. Sci. U.S.A.,* 1993, **90,** 1814–8.

104. Iwano, M., Kubo, A., Nishino, T., Sato, H., Nishioka, H., Akai, Y., Kurioka, H., Fujii,Y., Kanauchi, M., Shiki, H. and Dohi, K. Quantification of glomerular TGF-β1 mRNA in patients with diabetes mellitus. *Kidney Int.,* 1996, **49,** 1120–6.

105. Shankland, S.J. and Scholey, J.W. Expression of transforming growth factor β1 during diabetic renal hypertrophy. *Kidney Int.,* 1994, **46,** 430–42.

106. Kagami, S., Border, W.A., Miller, D.E. and Noble, N.A. Angiotensin II stimulates extracellular matrix protein synthesis through induction of transforming growth factor-β expression in rat glomerular mesangial cells. *J. Clin. Invest.,* 1994, **93,** 2431–7.

107. Border, W.A., Okuda, S., Languino, L.R. and Ruoslathi, E. Transforming growth factor-fl regulates production of proteoglycans by mesangial cells. *Kidney Int.,* 1990, **37,** 689–95.

108. Kasinath, B.S. Glomerular endothelial cell proteoglycans. Regulation by TGF-β1. *Arch. Biochem. Biophys.,* 1993, **305,** 370–7.

109. Nakamura, T., Miller, D., Rouslahti, E. and Border, W.A. Production of extracellular matrix by glomerular epithelial cells is regulated by transforming growth factor-β1. *Kidney Int.,*1992, **41,** 1213–21.

110. Ziyadeh, F.N., Sharma, K., Ericksen, M. and Wolf, G. Stimulation of collagen gene expression and protein synthesis in murine mesangial cells by high glucose is mediated by autocrine activation of transforming growth factor-β. *J Clin. Invest.,* 1994, **93,** 536–42.

111. Sharma, K., Jin, Y., Guo, J. and Ziyadeh, F.N. Neutralization of TGF-β by anti-TGF-β antibody attenuates kidney hypertrophy and the enhanced extracellular matrix gene expression in STZ-induced diabetic mice. *Diabetes,* 1996, **45,** 522–30.

112. Ketteler, M., Noble, N.A. and Border, W.A. Transforming growth factor-β and angiotensin II. The missing link from glomerular hyperfiltration to glomerulosclerosis. *Annu. Rev. Physiol.,* 1995, **57,** 279–95.

113. Bank, N. and Aynedjian, H.S. Role of EDRF (nitric oxide) in diabetic renal hyperfiltration. *Kidney Int.,* 1993, **43,** 1306–12.

114. Tolins, J.P., Shultz, P.J., Raij, L., Brown. D.M. and Mauer, S.M. Abnormal renal hemodynamic response to reduced renal perfusion pressure in diabetic rats, role of NO. *Am. J. Physiol.,* 1993, **265,** F886–95.

115. Tilton, R.G., Chang, K., Hasan, K.H., Smith, S.R., Petrash, J.M., Misko, T.P., Moore, W.M., Currie, M.G., Corbett, J.A., McDaniel, M.L. and Williamsson, J.R. Prevention of diabetic vascular dysfunction by guanidines. *Diabetes,* 1993, **42,** 221–32.

116. Flyvbjerg, A., Marshall, S.M., Frystyk, J., Hansen, K.W., Harris, A.G. and Ørskov, H. Octreotide administration in diabetic rats. Effects on renal hypertrophy and urinary albumin excretion. *Kidney Int.,* 1992, **41,** 805–12.

117. Doria, A., Fioretto, P., Avogaro, A., Carraro, A., Morocutti, A., Trevisan, R., Frigato, F., Crepaldi, G., Viberti, G.C. and Nosadini, R. Insulin resistance is associated with high sodium-lithium countertransport in essential hypertension. *Am. J. Physiol.,* 1991, **261,** E684–91.

118. Lopes de Faria, J.B.L., Jones, S.L., Macdonald, F., Chambers, J., Mattock, M.B. and Viberti, G.C. Sodium-lithium countertransport activity and insulin resistance in normotensive IDDM patients. *Diabetes,* 1992, **41,** 610–15.

119. Yip, J., Mattock, M., Sethi, M., Morocutti, A. and Viberti, G.C. Insulin resistance in family members of insulin-dependent diabetic patients with microalbuminuria. *Lancet,* 1993, **341,** 369–70.

120. McCance, D.R., Hanson, R.L., Pettitt, D.J., Jacobsson, L.T.H., Bennett, P.H., Bishop, D.T.

and Knowler, W.C. Diabetic nephropathy – a risk factor for diabetes mellitus in offspring. *Diabetologia*, 1995, **38**, 221–26.

121. Rossing, P., Tarnow, L., Nielsen, F.S., Hansen, B.V., Brenner, B.M. and Parving, H.H. Low birth weight. A risk factor for development of diabetic nephropathy? *Diabetes*, 1995, **44**, 1405–7.

122. Kofoed-Enevoldsen, A., Petersen, J.S. and Deckert, T. Glucosaminyl *N*-deacetylase in cultured fibroblasts. Comparison of patients with and without diabetic nephropathy, and identification of a mechanism for diabetes induced *N*-deacetylase inhibition. *Diabetologia*, 1993, **36**, 536–40.

123. Standl, E. and Stiegler, H. Microalbuminuria in a random cohort of recently diagnosed type 2 diabetic patients in the greater Munich area. *Diabetologia*, 1993, **36**, 1017–20.

124. Nelson, R.G., Knowler, W.C., McCance, D.R., Sievers, M.L., Pettitt, D.J., Charles, M.A., Hanson, R.L., Liu, Q.Z. and Bennett, P.H. Determinants of end-stage renal disease in Pima Indians with type 2 (non-insulin-dependent) diabetes mellitus and proteinuria. *Diabetologia*, 1993, **36**, 1087–93.

125. Nelson, R.G., Knowler, W.C., Pettitt, D.J., Hanson, R.L. and Bennett, P.H. Incidence and determinants of elevated urinary albumin excretion in Pima Indians with NIDDM. *Diabetes Care*, 1995, **18**, 182–7.

126. Schmitz, A., Hansen, H.H. and Christensen, T. Kidney function in newly diagnosed type 2 (non-insulin-dependent) diabetic patients, before and during treatment. *Diabetologia*, 1989, **32**, 434–9.

127. Vora, J.P., Dolben, J., Dean, J.D., Thomas, D., Williams, J.D., Owens, D.R. and Peters, J.R. Renal hemodynamics in newly presenting non-insulin dependent diabetes mellitus. *Kidney Int.*, 1992, **41**, 829–35.

128. Nowack, R., Raum, E., Blum, W. and Ritz, E. Renal hemodynamics in recent-onset type 2 diabetes. *Am. J. Kidney. Dis.*, 1992, **10**, 342–7.

129. Østerby, R., Gall, M.A., Schmitz, A., Nielsen, F.S., Nyberg, G. and Parving, H.H. Glomerular structure and function in proteinuric type 2 (non-insulin-dependent) diabetic patients. *Diabetologia*, 1993, **36**, 1064–70.

130. Gall, M.A., Nielsen, F.S., Smidt, U.M. and Parving, H.H. The course of kidney function in type 2 (non-insulin-dependent) diabetic patients with diabetic nephropathy. *Diabetologia*, 1993, **36**, 1071–8.

131. Nelson, R.G., Pettitt, D.J., Baird, H.R., Charles, M.A., Liu, Q.Z., Bennett, P.H. and Knowler, W.C. Prediabetic blood pressure predicts urinary albumin excretion after the onset of type 2 (non-insulin-dependent) diabetes mellitus in Pima Indians. *Diabetologia*, 1993, **36**, 998–1001.

Andrew J.M. Boulton and Rayaz A. Malik

17.1 INTRODUCTION

Diabetic polyneuropathy leads to considerable morbidity and mortality [1]. The most common manifestation is that of a distal symmetric, predominantly sensory neuropathy which is the major initiating factor for foot ulceration [2]. Although there is now a substantial body of evidence for the involvement of chronic hyperglycaemia [3–7], it is not known whether metabolic abnormalities directly cause nerve damage or whether they do so by first causing an alteration in nerve microvasculature, which the clustering of neuropathy with the classic microangiopathic complications suggests might be the case. This chapter presents the observational and experimental data supporting the microangiopathic origins of neuropathy.

17.2 HUMAN STRUCTURAL AND FUNCTIONAL NEUROVASCULAR ABNORMALITIES

The most compelling evidence for the importance of an acute vascular event in the aetiology of diabetic neuropathy comes from focal neuropathies of acute onset such as third cranial nerve palsy [8] and mononeuritis multiplex [9]. However, ischaemia secondary to large vessel arteriosclerosis had been implicated in neuropathy as early as 1893, when Pryce [8a] described areas of nerve degeneration in the posterior tibial nerve trunks supplied by severely atheromatous posterior tibial arteries with occlusion of smaller microscopic vessels. Subsequently, Woltman and

Wilder [10] also attributed neuropathy to arteriosclerosis of the vasa nervorum. Focal fascicular lesions characterized by reduced density of myelinated axons within fascicles in the posterior tibial nerve and the lumbosacral trunk were found in a autopsy study of 16 patients with diabetic neuropathy [11]. These lesions were found to be identical to those found in biopsies of nerves from non-diabetic subjects with vasculitis. From post-mortem studies, Dyck *et al.* [11a] also demonstrated that proximal multifocal lesions may summate to produce diffuse fibre loss distally in diabetic patients with distal symmetric neuropathy. In another morphometric and teased fibre study of sural nerve biopsies, Dyck *et al.* [11b] showed that fibre loss is multifocal in diabetic neuropathy, strongly implicating ischaemia as the primary cause. A study by Korthals *et al.* [12] showed that the epineurial vessel intimal area and numbers of intimal nuclei were significantly greater in diabetic subjects with neuropathy compared with healthy control subjects, although no correlation was found between this abnormality and the severity of neuropathy.

The first detailed study linking diabetic neuropathy to endoneurial capillary disease was undertaken by Fagerberg [13] who demonstrated the presence of thickening and hyalinization of vessel walls by a material staining positive with periodic acid-Schiff, which were later attributed to reduplication of the capillary basal lamina [14]. Several studies have confirmed the presence of endoneurial microangiopathy in diabetic patients without neuropathy [15, 16] and with mild [17] and chronic diabetic neuropathy [15, 18–22].

Endoneurial microangiopathy is characterized by basement membrane thickening, with endothelial cell hyperplasia and hypertrophy and pericyte cell degeneration. Recent studies have localized such abnormalities to the exact site of nerve fibre damage, the endoneurium. Here microangiopathy was found to be more severe in endoneurial compared with muscle or skin capillaries [15] and epineurial capillaries [19], i.e. the site of nerve fibre damage. Furthermore, endoneurial, but not muscle, skin or epineurial capillary disease was related to the severity of neuropathy [15, 19]. Endothelial cell hyperplasia has been found in endoneurial capillaries of diabetic patients with chronic sensorimotor neuropathy [23], in some cases leading to complete occlusion of small vessels [24]. In addition plugging of small vessels by degenerate cellular material and electron-dense protein in diabetic patients with a predominantly motor neuropathy has been demonstrated [25]. The frequency of closed endoneurial capillaries has been shown to be increased in patients with diabetic neuropathy and related to neuropathic severity employing semi-quantitative techniques [26]. However, this has not been confirmed in diabetic patients with mild neuropathy [17] nor has this been borne out in quantitative studies by assessing luminal size in the same group of patients by the same investigators [20].

Transperineurial capillary abnormalities have also been demonstrated in the form of endothelial cell hypertrophy and hyperplasia resulting in a reduction in luminal size which would be expected to further reduce endoneurial blood flow [27].

Thus a combination of epineurial arteriolar, transperineurial and endoneurial capillary abnormalities ultimately deprives the endoneurium of an adequate blood flow and hence oxygen. Accordingly endoneurial oxygen tension has been shown to be significantly reduced in diabetic patients with neuropathy [28]. Another mechanism by which this may be achieved is by endoneurial oedema. This has recently been demonstrated rather elegantly by using magnetic resonance spectroscopy in diabetic patients with and without neuropathy [29], although such an abnormality has not been borne out in structural studies which have assessed mean fascicular area [15, 21, 30, 31].

In human diabetic neuropathy there is a reduction in sural nerve oxygen tension [28] but elevation of pO_2 in foot veins due to arterio-venous shunting [32]. Recent work has demonstrated an impairment of nerve blood flow and the presence of active epineurial arterio-venous shunts in human diabetic neuropathy employing novel *in vivo* techniques of sural nerve photography and fluorescein angiography [32a]. More recently diabetic patients with insulin neuritis, a transient neuropathy that follows rapid improvement in glycaemic control [33], have shown widespread epineurial vessel abnormality. This includes severe arteriolar attenuation and venous distension and tortuosity with active arterio-venous shunts as well as a fine network of blood vessels resembling the 'new vessels' of the retina [34].

An acute onset neuropathy six weeks after lowering of blood glucose levels might be expected to be due to metabolic derangement and yet such dramatic vascular changes have been observed [34]. It is well recognized that arterio-venous shunting is a feature of the diabetic neuropathic leg [32] and it seems likely that the same mechanism takes place at the level of the nerve leading to nerve hypoxia. Loss of sympathetic fibres could result in arterio-venous shunting and this has been demonstrated in detailed electronmicroscopic studies assessing unmyelinated fibre counts in epineurial arterioles [35]. Indeed Doppler sonogram abnormalities and venous oxygenation abnormalities similar to those found in diabetic patients have been found in the limbs of non-diabetic subjects with quad-riplegia-total sympathetic denervation [36]. Exercise-induced conduction velocity increment has been demonstrated to be markedly reduced in diabetic patients with neuropathy compared to non-neuropathic diabetic patients and control subjects [36a]. This is not surprising as the epineurial vessels supplying the neuropathic nerve are severely diseased and consequently nerve blood flow is unlikely to increase after exercise [32a].

Several studies have suggested that haemo-rheological abnormalities may contribute to impaired blood flow brought about by micro-vascular disease [37] (see Chapter 13 for more detail). Fibrin deposition [25] and platelet clumping [38] have been observed in endo-neurial vessels in diabetic neuropathy. Recent work by Young *et al.* [38a] has demonstrated a good relationship between various haemo-rheological parameters and neuropathy. Furthermore a number of key factors such as platelet aggregation and fibrinogen levels have been related to endoneurial microan-giopathy [39]. More recently a prospective study has demonstrated that raised levels of von Willebrand factor activity, a marker of endothelial cell dysfunction predicts the development of diabetic neuropathy [40]. However, the exact causal relationship between deranged haemorheological factors and diabetic neuropathy remains to be clearly defined.

The symmetrical nature of distal, primarily sensory, diabetic neuropathy has been used as evidence against the microvascular hypothesis of nerve damage. This misconception arises when investigators have equated the vascular hypothesis for diabetic neuropathy with the type of neuropathological and indeed neurological lesions one would expect in patients with acute vascular occlusion of large vessels. However, we would argue that it would be perfectly reasonable to develop a diffuse symmetrical neuropathy secondary to microangiopathy if one considers the micro-angiopathy to be diffuse in nature and indeed

not characterized by acute occlusion but gradual impairment of blood flow.

The argument that vascular factors are important is particularly reinforced when one considers the predominantly distal nature of the neuropathy. Thus if one was postulating a metabolic causation it would be difficult to explain away a length-dependent pathology most prominent in the distal parts, particularly if a metabolic involvement is expected to be uniform, unless one was arguing that distal nerve was in some way more susceptible to damage given the same uniform metabolic insult. The only possible support for the latter would arise from the involvement of impaired axonal transport of various nerve growth factors which would be expected too affect distal nerve most prominently [41]. However, if one considers diabetic micro-angiopathy to be most pronounced in the endoneurium compared to epineurium [19], and particularly much more prominent in the distal tissues [42], then it would not be too difficult to comprehend a link between micro-angiopathy and neuropathy.

17.3 EXPERIMENTAL NERVE ISCHAEMIA

Because of numerous collateral anastomoses between the epineurial and endoneurial vascular systems, ligation of a single nutrient artery or nutrient arteries of a small segment results in only a partial or patchy ischaemia [43]. Similarly, injection of microspheres to selectively occlude endoneurial vessels supplying the sciatic nerve requires many microvessels to be occluded before fibre degeneration occurs [43]. Experimental ischaemia also results in an increase in basement membrane thickening, and an increase in the number of swollen pericytes and endothelial cells [44]. Such studies offer indirect evidence for the importance of microvascular disease in the genesis of nerve damage in diabetes. In recent years there have been a number of animal studies that further strengthen the case for microvascular/

hypoxic mechanisms in the pathogenesis of diabetic neuropathy.

Using a hydrogen clearance method, Tuck *et al.* [45] demonstrated that rats with experimental diabetic neuropathy have reduced nerve blood flow and oxygen tension. Cameron *et al.* [46] made the observation that a reduction in nerve blood flow of about 50% occurs as early as one week after the induction of diabetes and demonstrated that neuropathy could be prevented or corrected by vasodilator treatment that improves nerve blood flow [47, 48]. Oxygen supplementation [49] or hyperbaric oxygen rearing [50] has also been found to improve deterioration in nerve conduction velocity. Furthermore, in an hypoxic environment, normal rats develop electrophysiological [51] and morphological [52] abnormalities similar to those seen in experimental diabetes in the absence of hyperglycaemia. Central hypoxaemia also provokes neurological deficits similar to those seen in experimental diabetes [53].

Laser Doppler velocimetry has been employed to measure nerve blood flow [54, 55]. In a recent study, sciatic nerve laser Doppler flux in rats with experimental diabetes was found to be 80% of that of controls after four days of induction of diabetes. It fell steadily and formed a plateau at 40% of control values after four weeks [56]. Similar results were obtained in a previous study [55]. Treatment of diabetic rats with insulin prevented the reduction in nerve blood flow [56]. Nerve Doppler flux in BB rats with genetic diabetes of six weeks' duration was also significantly reduced compared to non-diabetic BB rats [56].

Recent studies, using an alternative method of measuring nerve blood flow by injection of radiolabelled microspheres, have shown an apparently contrary result of increased endoneurial and perineurial sciatic blood flow early after the onset of experimental diabetes [57]. More recent work from the same group has suggested that the reduced nerve blood flow measured by several groups in diabetic

animals may demonstrate an impaired hyperaemic response and not a true reduction in blood flow [58]. This argument is further developed in Chapter 10. Monafo *et al.* [58a] found that sciatic nerve blood flow was reduced in diabetic rats by using yet another method which involves intravenous injection of [^{14}C]butanol.

17.4 EVIDENCE FROM PHARMACEUTICAL STUDIES

Recently, a number of pharmacological agents that increase nerve blood flow have been found to improve nerve function in experimental diabetes. These include the calcium antagonist nifedipine [59], the alpha-adrenergic receptor blocker prazocin [60], the nicotinic acid derivative niceritrol [61], the angiotensin-converting enzyme (ACE) inhibitor lisinopril [48] and an angiotensin II receptor blocker [62]. Aminoguanidine, which prevents the generation of advanced glycation end-products has been postulated to prevent nerve ischaemia and improve nerve conduction [63] in streptozotocin diabetes by an action on nerve microvessels [64]. Glutathione, a free radical scavenger, has also been found to be partially effective in the prevention of diabetic neuropathy in experimental diabetes [63], possibly acting by improving nerve hypoxia [65]. Another recent study has also shown that treatment with the antioxidant probucol prevented nerve conduction deficit, reductions in endoneurial blood flow and oxygen tension in streptozotocin diabetic rats [66]. Gamma linolenic acid therapy has also been found to improve neuropathic symptoms and measures of nerve function [67].

There is some evidence that these changes may be due to improvement in nerve blood flow [54]. Recent observations of impaired nerve blood flow and the striking abnormalities of epineurial nutrient vessels in human diabetic neuropathy [32a], would support that therapeutic measures must be directed at improving nerve blood flow. In human diabetic neuropathy, large vessel revascularization has been shown to improve nerve conduction velocity in some studies [68] but not others [69]. Two preliminary studies have shown small but significant improvements in electrophysiological and quantitative sensory tests following 12 weeks of treatment with lisinopril [70, 71]. More recently, we have carried out a double-blind placebo-controlled clinical trial in 41 diabetic patients randomized to receive the ACE inhibitor trandalopril over 12 months and have shown improvement in nerve conduction velocity, sural nerve amplitude and vibration perception [72]. A recent study has shown that hypertension is closely linked to diabetic polyneuropathy [73], providing more support for vascular dysfunction in diabetic patients who develop neuropathy.

17.5   THE ROLE OF NITRIC OXIDE AND ENDOTHELIN

The potent vasoconstrictor endothelin has been implicated in the genesis of diabetic angiopathy and has been ascribed a role in the modulation of nerve blood flow [74].

The endothelial-derived vasodilator, nitric oxide, has also been implicated in the genesis of diabetic microangiopathy. However, this ubiquitous molecule is also involved in neurotransmission in sensory nerves [75] as well as transmission or modulation in non-adrenergic, non-cholinergic nerves [76] via so-called nitrergic transmission. This system appears to be involved in a wide variety of pathophysiological states, ranging from deranged gastrointestinal relaxation [77] and penile erection [78] to bladder function [79]. Such abnormalities could easily be linked to the manifestations of diabetic autonomic neuropathy whose clinical manifestations are therefore not surprisingly poorly correlated to the impairment of the conventional tests of autonomic nerve function.

17.6   CONCLUSIONS

Although multiple factors may be implicated in the pathogenesis of diabetic polyneuropathy, with the metabolic disturbance playing a pivotal role, there is now little doubt that microvascular abnormalities play an important part. A greater understanding of the mechanisms involved and particularly the involvement of vasoactive and vascular growth factors is urgently required. Any new knowledge must also be translated into the clinical situation so that we can ameliorate the impact of one of the most resistant complications of diabetes.

REFERENCES

1. Johnson, F.N. and Williams, R. Economic aspects of diabetic neuropathy and related diabetic complications. In *Diabetic Neuropathy*, (ed. A.J.M. Boulton), Marius Press, Exeter, 1997, pp. 77–98.
2. Boulton A.J.M. Late sequelae of diabetic neuropathy. In *Diabetic Neuropathy*, (ed. A.J.M. Boulton), Marius Press, Exeter, 1997, pp. 63–76.
3. Ward, J.D., Barnes, C.G., Fisher, D.J., Jessop, J.D. and Baker, R.W.R. Improvement in nerve conduction following treatment in newly diagnosed diabetics. *Lancet*, 1971, **i**, 428–30.
4. Pirart, J. Diabetes mellitus and its degenerative complications: a prospective study of 4400 patients observed between 1947 and 1973. *Diabetes Care*, 1978, **1**, 168–88, 252–63.
5. Ziegler, D., Mayer, P., Muhlen, H. and Gries, F.A. The natural history of somatosensory and autonomic nerve dysfunction in relation to glycaemic control during the first 5 years after diagnosis of type 1 (insulin-dependent) diabetes mellitus. *Diabetologia*, 1991, **34**, 822–9.
6. The Diabetes Control and Complications Trial Research Group. The effect of intensive diabetes therapy on the development and progression of neuropathy. *Ann. Intern. Med.*, 1995, **122**, 561–8.
7. Tesfaye, S., Stevens, L., Stephenson, J. and Ward, J.D. The prevalence of diabetic neuropathy and its relation to glycaemic control in insulin dependent subjects in Europe. *Diabetologia*, 1993, **36** (suppl 2), A176.

8. Asbury, A.K. Focal and multifocal neuropathies of diabetes. In *Diabetic Neuropathy*, (eds P.J. Dyck, P.K. Thomas, A.K. Asbury, A.I. Winegrad and D. Porte), W.B. Saunders, Philadelphia, 1987, pp. 45–55.

8a. Pryce, T.D. On diabetic neuritis, with a clinical and pathological description of three cases of diabetic pseudo-tabes. *Brain*, 1893, **16**, 416.

9. Raff, M.C., Sangalang, V. and Asbury, A.K. Ischaemic mononeuropathy multiplex associated with diabetes mellitus. *Arch. Neurol.*, 1968, **18**, 487–99.

10. Woltman, H.W. and Wilder, R.M. Diabetes mellitus pathological changes in the spinal cord and peripheral nerves. *Arch. Intern. Med.*, 1929, **44**, 576–603.

11. Johnson, P.C., Doll, S.C. and Cromey, D.W., Pathogenesis of diabetic neuropathy. *Ann. Neurol.*, 1986, **19**, 450–7.

11a. Dyck, P.J., Karnes, J.L., O'Brien, P., Okazaki, H., Lias, A. and Engelstad, J. The spatial distribution of fibre loss in diabetic polyneuropathy suggests ischaemia. *Ann. Neurol.*, 1986, **19**, 440–9.

11b. Dyck, P.J., Lais, A., Karnes, J.L., O'Brien, P. and Rizza, R. Fibre loss is primary and multifocal in sural nerves in diabetic polyneuropathy. *Ann. Neurol.*, 1986, **19**, 425–39.

12. Korthals, J.K., Gieron, M.A. and Dyck, P.J. Intima of epineurial arterioles is increased in diabetic polyneuropathy. *Neurology*, 1988, **38**, 1582–6.

13. Fagerberg, S.E. Diabetic neuropathy: a clinical and histological study on the significance of vascular affections. *Acta Med. Scand.*, 1959, **164** (suppl 345), 5–81.

14. Bischoff, A. Morphology of diabetic neuropathy. *Horm. Metab. Res.*, 1980, **9** (suppl), 18–28.

15. Malik, R.A., Newrick, P.G., Sharma, A.K., Jennings, A., Ah-See, A.K., Mayhew, T.M., Jakubowski, J., Boulton, A.J.M. and Ward, J.D. Microangiopathy in human diabetic neuropathy: relationship between capillary abnormalities and the severity of neuropathy. *Diabetologia*, 1989, **32**, 92–102.

16. Giannini, C. and Dyck, P.J. Basement membrane reduplication and pericyte degeneration precede development of diabetic polyneuropathy and are associated with its severity. *Ann. Neurol.*, 1995, **37**, 498–504.

17. Malik, R.A., Veves, A., Masson, E.A. *et al.* Endoneurial capillary abnormalities in mild human diabetic neuropathy. *J. Neurol. Neurosurg. Psychiat.*, 1992, **55**, 557–61.

18. Behse, F., Bucthal, F. and Carlsen, F. Nerve biopsy and conduction studies in diabetic neuropathy. *J. Neurol. Neurosurg. Psychiat.*, 1977, **40**, 1072–82.

19. Malik, R.A., Tesfaye, S., Thompson, S.D. *et al.* Endoneurial localisation of microvascular damage in human diabetic neuropathy. *Diabetologia*, 1993, **36**, 454–9.

20. Yasuda, H. and Dyck, P.J. Abnormalities of endoneurial microvessels and sural nerve pathology in diabetic neuropathy. *Neurology*, 1987, **37**, 20–8.

21. Britland, S.T., Young, R.J., Sharma, A.K. and Clarke, B.F. Relationship of endoneurial capillary abnormalities to type and severity of diabetic polyneuropathy. *Diabetes*, 1990, **39**, 909–13.

22. Dyck, P.J. and Giannini, C. Pathologic alterations in the diabetic neuropathies of humans: a review. *J. Neuropathol. Exp. Neurol.*, 1996, **55**, 1181–93.

23. Timperley, W.R., Ward, J.D., Preston, F.E., Duckworth, T. and O'Malley, B.C. Clinical and histological studies in diabetic neuropathy. *Diabetologia*, 1976, **12**, 237–43.

24. Williams, E., Timperley, W.R., Ward, J.D. and Duckworth, T. Electronmicroscopical studies of vessels in diabetic peripheral neuropathy. *J. Clin. Pathol.*, 1980, **33**, 462–70.

25. Timperley, W.R., Boulton, A.J.M., Davies Jones, G.A.B., Jarrat, J.A. and Ward, J.D. Small vessel disease in progressive diabetic neuropathy associated with good metabolic control. *J. Clin. Pathol.*, 1985, **38**, 1030–8.

26. Dyck, P.J., Hansen, S., Karnes, J. *et al.* Capillary number and percentage closed in human diabetic sural nerve. *Proc. Natl Acad. Sci. USA*, 1985, **82**, 2513–17.

27. Malik, R.A., Tesfaye, S., Thompson, S.D. *et al.* Transperineurial capillary abnormalities in the sural nerve of patients with diabetic neuropathy. *Microvasc. Res.*, 1994, **48**, 236–45.

28. Newrick, P.G., Wilson, A.J., Jakubowski, J., Boulton, A.J.M. and Ward, J.D. Sural nerve oxygen tension in diabetes. *Br.Med. J.*, 1986, **293**, 1053–4.

29. Eaton, R.P., Qualls, C., Bicknell, J., Sibbitt, W.L., King, M.K. and Griffey, R.H. Structure–function relationships within peripheral nerves in diabetic neuropathy: the hydration hypothesis. *Diabetologia*, 1996, **39**, 439–46.

30. Bradley, J., Thomas, P.K., King, R.H.M., Llewellyn, J.G., Muddle, J.R. and Watkins, P.J. Morphometry of endoneurial capillaries in diabetic sensory and autonomic neuropathy. *Diabetologia*, 1990, **33**, 611–18.

31. Giannini, C. and Dyck, P.J. Ultrastructural morphometric abnormalities of sural nerve endoneurial microvessels in diabetes mellitus. *Ann. Neurol.*, 1994, **36**, 408–15.

32. Boulton, A.J.M., Scarpello, J.H.B. and Ward, J.D. Venous oxygenation in the diabetic neuropathic foot: evidence of arterio-venous shunting? *Diabetologia*, 1982, **22**, 6–8.

32a. Tesfaye, S., Harris, N., Iakubowski, J., Mody, C., Wilson, R.M., Rennie, J.C. and Ward, J.D. Impaired blood flow and arterio-venous shunting in human diabetic neuropathy: a novel technique of nerve photography and fluorescein angiography. *Diabetologia*, 1993, **36**, 1266–74.

33. Llewelyn, J.G., Thomas, P.K., Fonesca, V., King, R.H.M. and Dandona, P. Acute painful diabetic neuropathy precipitated by strict glycaemic control. *Acta Neuropathol.*, 1986, **72**, 157–63.

34. Tesfaye, S., Malik, R., Harris, N., Jakubowski, J., Mody, C. and Ward, J.D. Arterio-venous shunting and proliferating new vessels in acute painful neuropathy of rapid glycaemic control (insulin neuritis). *Diabetologia*, 1996, **39**, 329–35.

35. Beggs, J., Johnson, P.C., Olafsen, A., Watkins, C.L. and Cleary, C. Transperineurial arterioles in human sural nerve. *J. Neuropathol. Exp. Neurol.*, 1991, **6**, 704–18.

36. Van-den-Hoogen, F., Brawn, L.A., Sherriff, S., Watson, N. and Ward, J.D. Arteriovenous shunting in quadriplegia. *Paraplegia*, 1986, **25**, 282–6.

36a. Tesfaye, S., Harris, N., Wilson, R.M. and Ward, J.D. Exercise-induced conduction velocity increment: a matter of impaired blood flow in diabetic neuropathy. *Diabetologia*, 1992, **35**, 155–9.

37. Greaves, M. and Preston, F.E. Haemostatic abnormalities in diabetes. In *Metabolic Aspects of Cardiovascular Disease*. Vol. 2. *Diabetes and Heart Disease*, (ed. J.R. Jarrett), Elsevier, Oxford, 1984, pp. 47–80.

38. O'Malley, B.C., Timperly, W.R., Ward, J.D., Porter, N.R. and Preston, F.E. Platelet abnormalities in diabetic neuropathy. *Lancet*, 1975, **ii**, 1274–6.

38a. Young, M.J., Bennett, J.L., Liderth, S.A., Veves, A., Boulton, A.J. and Douglas, J.T. Rheological and microvascular parameters in diabetic peripheral neuropathy. *Clin. Sci.*, 1996, **90**, 183–7.

39. Ford, I., Malik, R.A., Newrick, P.G., Preston, E.F., Ward, J.D. and Greaves, M. Relationship between haemostatic factors and capillary morphology in human diabetic neuropathy. *Thromb. Haemost.*, 1992, **68**, 628–33.

40. Plater, M.E., Ford, I., Dent, M.T., Preston, F.E. and Ward, J.D. Elevated von Willebrand factor antigen predicts deterioration in diabetic peripheral nerve function. *Diabetologia*, 1996, **39**, 336–43.

41. Thomas, P.K. Growth factors and diabetic neuropathy. *Diabet. Med.*, 1994, **11**, 732–9.

42. Walker, D., Malik, R.A., Boulton, A.J.M. and Rayman, G. Structural differences in skin between the arm and foot in normal subjects and diabetic patients. *Diabetologia*, 1996, **39**, A266, 1011.

43. Nukada, H. and Dyck, P.J. Microsphere embolization of nerve capillaries and fibre degeneration. *Am. J. Pathol.*, 1984, **115**, 275–87.

44. Benstead, T.J., Sangalang, V.E. and Dyck, P.J. Acute endothelial swelling is induced in endoneurial microvessels by ischaemia. *J. Neurol. Sci.*, 1990, **99**, 37–49.

45. Tuck, R.R., Schmelzer, J.D. and Low, P.A. Endoneurial blood flow and oxygen tension in the sciatic nerves of rats with experimental diabetic neuropathy. *Brain*, 1984, **107**, 935–50.

46. Cameron, N.E., Cotter, M.A. and Low, P.A. Nerve blood flow in early experimental diabetes in rats: relation to conduction deficits. *Am. J. Physiol.*, 1991, **261**, E1–8.

47. Cameron, N.E., Cotter, M.A. and Robertson, S. Essential fatty acid diet supplementation: effects on peripheral nerve and skeletal muscle function and capillarization in streptozotocin-induced diabetic rats. *Diabetes*, 1991, **40**, 532–9.

48. Cameron, N.E., Cotter, M.A. and Robertson, S. Angiotensin converting enzyme inhibition prevents the development of muscle and nerve dysfunction and stimulates angiogenesis in streptozotocin-diabetic rats. *Diabetologia*, 1992, **35**, 12– 18.

49. Low, P.A., Tuck, R.R., Dyck, P.J., Schmelzer, J.D. and Yao, J.K. Prevention of some electrophysiologic and biochemical abnormalities

with oxygen supplementation in experimental diabetic neuropathy. *Proc. Natl Acad. Sci. USA,* 1984, **81,** 6894–8.

50. Low, P.A., Schmelzer, J.D., Ward, K.K., Curran, G.L. and Poduslo, J.F. Effect of hyperbaric oxygenation on normal and chronic streptozotocin diabetic peripheral nerves. *Exp. Neurol.,* 1985, **99,** 201–12.

51. Low, P.A., Schmelzer, J.D., Ward, K.K. and Yao, J.K. Experimental chronic hypoxic neuropathy: relevance to diabetic neuropathy. *Am. J. Physiol.,* 1986, **250,** E94–9.

52. Benstead, T.J., Dyck, P.J. and Low, P.A. Chronic hypoxia induces selective maldevelopment of peripheral myelin in rat. *J. Neuropathol. Exp. Neurol.,* 1988, **47,** 599–608.

53. Smith, W.J., Diemel, L.T., Leach, R.M. and Tomlinson, D.R. Central hypoxaemia in rats provokes neurological defects similar to those seen in experimental diabetes mellitus: evidence for a partial role of endoneurial hypoxia in diabetic neuropathy. *Neuroscience,* 1991, **45,** 255–9.

54. Stevens, E.J., Lockett, M.J., Carrington, A.L. and Tomlinson, D.R. Essential fatty acid treatment prevents nerve ischaemia and associated conduction anomalies in rats with experimental diabetes mellitus. *Diabetologia,* 1993, **36,** 397–401.

55. Yasuda, H., Sonobe, M., Yamashita, M. *et al.* Effect of prostaglandin E1 analogue TFC 612 on diabetic neuropathy in streptozotocininduced diabetic rats: comparison with aldose reductase inhibitor ONO 2235. *Diabetes,* 1989, **38,** 832–8.

56. Stevens, E.J., Carrington, A.L. and Tomlinson, D.R. Nerve ischaemia in diabetic rats: timecourse of development, effect of insulin treatment plus comparison of streptozotocin and BB models. *Diabetologia,* 1994, **37,** 43–8.

57. Pugilese, G., Tilton, R.G. and Williamson, J.R. Glucose-induced metabolic imbalances in the pathogenesis of diabetic vascular disease. *Diabetes Metab. Rev.,* 1991, **7,** 35–59.

58. Chang, K., Ido, Y., Lejeune, W., Monafo, W. and Williamson, J. Invasive methodology is unsuitable for assessing nerve blood flow in diabetes. *Diabetes,* 1995, **44,** 255.

58a. Monafo, W.W., Eliasson, S.V., Shimazaki, S. and Sugimoto, H. Regional blood flow in resting and stimulated sciatic nerve of diabetic rats. *Exp. Neurol.,* 1988, **99,** 607–14.

59. Robertson, S., Cameron, N.E. and Cotter, M.A. The effect of calcium antagonist nifedipine on peripheral nerve function in streptozotocindiabetic rats. *Diabetologia,* 1992, **35,** 1113–17.

60. Cameron, N.E., Cotter, M.A., Ferguson, K., Robertson, S. and Radcliffe, M.A. Effects of chronic alpha-adrenergic receptor blockade on peripheral nerve conduction, hypoxic resistance, polyols, Na$^+$,K$^+$-ATPase activity and vascular supply in STZ-D rats. *Diabetes,* 1991, **40,** 1652–8.

61. Hotta, N., Kakuta, H., Fakasawa, H. *et al.* Effect of niceritrol on streptozotocin-induced diabetic neuropathy in rats. *Diabetes,* 1992, **41,** 587–91.

62. Maxfield, E.K., Cameron, N.E., Cotter, M.A. and Dines, K.C. Angiotensin II receptor blockade improves nerve function, modulates nerve blood flow and stimulates endoneurial angiogenesis in streptozotocin-diabetic rats. *Diabetologia,* 1993, **36,** 1230–7.

63. Bravenboer, B., Kappelle, A.C., Hamers, F.P.T., van Buren. T., Erkelens, D.W. and Gispen, W.H. Potential use of glutathione for the prevention and treatment of diabetic neuropathy in the streptozotocin induced diabetic rat. *Diabetologia,* 1992, **35,** 813–17.

64. Kihara, M., Schmelzer, J.D., Poduslo, J.F., Curran, G.L., Nickander, K.K. and Low, P.A. Aminoguanidine effects on nerve blood flow, vascular permeability, electrophysiology and oxygen free radicals. *Proc. Natl Acad. Sci. USA,* 1991, **88,** 6107–11.

65. Low, P.A. and Nickander, K.K. Oxygen free radical effects in sciatic nerve in experimental diabetes. *Diabetes,* 1991, **40,** 873–7.

66. Cameron, N.E., Cotter, M.A., Archibald, V., Dines, K.C. and Maxfield, E.K. Anti-oxidant and pro-oxidant effects on nerve conduction velocity, endoneurial blood flow and oxygen tension in non-diabetic and streptozotocin diabetic rats. *Diabetologia,* 1994, **37,** 449–59.

67. Horrobin, D. Gamma-linolenic acid in the treatment of diabetic neuropathy. In *Diabetic Neuropathy,* (ed. A.J.M. Boulton), Marius Press, Exeter, 1997, pp. 183–195.

68. Young, M.J., Bennett, J.L., Liderth, S.A., Veves, A., Boulton, A.J.M. and Douglas, J.T. Rheological and microvascular parameters in diabetic peripheral neuropathy. *Clin. Sci.,* 1996, **90,** 183–7.

69. Veves, A., Donaghue, V.M., Sarnow, M.R., Giurini, J.M., Campbell, D.R. and LoGerfo, F.W. The impact of reversal of hypoxia by

revascularization on the peripheral nerve function of diabetic patients. *Diabetologia,* 1996, **39,** 344–8.

70. Reja, A., Tesfaye, S., Harris, N. and Ward, J.D. Improvement in nerve conduction and quantitative sensory tests after treatment with lisinopril. *Diabet. Med.,* 1995, **12,** 307–9.

71. Al-Memar, A., Wimalaratna, H.S.K. and Millward, B.A. Lisinopril improves nerve function in insulin-dependent diabetic patients with neuropathy: a preferential effect on small fibres. *Diabet. Med.,* 1996, **S38,** P90.

72. Malik, R.A., Abbott, C.A., Williamson, S., Abu-Aisha, B. and Boulton, A.J.M. A double-blind placebo controlled trial of the effect of an ACE inhibitor trandalopril on diabetic polyneuropathy. *Diabet. Med.,* 1997, **14,** P157.

73. Forrest, K.Y.Z., Maser, R.E., Pambianco, G., Becker, D.J. and Orchard, T.J. Hypertension as a risk factor for diabetic neuropathy. *Diabetes,* 1997, **46,** 665–70.

74. Cameron, N.E., Dines, K.C. and Cotter, M.A. The potential contribution of endothelin-l to neurovascular abnormalities in streptozotocin diabetic rats. *Diabetologia,* 1994, **37,** 1209–15.

75. Duarte, I.D.G., Lorenzetti, B.B. and Ferreira, S.H. Acetylcholine induces peripheral analgesia by the release of nitric oxide. In *Nitric Oxide from L-Arginine: a Bioregulatory System. Proceedings of the Symposium on Biological Importance of Nitric Oxide,* (eds S. Moncada and E.A. Higgs), Excerpta Medica, Amsterdam, 1990, pp. 165–70.

76. Rand, M.J. Nitrergic transmission: nitric oxide as a mediator of non-adrenergic, non-cholinergic neuro-effector transmission. *Clin. Exp. Pharmacol. Physiol.,* 1992, **19,** 147–69.

77. Burleigh, D.E. N^g-nitro-L-arginine reduces nonadrenergic, noncholinergic relaxation of human gut. *Gastroenterology,* 1992, **102,** 679–83.

78. Ignarro, L.J., Bush, P.A., Buga, G.M., Wood, K.S., Fukuto, J.M. and Rajfer, J. Nitric oxide and cyclic GMP formation upon electrical field stimulation cause relaxation of corpus cavernosum smooth muscle. *Biochem. Biophys. Res. Commun.,* 1990, **170,** 843–50.

79. Persson, K., Igawa, Y., Mattiason, A. and Andersson, K.E. Effects of inhibition of the L-arginine/nitric oxide pathway in the rat lower urinary tract *in vivo* and *in vitro*. *Br. J. Pharmacol.,* 1992, **107,** 178–84.

Michael D. Flynn

18.1 INTRODUCTION

Of general hospital beds in the UK, 4% are occupied by diabetic patients; up to 28% of these diabetic admissions are for foot problems [1]. Of all diabetic subjects, 15% will develop a foot ulcer within their lifetime [2] with a prevalence in British studies of 5.3–7.4% [3, 4]. The scale of the clinical problem is such that 29% of all below-knee amputations are performed on diabetic patients, a figure which rises to 45% of all amputations with the inclusion of distal amputations [5]. Foot ulceration precedes more than 80% of all amputations [6].

Vascular disease alone is not the sole cause of clinical pathology in the diabetic foot [7]. The key clinical components in the pathogenesis of foot ulceration is the co-existence of both arterial disease and neuropathy which operate in conjunction with permissive behavioural and educational factors. The final common pathway to foot ulceration, tissue necrosis and amputation is microcirculatory failure.

This chapter reviews the pathogenesis of diabetic foot ulceration and the relationship of macro- and microvascular disease with other factors which contribute to diabetic foot pathology.

18.2 PATHOGENESIS: THE NEUROISCHAEMIC AND NEUROPATHIC FOOT

Many factors are implicated in the aetiopathogenesis of foot ulceration in diabetic subjects. These include: a reduced arterial pressure head, neuropathy, abnormal pressure loading and susceptibility to infection. The majority of these factors have implicit direct or indirect effects on the ability of the microcirculation to fulfil its normal function. Even in the absence of other factors, the diabetic foot skin microcirculation is recognized to have clearly defined functional and structural abnormalities which are compounded by the co-existence of neuropathy and significant large vessel disease.

In any diabetic population there is a high prevalence of arteriosclerotic peripheral vascular disease with a 50% excess of absent foot pulses demonstrated in the Framingham study [8]. Other studies confirm that peripheral vascular disease is a major factor in foot ulceration and subsequent amputation, and remains the key determining factor in clinical outcome [6, 9].

The pathophysiology of critical limb ischaemia was originally thought to be related to a low arterial pressure head or arterial occlusion: the tap was turned off and the supply of nutrients failed. It is now recognized that numerous secondary structural and functional abnormalities of the microcirculation contribute to the development of the clinical manifestation of critical limb ischaemia [10]. Thus it is important to distinguish between parameters which reflect major arterial perfusion and those reflecting the adequacy of the cutaneous circulation [11, 12].

In some diabetic individuals it is recognized that gangrene differs from non-diabetic critical ischaemia by lack of demarcation, patchy distribution, younger age and in some cases the presence of palpable pulses [13]. It is recognized that peripheral somatic and autonomic neuropathy is a key aetiological factor in foot ulceration in numerous cross-sectional and prospective studies [14, 15]. In the neuropathic foot, the absence of occlusive arterial disease directly implicates the microcirculation as a causative factor in foot ulceration. This concept was first crystallized as small vessel occlusion [16] but has now evolved to a more complex understanding of the role of the microcirculation in diabetic foot ulceration [17].

Thus in the majority of cases, the diabetic foot is classified as neuroischaemic. It is the combination of the two fundamental factors of neuropathy and peripheral vascular disease rather than either factor alone which contributes to the clinical problem of the diabetic foot. In the diabetic limb, the adverse clinical outcome is critically influenced by the presence of neuropathy and a microvascular circulation already damaged by diabetes.

The three main factors leading to diabetic foot ulceration – neuropathy, microangiopathy and large vessel disease – give rise to a similar array of abnormalities of microvascular function: limited vasodilatory reserve, impaired postural vasoconstriction, impaired pressure regulation and maldistribution of blood flow. A minor injury unnoticed in the insensitive neuropathic foot with subsequent infection initiates a chain of events. Limited vasodilatory reserve contributes to a diminished inflammatory response to trauma/infection and impaired wound healing. There is a greater propensity to oedema formation with impaired postural reflexes and pressure regulation and with increased microvascular permeability. Oedema enhances the risk of infection and ischaemia by increasing diffusion distance, increasing the risk of shoe trauma and possibly compromising capillary filling [17]. The failure of the microcirculation to respond to these demands is the final common pathway to tissue breakdown.

Other factors also contribute to foot ulceration. These include loss of joint position sense, limitation of joint mobility, foot deformity, high plantar foot pressures and the presence of callus under weight-bearing areas. These alone do not cause foot ulceration [3]. These factors have a clear interaction with microcirculatory abnormalities in the diabetic foot in common with duration of diabetes, glycaemic control, systolic pressure, smoking and the presence of other microvascular complications which are also predictive factors in amputation [18, 19].

18.3   THE MICROCIRCULATION OF THE FOOT

In the foot, nutritional capillaries which supply blood to the skin are organized into functional units, with each dermal papilla supplied by between one and three capillary loops, 4 μm apart and 200 μm long (up to 50 μm in the nail-bed). Capillary endothelium lies on a basement membrane which is at its thickest in the foot where it normally measures about 250 nm in width. This increased thickness probably reflects the high transmural pressure impinging on the vessel in the standing position. The basement membrane consists of several proteins and glycoproteins, many with a strong anionic charge with structural stability provided mainly by type IV collagen.

Blood is supplied to capillaries from side branches of the smallest arterioles (metarterioles), which are 10–15 μm in diameter and decrease to about 7 μm over a distance of 50–100mm. At the mouth of these side branches, the endothelium is thicker and the smooth muscle in the wall of the arteriole is replaced by two or more circularly disposed cells representing the precapillary sphincters. The arterioles are supplied by efferent non-myelinated vasoconstrictor nerve fibres. Arteriolar vasodilatation is achieved both by the relaxation of neurogenic vasoconstrictor tone and also by the direct action of locally generated vasodilator substances, such as endothelium-derived relaxation factor (EDRF).

The thermoregulatory function of the foot skin results in a more complex structural and functional organization with a large number of arteriovenous anastomoses. They are located about 1–1.5 mm beneath the skin surface [20] and are predominantly found in the nail-bed and digital pulps. No arteriovenous anastomoses are found on the dorsum of the foot [21].

18.4 REGULATION OF MICROVASCULAR BLOOD FLOW

The mechanisms which regulate blood flow in the microcirculation are necessarily complex, reflecting the dual function of the microcirculation in the foot (nutrition and thermoregulation) and the fact that the microcirculation must withstand an increase in hydrostatic pressure of 75–85 mmHg on standing.

The regulation of thermoregulatory flow is relatively clear, with a rapid neurogenic vasoconstriction in response to cooling and dilation in response to heating achieved by an alteration in sympathetic vasoconstrictor tone. The arteriovenous anastomoses are normally maintained with a high degree of vasoconstrictor tone and are relatively uninfluenced by non-thermoregulatory reflexes. Denervation results in an initial dilation of arteriovenous anastomoses for 10–14 days before the normally atonic smooth muscle in the wall of the arteriovenous anastomosis acquires some secondary intrinsic tonicity [22].

Capillary flow is predominantly regulated by varying pre-capillary arteriolar tone altering the balance of pre- and post-capillary resistance. The pre-capillary resistance vessels are under neurogenic control but, in contrast to arteriovenous shunts, the smooth muscle possesses intrinsic tone and has the capacity to autoregulate. Volume flow is regulated by

both modulation of the velocity and the duration of flow [23].

It is clear that additional control mechanisms have evolved in the foot to limit oedema formation. If these mechanisms did not exist, the increase in hydrostatic pressure on standing would cause hyperfiltration of fluid and peripheral oedema. In the dependent foot, the main physiological priority is the limitation of fluid filtration. Pre-capillary vasoconstriction limits the rise in capillary pressure when the limb is lowered below heart level and the expected increase in fluid exchange is limited in conjunction with a reduction in the rise in venous pressure achieved by the calf muscle pump. The mechanism of this pre-capillary vasoconstrictor response is thought to involve a local sympathetic axon reflex (the venoarteriolar response), which is dependent on an increase in venous pressure distending the veins [24]. It is abolished by local nerve blockade but not by blockade 3 cm more proximally or sympathectomy [25–27]. Any central neurogenic component would appear to be quite small.

A complementary explanation to account for pre-capillary vasoconstriction on dependency is a myogenic hypothesis [28]. Smooth muscle cells possess intrinsic myogenic tone and this inherent tone can be potentiated by vascular wall distension. Such vascular wall distension would be produced by increases in perfusion pressure and also by lowering a limb, which increases hydrostatic pressure and thus transmural pressure. Experimental evidence suggests that an increase in transmural pressure produces relatively little increase in total flow resistance but has a dramatic effect on the capillary bed, suggesting that the most responsive myogenic elements are in close approximation to the capillary [29].

In addition to these neurogenic and myogenic mechanisms, the endothelium modulates the contractile behaviour of pre-capillary resistance vessels. The release of EDRF appears to co-ordinate the relationship between flow and diameter in resistance vessels [30, 31]. EDRF is released in response to chemical stimuli, luminal hypoxia and an increase in vascular flow rate. It acts by altering smooth muscle cyclic GMP which in turn inhibits calcium influx into the cell and intracellular calcium release. The role of EDRF may be more marked in the microcirculation than in larger vessels because of the high endothelial/smooth muscle cell ratio and smaller vascular diameters.

18.5 THE ABNORMAL CIRCULATION IN THE DIABETIC FOOT

The haemodynamic hypothesis of the development of diabetic complications identifies that early functional changes, including capillary hypertension and hyperaemia, induce late structural changes in the microvessels which ultimately lead to loss of microvascular function, relative underperfusion under stress, loss of autoregulation and increased capillary permeability [32–34]. Functional abnormalities of the microcirculation can be detected soon after the diagnosis of diabetes related to metabolic abnormalities and may be reversible by tight metabolic control [35, 36] in contrast to the late functional abnormalities in long-term diabetic subjects which are irreversible [37].

In parallel with this progressive microvascular injury, there is damage to somatic and autonomic nerves. Peripheral denervation impairs both the neurogenic control of arteriovenous shunts and local axon reflexes such as the venoarteriolar reflex exposing the microcirculation to increased pressure and flow which may accelerate and compound intrinsic microvascular functional abnormalities.

Even in the absence of atherosclerosis, the delivery of blood to the microcirculation is probably abnormal due to the increased rigidity of the arteries [38]. The effect of large vessel disease on microvascular function has been best examined in non-diabetic ischaemic limbs. Nail-fold capillary velocity is increased in the dependent position in the presence of moderate ischaemia although falling in critical ischaemia. Resting laser Doppler flowmetry and transcutaneous oximetry are normal until the ankle–brachial pressure index falls below 0.3 [39], indicating the ability of the microcirculation to autoregulate. Peak hyperaemia is depressed and impaired postural regulation of flow is most abnormal in grossly ischaemic individuals where dependent cutaneous flow exceeds flow at heart level consistent with the clinical observation of dependent rubor. In non-diabetic subjects this has been shown to be related to capillary recruitment in limb-threatening ischaemia [40]. In significant proximal arterial obstruction there is maldistribution of flow between nutritional and arteriovenous shunt flow [41] also demonstrated using fluorescein studies where there is a heterogeneous distribution of microvascular flow in both time and region although skin capillary density is normal [42]. Postural vasoconstriction is impaired in the presence of rest pain or ankle:brachial pressure index of <0.5 [43]. This is perhaps related to the build-up of metabolites secondary to tissue ischaemia overcoming local myogenic and neurogenic reflexes as a compensatory mechanism to maintain nutritional skin flow in the presence of severe ischaemia. Post-reactive hyperaemia is severely impaired in ischaemic limbs with nutritional and arteriovenous shunt flow affected to a similar degree [41] with similar abnormalities being detected in maximum blood flow in heated skin and transcutaneous oximetry [43]. The changes are functional as they are reversed by angioplasty or surgery [44].

These abnormalities of increased flow at rest, loss of pressure regulation and impaired maximum hyperaemia seen in non-diabetic ischaemic limbs are similar to those seen in diabetic patients particularly with neuropathy [17]. They are an indication of a common pathogenic mechanism mediated via microcirculatory abnormalities. In addition to these microcirculatory abnormalities present in diabetic subjects, autoregulation is impaired. The development of occlusive arterial disease can reduce the pressure head which may exceed the capacity of the damaged diabetic microcirculation to autoregulate, and thus for a given degree of arterial obstruction potentially produce more severe clinical disease in a diabetic than a non-diabetic subject [45]. In subjects with peripheral vascular disease, examination of capillary flow demonstrated a normal resting total skin flow but a reduction in post-reactive hyperaemic flow in both diabetic and non-diabetic subjects [46]. Resting capillary flow was reduced most markedly in diabetic subjects during reactive hyperaemia with evidence of a local maldistribution of flow between the nutritional capillary circulation and non-nutritional flow.

In examining the abnormal circulation of the diabetic foot, it is useful to examine the structural changes documented in the microcirculation, functional changes, the effects of neuropathy and finally how microcirculatory disease contributes to the tissue necrosis.

18.6 CAPILLARY MORPHOLOGICAL CHANGES IN DIABETES

The capillaries in the skin can be observed *in vivo* in the toe nail-fold. Capillary abnormalities include increased tortuosity of the venous limb (more than three loops or undulations), 'glomerulus' deformities and congested dilated venous limbs with a venous–arterial limb ratio of greater than 3:1 [47, 48]. An 'ischaemic' pattern of capillary abnormality, with an arterial limb less than 6 μm in diameter is no more common in diabetic subjects [49]. A specific 'nodular apical elongation', unrelated to dilation of other parts [49] of the capillary, is described, but a later study found this abnormality in only one out of 40 subjects with diabetes of long duration with complications, perhaps because it was only recognized in capillaries which were otherwise normal [47].

In the dorsum of the foot, the axis of the capillary loop is tangential to the skin and only the apex of the capillary loop is visible. Healthy capillaries appear as a small dot or comma in each dermal papilla. With increasing ischaemia there is an increase in capillary diameter which may be aneurysmal, oedema develops and the capillaries become indistinct. When tissue viability is threatened, capillary haemorrhage is observed as red cells leak into the tissues. Finally, skin necrosis is impending when the dermal papillae become devoid of capillaries [50]. In diabetic subjects, including those with severe vascular disease, changes suggesting a loss of tissue viability are rare. The most severe change discovered in a systematic study was dilation of capillaries [51].This was more common in diabetic subjects than controls and most common in insulin-dependent diabetic (IDDM) subjects, diabetic subjects with the lowest toe/brachial pressure index and/or claudication and those with neuropathy. This simple method of direct observation of the microcirculation may be useful in the assessment of tissue viability [52].

18.7 CHANGES IN THE CAPILLARY BASEMENT MEMBRANE

Basement membrane thickening is not a specific marker of diabetes. It is considered as a late marker of microvascular disease and is probably best thought of as a proliferative response by vascular endothelium to a non-specific chronic injury [53]. In diabetic subjects, basement membrane thickening is a consistent finding in capillaries, arterioles and venules and is manifest by the deposition of a PAS-positive hyaline material in the endothelial basement membrane. Electron microscopy has revealed that the basement membrane is thickened and reduplicated and chemical analysis has revealed numerous modifications which include increased glycation of type IV collagen [54], a decreased sulphation of proteoglycans which results in a reduction of the normal charge barrier [55] and increased quantities of the plasma proteins immunoglobulin G_1, immunoglobulin M, complement 3 (C3) and albumin.

The pathogenesis of increased basement membrane thickening is incompletely understood. Most studies agree that basement membrane thickening increases with the duration of diabetes, age and the distance of the microvessel below the heart [56, 57]. Twin studies strongly suggest that genetic factors play a role in basement membrane thickening and plasma protein deposition within the basement membrane [58]. Hyperglycaemia is important [57] and studies in humans with accidentally chemically induced diabetes (i.e. no genetic component) demonstrate that a similar proportion develop muscle capillary basement membrane thickening as matched 'genetic' IDDM subjects. There is also limited evidence that normalization of glycaemia is associated with some regression of basement membrane thickening [57]. The assertion that haemodynamic factors are certainly important in the generation of basement membrane thickening [57] is supported by the observation that basement membrane thickness is progressively increased in association with exposure to increased vascular pressures, either physiologically (as when an infant begins to walk) or pathologically (right-heart failure).

Many possible pathological roles for a thickened basement membrane have been postulated, but most have been superseded by the recognition of the endothelium as a functioning cell. The microcirculation may be locked within a rigid basement membrane perhaps limiting hyperaemic responses to injury [58]. It may act as a barrier to the emigration of leucocytes. Increased basement membrane thickening is not thought to impinge on the capillary lumen [57].

18.8 IS THERE SMALL VESSEL DISEASE?

The term 'small vessel' disease [16] is used by many to describe the concept of occlusive disease in small arterioles. In some diabetic subjects the presence of palpable foot pulses and the patchy distribution of gangrene led to the conclusion that gangrene in diabetic patients occurs without occlusion of the large arterial trunks and, by implication, was due to occlusion of the 'small vessels'. The origin of this controversy is a study of 152 amputation specimens (92 diabetic), which described a specific diabetic vascular lesion involving endothelial proliferation sufficient to almost occlude the lumen of digital arteries and smaller vessels [59]. This report has not been confirmed, but asymmetrical thickening of the tunica intima is described [60] as is replication of the basement membrane with pericyte hyperplasia [61]. Endothelial hyperplasia may have been used inappropriately in the original report to describe intimal hyperplasia, which is the proliferation of smooth muscle originating in the subendothelium [62].

A study using a vascular casting technique demonstrated artherosclerotic occlusion of proximal small vessels in diabetic and non-diabetic subjects [63]. There was a similar degree of patchy occlusion of proximal digital arteries and terminal arterioles (<30 μm) in diabetic subjects and non-diabetic subjects, but the diabetic subjects had more extensive (70%) occlusion, particularly in arterioles of the fifth-order branches of the digital artery arcade (30–50 μm). The nature of these occlusions suggested that they were thrombotic secondary to stasis rather than embolic or secondary to atherosclerotic occlusion [63]. Limbs with ulcers (diabetic and non-diabetic) had more occluded vessels at all levels except the terminal arterioles. More vessels were occluded on the plantar surface and the first and fifth toe, which are areas exposed to local pressure and shoe trauma, and are the usual sites for diabetic 'ischaemic' ulceration [64]. The capillary bed distal to these occlusions was essentially intact and capillary loops were patent (sometimes dilated) right at the edge of an ulcer.

A recent study has examined the histology of diabetic foot ulcers in detail using biopsies taken from the margins of ulcers and limb amputations [65]. Inevitably, the wounds showed signs of acute and chronic inflammation consistent with infection being implicated as a secondary factor in diabetic foot ulcers. Larger vessels displayed a form of vascular sclerosis with intimal hyperplasia and medial fibrosis and in some cases completely occluding the vessel. Similar findings were described in the distant past [59], although in this and other studies similar changes have been noted in subjects with pressure ulcers [66]. The wounds were well vascularized with capillaries showing cuffing with laminin, collagen, fibronectin and fibrin similar to vessels described in normal forearm skin in diabetic subjects [67] as well as venous leg ulcers, ischaemic ulcers and pressure sores. The aetiology of this cuffing is unclear but the pattern is different from that described in venous ulceration and is most likely to be the response of fibroblasts to the release of inflammatory cytokines by activated neutrophils.

The question of whether capillary and precapillary vascular disease contributes to diabetic foot ulceration remains open to debate [66]. It is clear that the microvasculature remains patent in amputation specimens to a similar degree in diabetic and non-diabetic subjects. Diabetic subjects may be more prone to intravascular thrombosis at low flow rates due to abnormal rheology [67]. The superimposition of functional and structural microvascular abnormalities on a similar degree of arterial and arteriolar atherosclerosis in diabetic subjects may limit healing potential.

18.9 CHANGES IN THE CAPILLARY ENDOTHELIUM

There is no clinical evidence of endothelial loss in the skin of the diabetic foot, although acellular capillaries have been observed in foot muscle [56]. Endothelial damage can not be directly detected *in vivo* in the human microcirculation. Endothelial products in the circulation may act as indicators of generalized and widespread endothelial damage. Angiotensin-converting enzyme [68] and von Willebrand factor [69] are both elevated in diabetic subjects with microangiopathy. Albuminuria (or microalbuminuria) may also be considered as a marker of widespread vascular and microvascular endothelial incompetence [70].

Oedema may be related to endothelial dysfunction as the endothelium is involved in the regulation of vascular exchange function, with molecules passing either between or through endothelial cells. Increased vascular permeability is a feature of diabetes in the retina, kidney and skin [71]. Haemodynamic factors contribute to the regulation of vascular permeability, but glycosylation of endothelial components and the fibre matrix may alter effective pore size and charge density. The glycation of plasma albumin may contribute to its increased uptake (compared to native albumin) into micropinocytotic vesicles and passage through the endothelial barrier [72].

Many diabetic foot ulcers are initiated by the failure of a minor wound to heal. The endothelium is involved in the formation of new blood vessels (angiogenesis). This process whereby cells migrate from pre-existing capillaries to avascular tissue is important in wound healing. There is no direct evidence of excessive or reduced angiogenesis in the skin in diabetes, and evidence of delayed wound healing in diabetes is conflicting [73]. Angiogenesis is, however, stimulated by vasodilatation and increased capillary flow [74], both of which are impaired in diabetes [58, 75].

The synthetic function of the endothelium may be defective in diabetes. Prostanoids, synthesized by the endothelium, are important modulators of vascular tone and platelet aggregability although there is a lack of consensus as to how prostanoid function may be altered in diabetes [76–78]. The role of EDRF in the abnormal microvascular regulation observed in diabetes is currently speculative. The release of EDRF may be defective in diabetic microvascular disease [79] and thus the vessel may not be protected from vasoconstrictor substances released from aggregating platelets and may not respond normally to vasodilator neurotransmitters such as substance P. EDRF also plays an important role in reversing the myogenic response and, if EDRF synthesis is reduced, unopposed myogenic vasoconstriction may result in pathological underperfusion.

18.10 FUNCTIONAL CHANGES IN THE MICROCIRCULATION

Numerous functional changes in the microcirculation have been described. They include increased blood flow, widespread vascular dilation, increased vascular permeability, impaired vascular reactivity and limitation of hyperaemia. The concept of an early functional microangiopathy [80] originated from the recognition of an initially reversible loss of vascular tone and increased vascular permeability in the absence of detectable structural change. Functional changes such as reduced vascular reactivity and hyperaemia are present within two years of diagnosis and can be detected in children with diabetes [36, 81].

Vasodilation and increased blood flow are consistent observations in the diabetic foot. There is evidence for the increase in cardiac output which must accompany generalized vasodilatation. Regional blood flow is undoubtedly increased in the lower limb [82]. In complication-free diabetic subjects, toe nail-fold capillary flow is increased and direct observation confirms dilation of the capillary bed [83]. The mechanism of this increase in peripheral blood flow is unclear, but a number of possible mechanisms have been advanced. These include:

- reduced plasma renin activity and decreased vascular reactivity to angiotensin [84, 85]
- decreased vascular reactivity to catecholamines [86]
- plasma volume expansion [84, 86]
- increased prostaglandin production [87]
- a direct vasodilatory effect of growth hormone and glucagon [88, 89]
- acute hyperglycaemia acting to produce a direct vasodilation [90]
- tissue hypoxia [91, 92]
- a direct action of insulin on vascular smooth muscle [93]
- sympathetic neuropathy reducing vasoconstrictor tone.

Blood viscosity is increased in diabetic subjects [94], and thus the increased flow suggests either that perfusion pressure is increased and/or vascular resistance is reduced. The only direct human measurements to substantiate this hypothesis have been made in skin nail-fold capillaries. Capillary pressure is normal, using the relatively crude Landis technique [95], but there is evidence that on quiet standing capillary pressure may be raised in toe nail-fold capillaries in young male diabetic subjects [96]. The measurement of dynamic capillary pressure is more sensitive and has demonstrated increases in capillary pressure in diabetic subjects from early in the disease and related to the degree of hyperglycaemia [97].

The widespread dilation of blood vessels may be related to tissue hypoxia. Oxygen demand is 10% higher in diabetic subjects than controls and skin oxygen consumption is estimated to be 70% greater [98, 99]. A left shift in the oxygen dissociation curve due to metabolic changes within the erythrocyte with low levels of 2,3-diphosphoglycerate are present in the diabetic erythrocyte [91, 92]. These levels fall further during ketosis and during insulin administration, a manoeuvre which can induce rapid capillary dilation [100]. Glycated haemoglobin also has a higher affinity for oxygen than normal haemoglobin, although abnormal high-affinity haemoglobin alone does not produce microvascular disease in non-diabetic subjects [101]. The vascular smooth muscle in the pre-capillary sphincter which regulates pre-capillary resistance may be particularly sensitive to local metabolites and changes in oxygen tension [102, 103]. These vascular responses to hypoxia require an intact endothelium and are mediated by the release of EDRF [104] which may be important in the relationship of flow and diameter of resistance vessels [31, 105].

Vasodilatation may be related to an increased production and release of EDRF in response to greater shear stress impinging on the vessel wall, generated by increased plasma viscosity, increased erythrocyte aggregability [94, 106] and reduced erythrocyte deformability [107]. Increased EDRF production is only likely to be important early in the course of diabetes, before the endothelium is damaged and while the microcirculation retains the ability to respond to the increased shear stress. A disturbance of EDRF and other endothelial regulators of vascular tone may be of greater importance in the later development of widespread endothelial damage [70]. Endothelial factors may be implicated in the paradox which arises with increasing duration of diabetes. At this time, resting hyperaemia [108] co-exists with a reduced hyperaemic response manifest by underperfusion in response to circulatory stresses including injury [58, 75], pressure (reactive hyperaemia) [109] and possibly infection. The exact underlying mechanism behind these impaired hyperaemic responses is unknown.

Vascular permeability is increased [71] and direct observation of the skin in the diabetic foot also demonstrates evidence of tissue oedema. The observed increase in vascular permeability may relate to haemodynamic factors, structural change or alteration of charge density or endothelial cell fibre matrix and basement membrane. Histological studies have shown widened endothelial spaces in diabetic post-capillary venules and capillaries [110, 111] and immunohistochemical analysis of ulcer specimens demonstrates von Willebrand factor in the interstitial space [65].

18.11 NEUROPATHY AND MICROVASCULAR DISEASE

Neuropathy may contribute to foot ulceration directly or indirectly via secondary effects on the microcirculation. Clinical neuropathy is commonly observed in the diabetic foot and has both a somatic and an autonomic component. Somatic neuropathy renders the foot insensitive and more liable to minor trauma. Motor neuropathy promotes foot deformity [112] and alters pressure distribution under the feet [113] although abnormal foot pressures alone do not cause ulceration [114]. Impaired microcirculatory responses to trauma [58, 75] and reactive hyperaemic responses [110] may be important in conjunction with abnormal pressure loading. The loss of nocioceptive fibre function produces a loss of pain sensation and impaired neurogenic vasodilatation in response to trauma and to chemical stimuli (mediated via an axon reflex) [115, 116]. Such changes are present in the dorsum of the foot at an early stage of clinical neuropathy [117].

The clinical entity of diabetic autonomic neuropathy is characterized by abnormalities of skin temperature and sweating [118]. Absent or diminished vasomotor function is a prerequisite for neuropathic foot ulceration [119]. There are several possible mechanisms by which autonomic neuropathy could interact with the microcirculation. The mechanism may be independent of a direct effect on the microcirculation, such as a loss of sudomotor function, which may predispose to skin fissuring and the entry of infection. Peripheral autosympathectomy damages the neurogenic control mechanisms which regulate capillary and arteriovenous shunt flow and results in an increase in arteriovenous shunt flow and loss of pre-capillary vasoconstriction. The neurogenic venoarteriolar reflex, thought to be a sympathetic axon reflex [24–27], is an important oedema prevention mechanism and limits the exposure of the capillary to the increase in hydrostatic pressure on standing. The failure of this reflex may accelerate capillary structural damage and basement membrane thickening, due to chronic exposure to increased intravascular pressures [57].

An early clinical observation in diabetic neuropathy was the presence of both abnormally warm and abnormally cold feet, with both the failure of vasoconstriction in response to body cooling and the failure of vasodilatation in response to body warming. The cold neuropathic foot was initially attributed to the selective destruction of sympathetic vasodilator fibres [120]. It is now accepted that denervated peripheral vessels exhibit autonomous tone and the cutaneous vessels become hypersensitive to local cold and circulating catecholamines [121]. Both hyper- and underactivity of the sympathetic nervous system have been detected using the galvanic skin response and quantitative tests of sudomotor function [122]. Partial sympathectomy may promote the hyperactive state with later diminution of function because of complete autosympathectomy. Increased sweating may occur because of sprouting of surviving axons to replace lost fibres and a similar process of multi-innervation may relate to blood vessels.

There is no doubt, however, that most neuropathic feet are warm and that regional and total skin blood flow is increased [82]. The partition of this increased blood flow within the microcirculation is abnormal with increased arteriovenous shunt flow as a consequence of peripheral autonomic denervation. This hypothesis is supported by several sources. The venous system in the diabetic lower limb is histologically 'arterialized', which is compatible with an increased flow of blood at higher than normal pressure passing through open arteriovenous shunts. Arteriographic studies reported a very rapid passage of contrast medium into the venous side of the circulation and further indirect evidence was obtained by measuring a high partial pressure of oxygen in the foot veins of diabetic subjects with neuropathy [122]. This suggests that saturated blood passes directly into the venous circulation of the leg, bypassing the capillary circulation. A study using radiolabelled microspheres demonstrated that vascular channels of greater than 20 μm diameter were present in the feet of subjects with neuropathic ulcers [123]. These were assumed to be dilated arteriovenous shunts, which can reach 60 μm in diameter.

Measurements with Doppler ultrasound demonstrate increased pulse wave velocity in subjects with foot ulceration [124], related to the high frequency of arterial wall calcification [125, 126] and an abnormal frequency spectrum analysis in limb of subjects with ulceration [124, 125]. Peripheral arterial flow was increased with a greater than normal forward systolic flow component accompanied by continuous forward flow in diastole. The loss of the normal reverse flow component was attributed to a reduction in peripheral resistance, as is seen in increased arteriovenous shunting. Other studies in diabetic subjects with neuropathy using venous occlusion plethysmography [82] and laser Doppler flowmetry [83, 127] have demonstrated increased skin blood flow in the toe pulps where arteriovenous shunts are common. Similar abnormalities are seen in diabetic subjects apparently free of peripheral or autonomic neuropathy, indicative of isolated peripheral sympathetic damage despite normal cardiovascular autonomic function tests.

Postural vasoconstriction is impaired in the feet of diabetic subjects with peripheral and/or autonomic neuropathy compatible with a loss of the local sympathetic axon reflex (venoarteriolar reflex) [127]. This hyperperfusion on dependency is thought predominantly to involve flow through arteriovenous shunts. This may increase venous pressure and contribute to a reduction in skin capillary flow and increased fluid filtration.

18.12   CAPILLARY FLOW IN THE DIABETIC FOOT

The capillary component of flow comprises approximately 10% of total skin flow, the remainder passing via arteriovenous shunts [128]. Direct measurement of capillary blood flow has demonstrated that, when the foot is at heart level, capillary flow is increased in subjects with neuropathy compared to normal control subjects [83]. Total skin blood flow in the toe pulps by laser Doppler flowmetry was increased in diabetic control subjects and further increased in diabetic subjects with neuropathy [83]. This study suggests that the increase in arteriovenous shunt flow does not grossly compromise capillary flow. It is unclear if the capillary flow is increased appropriately for the increase in skin temperature measured in both the diabetic neuropathy group and the diabetic control group. A further review suggests an abnormal distribution of flow. In the feet of insulin-dependent diabetic subjects free from macroangiopathy, capillary blood cell velocity and peak capillary blood cell velocity after reactive hyperaemia was reduced in subjects both with and without late complications [129]. The measurement of total skin blood flow in the toe nail-fold by laser Doppler flowmetry was similar in patients and control subjects with the ratio of capillary to total skin blood flow being reduced, indicating a maldistribution of flow. Skin temperatures were not increased in the diabetic groups.

When the foot is lowered below heart level in normal subjects, both capillary and arteriovenous shunt flow are substantially diminished to protect the microcirculation from the effects of the increase in hydrostatic pressure [23]. In diabetic subjects, this mechanism is impaired particularly in subjects with overt neuropathy [127]. This is compatible with a failure of neurogenic vasoconstriction to the shunt circulation. The failure to restrict arteriovenous shunt flow on dependency would be expected to lead to the development of oedema. Neuropathic oedema is uncommon despite the high prevalence of diabetic somatic and autonomic neuropathy. This suggests that fluid filtration in the diabetic capillary bed may be restricted by other mechanisms. In the standing position there is a profound reduction in capillary flow [130]. In the presence of neuropathy, this suggests that a secondary myogenic mechanism may effect pre-capillary vasoconstriction.

Some studies of the abnormal microcirculation have been made in the skin of the upper limb. The available evidence suggests that these abnormalities are global and applicable to the foot skin. A recent study has demonstrated significantly worse abnormalities in the feet when compared with the hands. In the hand, capillary blood velocity and laser Doppler velocimetry were normal whereas there were reduced reactive hyperaemic responses in the toes [46].

18.13   DO CLOSED CAPILLARIES CONTRIBUTE TO ISCHAEMIA IN THE SKIN OF THE FOOT?

The evidence for this is scanty and is mainly derived by extension from changes seen in the eye where acellular (non-blood-filled) capillaries are observed [131]. Similar acellular capillaries in skeletal muscle are more frequently observed in diabetic subjects [132] and increase in frequency from the neck to the foot [56]. Such acellular capillaries are associated with an increase in the amount of pericyte cell debris within the basement membrane. The circumferential coverage of the capillary wall with pericytes in samples taken from foot muscles in diabetic subjects was the same as in normal controls, and intact cell processes were seen within a few of the acellular capillaries. This suggests that, although pericytes are damaged in the diabetic foot, turnover is increased so that overall pericyte numbers are maintained. The cause of acellular capillaries is unknown in muscle, but has been attributed to intracapillary thrombosis [69]. It appears that, in contrast to the retina, acellular capillaries can be revascularized in the foot. Histological studies of muscle capillaries do not demonstrate any luminal narrowing in capillaries, even when marked basement membrane thickening [56, 57] or a reduction in capillary circumference is present.

Histological study in the skin has provided no evidence of acellular capillaries. A reduction in capillary lumen has been reported in foot skin [133]. In the skin of the arm, a similar reduction of luminal area is associated with vascular complications of diabetes but not disease duration [134]. Direct observation of capillaries in the skin of ischaemic feet does not show any loss of blood-filled capillaries until skin necrosis is imminent [50].

In the great toe nail-fold of diabetic subjects without clinical evidence of vascular disease but with severe neuropathy, there is no evidence of capillary closure [83]. Histological studies of the margins of diabetic foot ulcers show that in general they are well vascularized, although there was narrowing or occlusion of some large blood vessels due to vessel wall thickening in both the ulcer margin and occasionally in the surrounding skin. Although numbers were small, the changes were present in 6/14 neuropathic ulcers and 4/5 neuroischaemic ulcers [65]. The authors speculate that some vessels may have undergone thrombosis and recanalized. No comment was made on closure of capillaries.

Although there is no evidence of capillary closure, it is possible that the foot capillary bed is not perfused in end-stage disease, either because of pre-capillary vascular disease or intracapillary thrombosis secondary to deranged rheology.

18.14   CLINICAL IMPLICATIONS

In established foot disease, bed rest which elevates the foot to heart level is an established treatment. Studies of the microcirculation demonstrate that this helps to optimize nutritional capillary flow and reduces oedema. Clinical observation suggests that this increases healing potential.

The involvement of the microcirculation in the pathogenesis of foot disease raises the possibility of pharmacological manipulation to optimize microcirculatory flow. The haemodynamic hypothesis suggests that capillary hypertension promotes structural damage, and thus vigorous antihypertensive treatment early in the course of the disease may reduce capillary pressure and limit damage. Care must be exercised in the choice of antihypertensive agent, because beta blockade, particularly in the presence of proximal vascular disease, may reduce perfusion pressure to the microcirculation. Nifedipine promotes peripheral oedema formation by attenuating postural vasoconstriction [135].

Glycaemic control is important in the development of diabetic microangiopathy [136] but the optimum means and degree of control awaits clarification particularly in type 2 diabetes. Microvascular autoregulatory responses are significantly impaired in uncomplicated diabetic subjects with poor control compared to matched subjects with good control. Insulin itself is a powerful vasoactive substance and can provoke postural hypotension [137], reduce plasma volume, increase albumin loss from the circulation [138] and act as a vasodilator on resistance and capacitance vessels [139]. Strict metabolic control has no effect on subcutaneous blood flow measured by the xenon washout technique [37]. Cutaneous blood flow is redistributed by nine days of continuous subcutaneous insulin infusion in patients with poor control, with an increase in capillary blood velocity and a fall in venous oxygen tension in the finger suggesting a reduction in arteriovenous shunting [140]. This is probably an effect of insulin *per se*, as acute experiments show increased capillary flow at high intravenous insulin infusion rates without changes in blood glucose [141]. In diabetic subjects with neuropathy, the acute infusion of insulin following withdrawal of oral hypoglycaemic agents resulted in a 225% increase in the capillary component of blood flow and marked capillary dilation without any similar change in shunt flow [142]. Low molecular weight heparin has been shown to improve the nutritional capillary circulation and clinical outcome in patients with neuroischaemic foot ulcers with arterial and total skin microcirculation remaining unchanged [143].

A further recent observation of clinical significance is that the tissue breakdown which occurs under the abnormal build up of callus may be related not to pressure and shear stresses but to an increase in capillary fragility [144].

18.15 CONCLUSIONS

The failure of the microcirculation is the terminal definitive event in the pathogenesis of foot ulceration, gangrene and amputation in both diabetic and non-diabetic subjects. In critical ischaemia the restriction of blood supply secondary to proximal arterial occlusion induces numerous secondary effects on the microcirculation. These functional abnormalities are similar to those which can be detected in the diabetic foot. Many of these are present in early diabetes but become more significant with the development of common complications of diabetes such as neuropathy.

Thus ulceration of the neuroischaemic diabetic foot is a manifestation of the synergy of intrinsic microcirculatory abnormalities of diabetes, those secondary to neuropathy and to proximal arterial disease. It is therefore not surprising that diabetic foot disease is a major and common clinical problem. A clear understanding of these mechanisms is essential to rational treatment and to preventive therapy.

REFERENCES

1. Williams, D.R.R. Hospital admissions of diabetic patients: information from hospital activity analysis. *Diabet. Med.*, 1985, **2**, 27–32.
2. Palumbo, P.J. and Melton, L.J. Peripheral vascular disease and diabetes. In *Diabetes in America*, (eds M.J. Harris and R.F. Hamman), NIH Publication 85-1468. US Government Printing Office, Washington, 1985, pp. 1–21.
3. Veves, A., Murray, H.J., Yound, M.J. and Boulton, A.J.M. The risk of foot ulceration in diabetic patients with high foot pressure: a prospective study. *Diabetologia*, 1992, **35**, 660–3.
4. Walters, D.P., Gatling, W., Mullee, M.A. and Hill, R.D. The distribution and severity of diabetic foot disease: a community study with comparison to a non diabetic group. *Diabet. Med.*, 1992, **9**, 354–8.
5. Connor, H. The economic impact of diabetic foot disease. In *The Foot in Diabetes*, (eds H. Connor, A.J.M. Boulton and J.D. Ward), John Wiley, Chichester, 1987, pp. 145–9.
6. Percoraro, R.E., Reiber, G.E. and Burgess, E.M. Pathways to diabetic limb amputation: basis for prevention. *Diabetes Care*, 1990, **13**, 513–21.
7. Le Quesne, L.P. Surgical aspects of the diabetic foot. In *The Foot in Diabetes*, (eds H. Connor, A.J.M. Boulton and J.D. Ward), John Wiley, Chichester, 1987, pp. 69–79.
8. Abbott, R.D., Brand, F.N. and Kannell, W.B. Epidemiology of some peripheral arterial findings in diabetic men and women: experiences from the Framingham study. *Am. J. Med.*, 1990, **88**, 376–81.
9. Siitonen, O.I., Niskanen, L.K., Laasko, M., Siitonen, J.T. and Pyorala, K. Lower extremity amputation in diabetic and non-diabetic patients: a population based study in Eastern Finland. *Diabetes Care*, 1993, **16**, 16–20.

10. Lowe, G. Pathophysiology of critical limb ischaemia. In *Critical Leg Ischaemia. Its Pathophysiology and Management*, (eds J.A. Dormandy and G. Stock), Springer Verlag, Berlin, 1990, pp. 17–38.

11. Cina, C., Katsamouris, A., Megreman, J. and Brewster, D.C. Utilty of transcutaneous oxygen measurements in peripheral arterial occlusive disease. *J. Vasc. Surg.*, 1984, **1**, 362–71.

12. Oishi, C.S., Fronek, A. and Golbranson, F.L. The role of non-invasive vascular studies in determining the levels of amputation. *J. Bone. Joint. Surg.*, 1988, **70A**, 1520–30.

13. Kramer, D.W. Diabetic grangrene: incidence and pathogenesis: an analysis of 58 cases amongst 1008 diabetics. *Circulation*, 1932, **4**, 503–14.

14. Boulton, A.J.M. The diabetic foot: neuropathic in aetiology? *Diabet. Med.*, 1990, **7**, 852–8.

15. Young, M.J., Breddy, J.L., Veves, A. and Boulton, A.J.M. The prediction of neuropathic foot ulceration using vibration perception thresholds. *Diabetes Care*, 1994, **17**, 557–61.

16. Dry, T.J. and Hines, E.A. The role of diabetes in the development of degenerative vascular disease with special reference to the evidence of retinitis and peripheral neuritis. *Ann. Intern. Med.*, 1941, **14**, 1893–902.

17. Flynn, M.D. and Tooke, J.E. Aetiology of diabetic foot ulceration : a role for the microcirculation. *Diabet. Med.*, 1992, **8**, 320–9.

18. Selby, J.V. and Zhnag, D. Risk factors for lower extremity amputations in persons with diabetes. *Diabetes Care*, 1995, **18**, 509–16.

19. Moss, S.E., Klein, R. and Klein, B. The prevalence and incidence of lower extremity amputation in a diabetic population. *Arch. Intern. Med.*, 1992, **152**, 610–5.

20. Mescon, H., Hurley, J. and Moretti, G. The anatomy and histochemistry of the arteriovenous anastomosis in human digital skin. *J. Invest. Dermatol.*, 1956, **27**, 133–44.

21. Grant, R.T. and Bland, E.F. Observations on arteriovenous anastomoses in human skin and in the bird's foot with special reference to reaction to cold. *Heart*, 1931, **15**, 385–411.

22. Clark, E.R. and Clark, E.L. Observations on living preformed blood vessels as seen in a transparent chamber inserted in the rabbit's ear. *Am. J. Anat.*, 1932, **49**, 441.

23. Flynn, M.D., Hassan, A.A.K. and Tooke, J.E. Effect of postural change and thermoregulatory stress on the capillary microcirculation of the human toe. *Clin. Sci.*, 1989, **76**, 231–6.

24. Gaskell, P. and Burton, A.C. Local postural vasomotor reflexes arising from the limb veins. *Circ. Res.*, 1953, **1**, 27–9.

25. Henriksen, O. Effect of chronic sympathetic denervation upon local regulation of blood flow in human subcutaneous tissue. *Acta Physiol. Scand.*, 1976, **97**, 377–84.

26. Henriksen, O. Local reflex in microcirculation in human subcutaneous tissue. *Acta Physiol. Scand.*, 1976, **97**, 447–56.

27. Henriksen, O. and Sejrsen, P. Local reflex in microcirculation in human cutaneous tissue. *Acta Physiol. Scand.*, 1976, **98**, 227–31.

28. Folkow, B. Autoregulation in muscle and skin. *Circ. Res.*, 1964, **14, 15** (suppl. l), I19–24.

29. Folkow, B. Description of the myogenic hypothesis. *Circ. Res.*, 1964, **14, 15** (suppl. l), I279–85.

30. Griffith, T.M., Edwards, D.H., Davies, R.L.I., Harrison, T.J. and Evans, K.T. EDRF co-ordinates the behaviour of vascular resistance vessels. *Nature*, 1987, **329**, 442–5.

31. Aalkjaer, C., Heagerty, A.M., Swales, J.D. and Thurston, H. Endothelial-dependent relaxation in human subcutaneous resistance vessels. *Blood Vessels*, 1987, **24**, 85–8.

32. Parving, H.H., Viberti, G., Keen, H., Christiansen, J.S. and Lassen, N.A. Haemodynamic factors in the genesis of diabetic microangiopathy. *Metabolism*, 1983, **32**, 943–9.

33. Zatz, R. and Brenner, B.M. Pathogenesis of diabetic microangiopathy. The haemodynamic view. *Am. J. Med.*, 1986, **80**, 443–53.

34. Tooke, J.E. Microvascular haemodynamics in diabetes mellitus. *Clin. Sci.*, 1986, **70**, 119–25.

35. Tooke, J.E., Lins, P.E., Ostergren, J. and Fagrell, B. Skin microvascular autoregulatory responses in type 1 diabetes: the influence of duration and control. *Int. J. Microcirc. Clin. Exp.*, 1985, **4**, 249–56.

36. Ewald, U., Tuvemo, T. and Rooth, G. Early reduction of vascular reactivity in diabetic children detected by transcutaneous oxygen electrode. *Lancet*, 1981, **i**, 1287– 8.

37. Kastrup, J., Mathiesen, E.R., Saurbrey, N., Norgaard, T., Parving, H.H. and Lassen, N.A. Effect of strict metabolic control on regulation of subcutaneous blood flow in insulin-dependent diabetic patients. *Diabet. Med.*, 1987, **4**, 30–6.

38. Walmsley, D. and Wiles, P.G. Myogenic micro-

vascular responses are impaired in long-duration type 1 diabetes. *Diabet. Med.*, 1990, **7**, 222–7.

39. Ubbink, D.T., Jacobs, M.J., Slaaf, D., Tangelder, G.J. and Reneman, R.S. Microvascular reactivity differences between two legs of patients with unilateral lower limb ischaemia. *Eur. J. Vasc. Surg.*, 1992, **6**, 269–75.

40. Ubbink, D.T., Jacobs, M.J., Slaaf, D.W., Tangelder, G.J. and Reneman, R.S. Capillary recruitment and pain relief on leg dependency in patients with severe lower limb ischaemia. *Circulation,* 1992, **85**, 223–9.

41. Bonogard, O. and Fagrell, B. Discrepancies between total and nutritional skin microcirculation in patients with peripheral arterial occlusive disease. *Vasa,* 1990, **19**, 105–11.

42. Junker, M., Frey-Schnewlin, G. and Bollinger, A. Microvascular flow distribution and transcapillary diffusion at the forefoot in patients with peripheral ischaemia. *Int. J. Microcirc. Clin. Exp.*, 1989, **8**, 3–24.

43. Ubbink, D.T., Jacobs, M.J., Tangelder, G.J., Slaaf, D.W. and Reneman, R.S. Posturally induced microvascular constriction in patients with different stages of leg ischaemia: effects of local heating. *Clin. Sci.,* 1991, **81**, 43–9.

44. Jacobs, M.J., Beches, R.C., Jorning, P.J., Slaaf, D.W. and Reneman, R.S. Microvascular haemodynamics before and after vascular surgery in severe limb ischaemia. *Eur. J. Vasc. Surg.,* 1990, **4**, 525–9.

45. Ubbink, D.T., Kitslaar, P.J.E., Tordoir, J.H.M., Reneman, R.S. and Jacobs, M.J.H.M. Skin microcirculation in diabetic and non diabetic patients at different stages of lower limb ischaemia. *Eur. J. Vasc. Surg.,* 1993, **7**, 659–66.

46. Jorneskog, G., Brismar, K. and Fagrell, B. Skin capillary circulation is more impaired in the toes of diabetic than non-diabetic patients with peripheral vascular disease. *Diabet. Med.,* 1995, **12**, 36–41.

47. Chazan, B.I., Balodimos, M.C., Lavine, R.L. and Koncz, L. Capillaries of the nailfold of the toe in diabetes mellitus. *Microvasc. Res.,* 1970, **2**, 504–7.

48. Landau, J. and Davis, E. The small blood-vessels of the conjunctiva and nailbed in diabetes mellitus. *Lancet,* 1960, **ii**, 731–4.

49. Terry, E.N., Messina, E.J., Schwartz, M.S., Redisch, W. and Steele, J.M. Manifestation of diabetic microangiopathy in nailfold capillaries. *Diabetes* ,1967, **16**, 595–7.

50. Fagrell, B., Hermansson, H.L., Karlander, S.G. and Ostergren, J. Vital capillary microscopy for assessment of skin viability and microangiopathy in patients with diabetes mellitus. *Acta Med. Scand.,* 1984, **687**, 25–8.

51. Karlander, S.G., Hermansson, I.L. and Hellstrom, K. Nutritive toe skin capillaries in middle aged patients with diabetes mellitus. *Diabet. Metab.,* 1985, **11**, 165–9.

52. Fagrell, B. How best to evaluate skin viability and the effect of therapy in patients with peripheral obliterative arterial disease. *Vasc. Med. Rev.,* 1990, **1**, 59–68.

53. Vrackow, R. Skeletal muscle capillaries in diabetics. A quantitative analysis. *Circulation,* 1970, **41**, 271–83.

54. Uitto, J., Peredja, A.J. and Grant, G.A. Glycosylation of human glomerular basement membrane collagen. *Connect. Tissue Res.,* 1982, **10**, 45–54.

55. Rohrbach, D.H., Wagner, C.W., Star, V. and Martin, G.R. Alterations in basement membrane (heparan sulphate) proteoglycan in diabetic mice. *Diabetes,* 1982, **31** (suppl. 2), 185–8.

56. Tilton, R.G., Faller, A.M., Burkhardt, J.K., Hoffman, P.L., Kilo, C. and Williams, J.R. Pericyte degeneration and acellular capillaries are increased in the feet of human diabetics. *Diabetologia,* 1985, **28**, 895–900.

57. Williamson, J.R., Tilton, R.G., Chang, K. and Kilo, C. Basement membrane abnormalities in diabetes mellitus: relationship to clinical microangiopathy. *Diabetes Metab. Rev.,* 1988, **4**, 339–70.

58. Rayman, G., Williams, S.A., Spencer, P.D., Smaje, L.H., Wise, P.H. and Tooke, J.E. Impaired microvascular hyperaemic response to minor skin trauma. *BMJ,* 1986, **292**, 1295–8.

59. Goldenberg, S., Morris, A., Joshi, R.A. and Blumenthal, H.T. Non atheromatous peripheral vascular disease of the lower extremity in diabetes mellitus. *Diabetes,* 1959, **8**, 261–73.

60. Ferrier, T.M. Comparative study of arterial disease in amputated lower limbs from diabetics and non-diabetics. *Med. J. Aust.,* 1967, **1**, 5–11.

61. Banson, B.B. and Lacy, P.E. Diabetic microangiopathy in human toes, with emphasis on

the ultrastructural change in dermal capillaries. *Am. J. Pathol.*, 1964, **45**, 41–58.

62. LoGerfo, F.W. and Coffman, J.D. Vascular and microvascular disease of the foot in diabetes. Implications for foot care. *N. Engl. J. Med.*, 1984, **311**, 1615–19.

63. Conrad, M.C. Abnormalities of the digital vasculature as related to ulceration and gangrene. *Circulation*, 1968, **38**, 568–81.

64. Edmonds, M.E. Experience in a multidisciplinary diabetic foot clinic. In *The Foot in Diabetes*, (eds H. Connor, A.J.M. Boulton and J.D. Ward), John Wiley, Chichester, 1987, pp. 121–33.

65. Ferguson, M.W.J., Herrick, S.E., Spencer, M.J., Shaw, J.E., Boulton, A.J.M. and Sloan, P. The histology of diabetic foot ulcers. *Diabet. Med.*, 1996, **13**, S30– 33.

66. Blumenthal, H.T. More on microvascular disease of the foot in diabetes. *N. Engl. J. Med.*, 1985, **312**, 696.

67. Colwell, J.A. and Haluska, P.V. Platelets, prostaglandins and coagulation in diabetes mellitus. *Mt. Sinai. J. Med.*, 1983, **49**, 215–22.

70. Deckert, T., Feldt-Rasmussen, B., Borch-Johnsen, K., Jensen, T. and Kofoed-Enevoldsen, A. Albuminuria reflects widespread vascular damage: the Steno hypothesis. *Diabetologia*, 1989, **32**, 219–26.

71. Bollinger, A., Frey, J., Jager, K., Furrer, J., Seglias, J. and Siegenthaler, W. Patterns of diffusion through skin capillaries in patients with long term diabetes. *N. Engl. J. Med.*, 1982, **307**, 1305–10.

72. Williams, S.K., Devenny, J.J. and Bitensky, M.W. Micropinocytic ingestion of glycosylated albumin by isolated microvessels: possible role in pathogenesis of diabetic microangiopathy. *Proc. Natl Acad. Sci. USA*, 1981, **78**, 2393–7.

73. McMurray, J.F. Wound healing in diabetes mellitus: better glucose control for better wound healing in diabetes. *Surg. Clin. N. Am.*, 1984, **64**, 779–94.

74. Hudlicka, O. Development of microcirculation: capillary growth and adaptation. In *Handbook of Physiology*, (eds E.M. Renkin and C.C. Michel), Williams & Wilkins, Baltimore, 1984, pp. 165–216.

75. Walmsley, D., Wales, J.K. and Wiles, P.G. Reduced hyperaemia following skin trauma: evidence for an impaired microvascular response to injury in the diabetic foot. *Diabetologia*, 1989, **32**, 736–9.

76. Dollery, C.T., Friedman, L.A., Hensby, C.N. *et al.* Circulating prostacyclin may be reduced in diabetes. *Lancet*, 1979, **ii**, 1365.

77. Johnson, M., Harrison, H.E., Raftery, A.T. and Elder, J.B. Vascular prostacyclin may be reduced in diabetes in man. *Lancet*, 1979, **i**, 3225–6.

78. Davis, T.M.E., Mitchell, M.D., Dornan, T.L. and Turner, R.C. Plasma 6-keto-PGFl alpha concentrations. *Lancet*, 1980, **i**, 373.

79. Schultz-Ehrenburg, U. and Weindorf, N. Function diagnostics of diabetic microangiopathy by TCPO: stimulation tests. *Int. J. Microcirc. Clin. Exp.*, 1986, **201**, M27.

80. Ditzel, J. Functional microangiopathy in diabetes mellitus. *Diabetes*, 1968, **17**, 388–97.

81. Shore, A.C., Price, K.J., Tripp, J.H. and Tooke, J.E. Impaired microvascular hyperaemia in children with diabetes mellitus. *Clin. Sci.*, 1989, **76** (suppl. 20), 15.

82. Archer, A.G., Roberts, V.C. and Watkins, P.J. Blood flow patterns in painful diabetic neuropathy. *Diabetologia*, 1984, **27**, 563–7.

83. Flynn, M.D., Edmonds, M.E., Tooke, J.E. and Watkins, P.J. Direct measurement of capillary blood flow in the diabetic neuropathic foot. *Diabetologia*, 1988, **31**, 652–66.

84. Christlieb, A.R. Renin angiotensin and norepinephrine in alloxan diabetes. *Diabetes*, 1974, **23**, 962–70.

85. Christlieb, A.R., Janka, H.V., Kraus, B. *et al.* Vascular reactivity to angiotensin 11 and to norepinephrine in diabetic subjects. *Diabetes*, 1976, **25**, 268–74.

86. Brochner-Mortensen, J. Glomerular filtration rate and extracellular fluid volumes during normoglycaemia and moderate hyperglycaemia in diabetes. *Scand. J. Clin. Lab. Invest.*, 1973, **32**, 311–16.

87. Haluska, P.V., Lurie, D. and Colwell, J.A. Increased synthesis of prostaglandin-E-like material by platelets from patients with diabetes mellitus. *N. Engl. J. Med.*, 1977, **297**, 1306–10.

88. Christiansen, J.S., Gammelgaard, J., Orskov, H. *et al.* Kidney function and size in normal subjects before and during growth hormone administration for one week. *Eur. J. Clin. Invest.*, 1981, **11**, 487–90.

89. Parving, H.H., Christiansen, J.S., Noer, I., Tronier, B. and Mogensen, C.E. The effect of

glucagon infusion on kidney function in short-term insulin-dependent juvenile diabetics. *Diabetologia*, 1980, **19**, 350–4.

90. Brochner-Mortensen, J. The glomerular filtration rate during moderate hyperglycaemia in normal man. *Acta Med. Scand.*, 1973, **194**, 31–7.

91. Ditzel, J., Jaeger, P. and Kjaergaard, J.J. Haemoglobin Alc and red cell oxygen releasing capacity in relation to early microvascular responses in ambulatory diabetics. *Adv. Microcirc.*, 1979, **8**, 1–13.

92. Ditzel, J. Affinity hypoxia as a pathogenic factor of microangiopathy with particular reference to diabetic retinopathy. *Acta Endocrinol.*, 1980, **94**, 39–55.

93. Liang, C.S. *et al.* Insulin infusion in conscious dog. Effects on systemic and coronary haemodynamics, regional blood flows and plasma catecholamines. *J. Clin. Invest.*, 1982, **69**, 1321–6.

94. McMillan, D.E. The effect of diabetes on blood flow properties. *Diabetes*, 1983, **32** (suppl. 2), 56–63.

95. Tooke, J.E. Capillary pressure disturbance in young diabetics. *Diabetes*, 1983, **29**, 818–19.

96. Rayman, G., Williams, S.A., Hassan, A.A.K., Gamble, J. and Tooke, J.E. Capillary hypertension and overperfusion in the feet of young diabetics. *Diabet. Med.*, 1985, **2**, 304A.

97. Sandeman, D.D., Shore, A.C. and Tooke, J.E. Relation of capillary pressure in patients with insulin dependent diabetes to complications and metabolic control. *N. Engl. J. Med.*, 1992, **327**, 760–4.

98. Corcoran., C.A. and Yudkin, S. Loss of spontaneous variability of fingertip anastomotic blood flow in diabetic autonomic neuropathy. *Clin. Sci.*, 1987, **72**, 557–67.

99. Horstman, P. The oxygen consumption in diabetes mellitus. *Acta Med. Scand.*, 1951, **139**, 326–30.

100. Flynn, M.D., Booleel, M., Flynn, H.M., Carter, G.D., Tooke, J.E. and Watkins, P.J. Improved skin perfusion in the diabetic neuropathic foot with euglycaemia induced by short term insulin infusion. *Diabetologia*, 1987, **30**, 520A.

101. Koenig, R.J. and Cerami, A. Haemoglobin Alc and diabetes mellitus. *Annu. Rev. Med.*, 1980, **31**, 8–13.

102. Altura, B.M. Chemical and humoral regulation of blood flow through the precapillary sphincter. *Microvasc. Res.*, 1971, **3**, 361–84.

103. Ditzel, J. and Standl, E. The problem of tissue oxygenation in diabetes mellitus. Its relation to the early functional changes in the microcirculation of diabetic subjects. *Acta Med. Scand.*, 1975, **578** (suppl.), 49–58.

104. Harder, D.R. Pressure induced myogenic activation of cat cerebral arteries is dependent on intact endothelium. *Circ. Res.*, 1987, **60**, 102–7.

105. Griffith, T.M., Edwards, D.H., Davies, R.L., Harrison, T.J. and Evans, K.T. EDRF coordinates the behaviour of vascular resistance vessels. *Nature*, 1987, **329**, 442–5.

106. Barnes, A.J. Rheology of diabetes mellitus. In *Clinical Blood Rheology*, vol. 11, (ed. G.D.O. Lowe), CRC Press, Boca Raton, 1988, pp. 163–87.

107. Ernst, E. and Matrai, A. Altered red and white blood cell rheology in type II diabetes. *Diabetes*, 1986, **35**, 1412–15.

108. Rayman, G., Hassan, A. and Tooke, E. Blood flow in the skin of the foot related to posture in diabetes mellitus. *BMJ*, 1986, **292**, 87–90.

109. Newrick, P.G., Cochrane, T., Betts, R.P., Ward, I.D. and Boulton, A.I.M. Reduced hyperaemic response under the diabetic neuropathic foot. *Diabet. Med.*, 1988, **5**, 570–3.

110. Chavers, B., Etzwiler, D. and Michael, A.F. Albumen deposition in dermal capillary basement membrane in insulin dependent diabetes mellitus: a preliminary report. *Diabetes*, 1981, **30**, 275–8.

111. Braverman, I.M., Sibley, J.M. and Keh, A. Ultrastructural analysis of the endothelial–pericyte relationship in diabetic cutaneous vessels. *J. Invest. Dermatol.*, 1990, **95**, 147–53.

112. Harrison, M.J.G. and Faris, I.B. The neuropathic factor in the aetiology of diabetic foot ulcers. *J. Neurol. Sci.*, 1976, **28**, 217–23.

113. Ctercteko, G.C., Dhanedran, M., Hutton, W.C. and LeQuesne, L.P. Vertical forces acting on the feet of diabetic patients with neuropathic ulceration. *Br. J. Surg.*, 1981, **68**, 608–14.

114. Masson, E.A., Hay, E.M., Stockley, I., Veves, A., Betts, R.P. and Boulton, A.J.M. Abnormal foot pressures alone may not cause ulceration. *Diabet. Med.*, 1989, **6**, 426–8.

115. Parkhouse, N. and Le Quesne, P.M. Impaired neurogenic vascular response in patients with diabetes and neuropathic foot lesions. *N. Engl. J. Med.*, 1988, **318**, 1306–9.

116. Aronin, N., Leeman, S.L. and Clements, R.S. Diminished flare response in neuropathic diabetic patients. Comparison of effects of substance P, histamine, and capsaicin. *Diabetes*, 1987, **36**, 1139–43.

117. Walmsley, D. and Wiles, P.G. Early loss of neurogenic inflammation in the human diabetic foot. *Clin. Sci.*, 1991, **80**, 605–10.

118. Ewing, D.J. and Clarke, B.F. Autonomic neuropathy: its diagnosis and prognosis. In *Clinics in Endocrinology and Metabolism* (ed. P.J. Watkins), W.B. Saunders, London, Philadelphia, Toronto, 1986, pp. 855–88.

119. Edmonds, M.E., Nicoliades, K.H. and Watkins, P.J. Autonomic neuropathy and diabetic foot ulceration. *Diabet. Med.*, 1986, **3**, 56–9.

120. Martin, M.M. Involvement of autonomic nerve fibres in diabetic neuropathy. *Lancet*, 1953, **i**, 560–65.

121. Moorhouse, J.A., Carter, S.A. and Doupe, J. Vascular responses in diabetic peripheral neuropathy. *BMJ*, 1966, **1**, 883–8.

122. Boulton, A.J.M., Scarpello, J.H.B. and Ward, J.D. Venous oxygenation in the diabetic neuropathic foot: evidence of arteriovenous shunting? *Diabetologia*, 1982, **22**, 6–8.

123. Partsch, H. Gestorte Gefassregulation bei ulzero-mutilier-enden Neuropathien der unteren Extremitiiten. *Vasa*, 1978, **7**, 119–25.

124. Scarpello, J.H.B., Martin, T.R.P. and Ward, J.D. Ultrasound measurements of pulse-wave velocity in the peripheral arteries of diabetic subjects. *Clin. Sci.*, 1980, **58**, 53–7.

125. Edmonds, M.E., Morrison, N., Laws, J.W. and Watkins, P.J. Medical arterial calcification in diabetes mellitus. *BMJ*, 1982, **284**, 928–30.

126. Corbin, D.O.C., Young, R.J., Morrison, D.C. *et al.* Blood flow in the foot, polyneuropathy and foot ulceration in diabetes mellitus. *Diabetologia*, 1987, **30**, 468–73.

127. Rayman, G., Hassan, A. and Tooke, J.E. Blood flow in the skin of the foot related to posture in diabetes mellitus. *BMJ*, 1986, **292**, 87–90.

128. Coffman, J.D. Total and nutritional blood flow in the finger. *Clin. Sci.*, 1972, **42**, 243–50.

129. Jorneskog, G., Brismar, K. and Fagrell, B. Skin capillary circulation severely impaired in toes of patients with IDDM, with and without late diabetic complications. *Diabetologia*, 1995, **38**, 474–80.

130. Flynn, M.D., Watkins, P.J. and Tooke, J.E. The first demonstration of capillary underperfusion in the diabetic neuropathic foot. *Diabet. Med.*, 1990, **7** (Suppl. 2), 36A.

131. Garner, A. Pathology of diabetic retinopathy. *Br. Med. Bull.*, 1970, **26**, 137– 42.

132. Vrackow, R. and Benditt, E.P. Capillary basal lamina thickening. Its relationship to endothelial cell death and replacement. *J. Cell. Biol.*, 1970, **47**, 281–5.

133. Rayman, G., Malik, R.A., Sharma, A.K. and Day, J.L. Microvascular response to tissue injury and capillary ultrastructure in the foot skin type 1 diabetic patients. *Clin. Sci.*, 1995, **89**, 467–74.

134. Ajjam, Z.S., Barton, S., Corbett, M., Owens, D. and Marks, R. Quantitive evaluation of the dermal vasculature of diabetics. *Q. J. Med.*, 1985, **215**, 229–39.

135. Williams, S.A., Rayman, G. and Tooke, J.E. Dependent oedema and attenuation of postural vasoconstriction associated with nifedipine therapy for hypertension in diabetic patients. *Eur. J. Pharmacol.*, 1989, **37**, 333–5.

136. Hanssen, K.F., Dahl-Jorgensen, K., Lauritzen, T., Feldt-Rasmussen, B., Brinchmann-Hansen, O. and Deckert, T. Diabetic control and microvascular complications: the near normoglycaemic experience. *Diabetologia*, 1986, **29**, 677–84.

137. Page, M.M.C.B., Smith, R.W.B. and Watkins, P.J. Cardiovascular effects of insulin. *BMJ*, 1976, **1**, 430–32.

138. Gundersen, H.J.C. and Christensen, N.J. Intravenous insulin causing loss of intravascular water and albumin and increased adrenergic nervous activity in diabetics. *Diabetes*, 1977, **26**, 551–7.

139. Takata, S., Yamamoto, M., Yagi, S., Noto, Y., Ikeda, T. and Hattori, N. Peripheral circulatory effects of insulin in diabetes. *Angiology*, 1985, **36**, 110–15.

140. Tymms, D.J. and Tooke, J.E. The effect of continuous subcutaneous insulin infusion (CSII) on microvascular blood flow in diabetes mellitus. *Int. J. Microcirc. Clin. Exp.*, 1988, **7**, 347–56.

141. Tooke, J.E., Lins, P.E., Ostergren, J., Adamson, U. and Fagrell, B. The effects of intravenous insulin infusion on skin microcirculatory flow in type 1 diabetes. *Int. J. Microcirc. Clin. Exp.*, 1985, **4**, 69–83.

142. Flynn, M.D. and Tooke, J.E. Microcirculation

and the diabetic foot. *Vasc. Med. Rev.*, 1990, **1,** 121–138.

143. Jornskog, G., Brismar, K. and Fagrell, B. Low molecular weight heparin seems to improve local capillary circulation and healing of chronic foot ulcers in diabetic patients. *Vasa,* 1993, **22,** 137–42.

144. Brash, P.D. and Tooke, J.E. Increased capillary fragility in the diabetic foot. *Diabetologia,* 1996, **39** (Suppl. 1), 104.

INDEX

Numbers in **bold** refer to figures; numbers in *italic* refer to tables.

Acellular capillaries 283, 287
Acetylcholine (ACh), vascular
    responses to 198–200
Acute phase response and insulin
    resistance 122–5
  relationships of acute phase
    markers and cytokines with
    antibody titres and obesity
    measures *126*
Adenosine-triphosphatase (ATP)
  myocardial, peripheral nerve and
    retinal levels 178–9
  synthesis and redox cycling of
    NAD(H) 170–1
Adhesion molecule expression 225
Adipose tissue 125–7
Advanced glycosylation
    endproducts (AGEs) 23–6, 41,
    203, **204**, 238
  adhesion molecule expression 225
  contribution to nephropathy 52,
    257
  degree of retinopathy 239
AGE-modified proteins 239
AGE-specific cell–surface receptor
    (AGE-R) 24, 203, **204**, 239
Albuminuria 3, 14, 53, 96, 249, 283
  intensive insulin therapy 55
  myocardial infarction risk 98
  prevention 28
  see also Microalbuminuria
Aldose reductase activity 238
  utilization of NADPH 172
Aldose reductase inhibitors 165,
    167, 203, 238, 257
Alpha-blockers 116, 270
Ambulatory blood pressure 53
American Diabetes Association
  dietary recommendations
    dyslipidaemia 83
    hypertension 53
    hypertriglyceridaemia guidelines
    81, 82
    LDL cholesterol recommendations
    81
Aminoguanidine 174, 203, 258, 270
Amputations, foot disease 277

Angina, prevalence 10
Angiotensin gene polymorphisms
    253
  'insertion/deletion' (I/D)
    polymorphism 253
Angiotensin-converting enzyme
    (ACE) 222, 283
Angiotensin-converting enzyme
    (ACE) inhibitors 45, 52, 56,
    116, 222, 252, 270, 271
  combination with calcium
    antagonist 58
  effects on lipid and lipoprotein
    levels *81*
  versus calcium antagonists 57
Antioxidants 204–6
Apolipoprotein B (ApoB) 78
  glycation 49, *50*
Apoptosis
  microvascular endothelial cells
    227
  of pericytes 240
Arachidonic acid products,
    alterations 50
Arteriovenous shunting 188, 190,
    268, 286, 287
Atenolol 58, 252
Atherogenic lipoprotein profile 76
Atherosclerosis
  lipids and lipoproteins 72–6
  related disease 66
  see also Cardiovascular disease;
    Cerebrovascular disease;
    Coronary artery disease
Atherosclerosis Risk in
    Communities (ARIC) Study
    38, 39
Atherosclerotic process
  atherogenesis 21–2
  in diabetes 22–9
    the AGE hypothesis 23–6
    cytokines and growth factors 26
    future perspectives 30–1
    heparan sulphate proteoglycan
    (HSPG) depletion 27–9
    inositol depletion 26, 27

vascular endothelial growth
    factor (VEGF) 29
'Atheroselectin' 30
Atherothrombotic risk 97
Atorvastatin 84
Autonomic nerve damage 280
Autoregulation
  abnormal, in foot 281, 288–9
  failure 151
  in retina 235, 237
Axon reflex, local sympathetic 279

Background retinopathy 147, 233,
    234
Basal myocardial contractile
    function 178
Basement membrane
  components and permselectivity
    51–2
  extracellularly deposited
    collagens 28
  HSPG depletion 27, 28, 225–6
  thickening 163, 189, 190, 215–16,
    281–2
  correlation with hyperaemic skin
    response 222
  glomerulus 250
Bcl-1 polymorphism 99
BECAIT study 87
Bed rest, foot disease 288
Bedford Study 97
'Berksonian bias' 7–8
Beta-blockers 58, 252
  care in choosing 116, 288
  effects on lipid and lipoprotein
    levels *81*
Beta-thromboglobulin 102
Bezafibrate Infarction Prevention
    Study 84
Bias, epidemiological studies 7–8
Bile acid sequestrant resins 84–5
Blindness, prevalence in NIDDM
    following change of therapy
    148
Blood flow, changes in 213–16
  foot 279–81, 284
  limb 188, 198–9, 200

Blood flow, changes in *cont.*
  nerve 162, 270
  pathological significance 163–4
  potential causes of increased
      microvascular 220
  renal 162
  retinal 162, 189, 235–8
  white cell and platelet
      abnormalities 215–16
Blood flow-mediated, endothelium-
    dependent dilation 200–2
Blood pressure, measuring 53
Body mass index 98
Bradykinin 220
British Regional Heart Study 116
Bypass Angioplasty
    Revascularisation
    Investigation 66

C-reactive protein 123, 124, 125, 127
Calcium
  enhanced platelet [Ca^{2+}] 48
  metabolism, abnormal cellular
      30–1
Calcium antagonists 56–7, 270
combination with ACE inhibitor 58
  effects on lipid and lipoprotein
      levels *81*
Callus formation 289
Capillary
  endothelial changes, diabetic foot
      283–4
  morphological changes, skin 281
  occlusion in retinopathy 216,
      240–1
  permeability, changes in diabetes
      224–7
    determinants of permeability
        224–5
    molecular basis for increased
        permeability 225–7
  pressure 192
    in diabetic glomerulus 251–2
    nail-fold capillaries 190, **191**,
        284
    origins of capillary
        hypertension 221–2
Captopril 56, 252
Carbohydrate intolerance 46
Cardiovascular disease (CAD)
  and hyperinsulinaemia 47–8
  increased risk in diabetes 37–9
  see also Cerebrovascular disease
      (CVD); Coronary heart
      disease (CHD); Peripheral
      vascular disease (PVD)
CARE Study *84*
Central obesity 45, 115

Cerebrovascular disease (CVD) 7,
    22, 37, 38, 39–40, 46
  definition 11
  epidemiology
    population-based studies 12
    practice-based studies 11–12
    world-wide comparisons 12
Chicago Heart Association
    Detection in Industry Study
    38
Chlamydia pneumoniae 125
Chlorpropamide 55
Chlorthalidone 55
Cholesterol 72–4
  content, vessel walls, correlation
      with heparan sulphate 28
  daily intake 67
  reverse cholesterol transport and
      HDL 71–2
  serum, predictor of macrovascular
      disease 78
  total cholesterol:HDL ratio 73
Cholestyramine 84–5, 206
Chylomicrons 67, 68
  chylomicron remnant particles 68
Ciglitazone 55
Clofibrate 85
Clot formation, attenuation of 49
Coagulation 93, 94, 97–100
Coagulopathy 93–105
  diabetes and atherothrombotic
      risk 97
  diabetes as hypercoagulable state
      95–6, 104
    biochemical evidence 96
  diabetic hypertensive persons 48–9
  effect of hyperglycaemia 41
  mechanisms in thrombosis 93–5
Cold neuropathic foot 286
Colestipol 84–5
Collaborative Atorvastatin Diabetes
    Study (CARDS) 84
Collagens
  increase in extracellular
      deposition 28
  type IV 51, 222, 223
Continuous subcutaneous insulin
    infusion (CSII)
  improvement in cutaneous blood
      flow 289
  retinopathy/nephropathy
      progression 142–3, **144**
Coronary artery bypass graft 66
Coronary heart disease (CHD) 7, 37,
    45–6, 65, 66
  definition 9–10
  epidemiology
    population-based studies 10–11
    practice-based studies 10

and insulin resistance 116–17
  relationship with cholesterol 72
Critical limb ischaemia 277
Cytokines 113
  atherosclerotic process 26, *27*
  and insulin resistance 122–5, 127
  relationships with antibody titres
      and obesity measures 125,
      126
Cytomegalovirus 125
Cytosolic free $NADH/NAD^+$ ratio
    165–6, 256, 258
Cytosolic reductive stress
  energy metabolism and regulation
      of blood flow 166–71, 172
    oxidation of cytosolic NADH
        167, **168**
    redox cycling of NAD(H) and
        ATP synthesis 170–1
  metabolic consequences 173–9
    de novo synthesis of
        diacylglycerol and activation
        of protein kinase C 176–7
    ischaemic injury and metabolic
        suppression, paradoxical
        responses 178–9
    vascular consequences, non-
        vascular versus vascular cells
        177–8
    vascular endothelial growth
        factor (VEGF) 175–6

Deep vein thrombosis 95
Diabetes Atherosclerosis
    Intervention Study (DAIS) 83,
    84
Diabetes Control and Complications
    Trial (DCCT) 4, 14, 65, 93,
    137, 150, 161, 164–5, 235
  albuminuria/microalbuminuria
      reduction 55
  ancillary study 220
  details of trial 144–6, 147, *149*
  efficacy, intensive glycaemic
      control *149*
  LDL cholesterol reduction 82
Diabetic
  foot *see* Foot problems
  nephropathy *see* Nephropathy
  neuropathy *see* Neuropathy
  retinopathy *see* Retinopathy
Diaclyglcerol (DAG), *de novo*
    synthesis 176–7, 241
Dietary recommendations
  dyslipidaemia 83
  hypertension 53
Diffuse intercapillary sclerosis 52
Dihydropyridine 57
Divalent cation flux, abnormality 31

Doppler ultrasound
  ACh-induced increases, forearm blood flow 200
  investigating flow-mediated responses 201
  nerve blood flow studies 270
  pulse wave velocity, foot ulceration subjects 286
  PVD detection 8, 9
  red cell velocity and vessel diameter, retina 235, 237
Dyslipidaemia 37, 45, 65–87
  atherosclerosis-related disease 66
  and insulin resistance 115
  lipid and lipoprotein
    metabolism in diabetes 76–9
    transport, physiology 66–76
  management 79–87
    approach to lipid-lowering therapy 87
    choice of lipid-lowering drugs 84–7
    glycaemic control 82
    hypolipidaemic drugs 83–4
    lifestyle measures 82–3
    screening 79–81
    treatment targets 81–2
  platelet aggregation 48
  primary *80*
  secondary *81*

E-selectin 30
ECTIM study 100, 102
Enalapril 57
End-stage renal disease 52, 53, 250
Endoneurial microangiopathy 267–8, 269
Endothelial cells
  glomerulus 51, 52
  injury and atherosclerosis 21
  markers of cell dysfunction 197, **198**
Endothelial-derived relaxing factor
  see Nitric oxide (NO)
Endothelin 52
  concentrations 30
  impaired vasoconstriction 221
  role in neuropathy 271
Endothelium 197–206, 223, 224
  diabetic milieu and endothelial function 202–6
  hypertension 50–1
  endothelium-dependent constrictors 202
  dilation, flow-mediated 200–2
  insulin resistance 121–2
  vascular responses to ACh 198–200

Epidemiology 7–15
  cerebrovascular disease (CVD) 11–12
  coronary heart disease (CHD) 9–11
  microvascular disease 12, 13–14
  peripheral vascular disease (PVD) 8–9
  predicting the future 14–15
Epineurial capillary abnormalities 268, 269
Euglobulin clot analysis 100, 101
Euglycaemic hyperinsulinaemic clamp 114
Eurodiab IDDM Complications Study 13, 14
European Concerted Action on Thrombosis (ECAT) study 122
European Working Group on NIDDM 81
Exercise, dyslipidaemia 83
Exercise-induced conduction velocity increment 269
Extracellular matrix changes 174–5

Factor VII levels 48, 99–100
  determinants of concentrations 99
  genetics of 100
  and vascular disorders 100
Factor VIII levels 48
Fasting
  cholesterol, triglyceride and HDL cholesterol 79
  hyperinsulinaemia 45, 47, 114
Fatty acids 46, 68
  see also Non-esterified fatty acid (NEFA) metabolism abnormalities
Fatty streaks 21, 66
Fenestrae 224
Fenofibrate 84
Fibrates 74, 83, 84, 85–6
Fibrin deposition, endoneurial vessels 269
Fibrinogen
  genetics of 98–9
  and insulin resistance 119
  levels 41, 48, 97–8, 214, 220
    determinants of plasma 98
Fibrinolysis
  fibrinolytic activity
    abnormal 41, 49, 96
    determinants of 101
  fibrinolytic cascade **94–5**
  in NIDDM and IDDM subjects 100–1
  and vascular disorders 101
Fibrinopeptide A (FPA) 96

Fibronectin expression 28
Fibrous plaques 21
FINNVASC study 95
Fish-oil 85, 86
Fluorescein angiography, retina **234**, 235
Foam cells 21, 41, 50
  formation, monocyte role 72–3
  uptake of LDL 49
Focal fascicular lesions 267
Foot disease
  clinical implications 288–9
  historical perspective 3, 4
  microcirculation of foot 278–9
    abnormal in diabetes 280–1
    capillary flow, diabetic foot 287
    changes in capillary endothelium 283–4
    contribution of closed capillaries to ischaemia 287–8
    functional changes in 284–5
    regulation of blood flow 279–80
  neuropathy and microvascular disease 285–7
  pathogenesis, neuroischaemic and neuropathic foot 277–8
  small vessel disease 282–3
Framingham Study 37, 38, 39, 66, 74, 78, 97
Friedewald equation 79, 82

Gamma linolenic acid therapy 270
Gangrene 282
Gemfibrozil 74, 83
Genetic
  determinants, diabetic nephropathy 251
  predisposition
    hypertension and metabolic abnormalities 46
    microalbuminuria 22
Genetics
  of factor VII 100
  of fibrinogen 98–9
  of PAI-1 101–2
  of renin–angiotensin system 253
Gestational diabetes 199, 200
Globulin levels 214, 220
Glomerular
  extracellular matrix, derangement of 254–6
  filtration rate (GFR) 251–2
  macromolecular permeability 253–4
Glomerulosclerosis 3
  analogy with atherosclerosis 51–3
Glucokinase mutations 139

Glucose
    hypothesis 137–8
    pathogenesis of microangiopathy,
        indirect evidence
        incriminating 138–42
    pathways, diabetic angiopathy
        22–9
Glucose intolerance 137
    hypertension 46
    role of glycaemia as
        cardiovascular risk factor
        39–40
    studies 138–9
Glutathione, neuropathy prevention
    270
Glutathione reductase, utilization of
    NADPH 172
Glyburide 55
Glycaemia, role in pathogenesis of
        microangiopathy 137–54
    glucose hypothesis 137–8
    hypoglycaemia 152–3, 237
    interventional studies 142–6
    missing links 153–4
    observational studies 140–2
    tight control in NIDDM 146–50
    see also Hyperglycaemia
Glycaemic index 141
'Glycaemic re-entry' 137, 150–2
Growth factors
    involved
        atherosclerotic process 26
        retinopathy 242
    mesangial cell synthesis 52
Growth hormone and IGF-1 259
Growth retardation, fetal 120

Haemodynamic
    changes
        nephropathy 251–3
        retinopathy 235–8
        spontaneously/experimentally-
            induced diabetes 162
    hypothesis, diabetic
        microangiopathy 189–91
        direct support for 190–1
HbA1c values 40
    macrovascular complications 22
        predictor of vascular death *23*
    microvascular complications 14,
        141, 146–7
        following intensive insulin
            therapy 150
Heart Protection Study 84
Helicobacter pylori 125
Helsinki Heart Study 73–4, 83
Helsinki Policemen Study 39
Heparan sulphate protoglycan
    (HSPG) **254**

depletion 27–9
    glomerular basement
        membranes 225–6, 255–6, 258
Heparin, low molecular weight 289
High-density lipoproteins (HDL) 46
    HDL cholesterol 73–4
    physical and chemical
        characteristics **68**
    and reverse cholesterol transport
        70, 71–2
Historical perspective 3–4
HMG-CoA reductase inhibitors 73,
    83, 84, 86, 87
Honolulu Heart Study 97
Hydrochlorothiazide 55
Hydroxyl radical 206
Hypercholesterolaemia 51
Hyperglycaemia 37–42, 104, 137
    cardiovascular disease, increased
        risk 37–9, 46
    clinical implications 41–2
    in pathogenesis of
        microangiopathy 137–54
        atherosclerosis 41
        degree of, relationship to
            microvascular complications
            139–40
        interventional studies 142–6
        observational studies 140–2
    retinal blood flow 237
    vascular cellular consequences
        161–79
        direct effect on retinal cells
            238–41
        endothelial dysfunction 50–1,
            203
        functional and structural
            vascular responses 161–2
        metabolic imbalances in
            mediating 164–6
        studies, spontaneous or
            experimentally induced
            diabetes 162–3
Hyperinsulinaemia 121
    and cardiovascular disease 40–1,
        45, 46, 47–8, 116–17
Hyperlipidaemia, type III 74
Hyperpermeability hypothesis
    191–3
Hypertension 37, 41, 45–58, 164
    capillary 190
        origins of 221–2
        see also Capillary: pressure
    coagulation abnormalities 48–9
    endothelial dysfunction 50–1
    hyperinsulinaemia and
        cardiovascular disease 47–8
    and insulin resistance 115–16
    and kidney disease 51–3, 253

microalbuminuria 22
non-esterified fatty acid (NEFA)
    metabolism abnormalities 50
platelet abnormalities 48
prevalence 12, *13*, 25, 45–6, 138
treatment 53–8, 65
    goals of therapy 53
    and insulin resistance 116
    non-pharmacological therapy
        53, 55
    pharmacological therapy 55–8
    suggested approach **54**
Hypertriglyceridaemia 41, 51, 74,
    75–6, 115
    NIDDM patients 76, 77
    treatment guidelines 81, 82
Hypoglycaemia and
    microangiopathy 152–3
    retinal blood flow 237
Hypoglycaemic coma 139–40
Hypothyroidism 79

Impaired glucose tolerance *see*
    Glucose intolerance
Infections 125–7
Inositol depletion 26, 27
'Insertion/deletion' (I/D)
    polymorphism 253
Insulin
    effects, components of large blood
        vessels 30, 31
    neuritis 268
Insulin resistance 4, 30, 31, 45, 46,
        65, 113–28, 202
    and coronary heart disease
        (CHD) 116–17
    definition 114
    dyslipidaemia and hypertension
        115–16
    endothelial dysfunction 121–2,
        223
    fibrinogen 98, 119
    and metabolic syndrome 114–15
    microalbuminaemia 119
    new paradigm for 127–8
    NIDDM patients 77
    obesity and physical activity,
        relevance 115
    plasminogen activator inhibitor–1
        (PAI–1) 117
    pro-inflammatory cytokines 122–5
    pro-insulin–like molecules 117,
        118–19
    role of infections and adipose
        tissue 125–7
    role in nephropathy development
        259
    small baby syndrome 119–21

Insulin therapy 3, 4, 55
   intensive versus conventional, retinopathy/nephropathy progression 142–6, 235
   NIDDM and IDDM studies *149*
   NIDDM studies 147–50
Insulin-dependent diabetes (IDDM) 4
   cardiovascular disease (CAD) 10, 22, 66
   coagulopathy
      factor VII levels 99–100
      fibrinogen levels 97–8
      fibrinolysis 100–1
      prothrombotic risk factors 96
   lipid and lipoprotein
      levels, glycaemic control 82
      metabolism 78
   maximal microvascular hyperaemia, limitation 222
   nephropathy 52, 53, 259–60
   peripheral vascular disease (PVD) 9
   retinopathy 13, 140–1
   small baby syndrome 120
   venous occlusion plethysmographic studies 199
Insulin-like growth factor (IGF–1) 47–8, 259
   increased levels, retinopathy progression 151, 152, 242
Interendothelial cell junction 224–5, 227
Interleukin–6 (IL–6) 123, 124, 128
   administration 127
   expression, adipose tissue 113, 125
Intermediate density lipoprotein (IDL)
   concentrations 41
   physical and chemical characteristics **68**
International Atherosclerosis Project 66
Interstitial fluid, insulin concentrations 121–2
Ischaemic injury
   critical limb ischaemia 277
   cytosolic reductive stress 178
   experimental nerve 269–70
   ulceration sites 283
Ischaemic stress, hypoglycaemia 153
Isoprostanes 205

Kallikrein synthesis 220
Kumamoto study, intensive insulin, NIDDM patients 147, **148**, *149*

Lactate/pyruvate ratio 167, 169, 171
   retinal pigment epithelial cells 177
LDL receptor pathway **71**
LDL receptor–related protein 68
Leucocytes 30, 215
   capillary occlusion by 216, 240–1
Lifestyle measures, dyslipidaemia treatment 82–3
Limb
   blood flow changes 188, 198–9, 200
   ulcers 282–3
Lipid peroxides 205
Lipid-lowering therapy 206
Lipids
   and atherosclerosis 72–6
   metabolism in diabetes 76–9
Lipoprotein lipase (LPL) 46, 115
Lipoproteins 67
   and atherosclerosis 72–6
   lipoprotein A (LpA) 49, **68**, 76, 79
   metabolism **69–70**
      endogenous pathway 70–1
      exogenous pathway 67, 68
      HDL and reverse cholesterol transport 71–2
      IDDM patients 78
      levels in relation to macrovascular disease 78–9
      NIDDM patients 76–8
   physical and chemical characteristics **68**
   structure **67**
   see also High density lipoprotein (HDL); Intermediate density lipoprotein (IDL); Low density lipoprotein (LDL); Very low density lipoprotein (VLDL)
Lisinopril 57, 58
   nerve function improvement 270
LOCAT study 87
Longterm Intervention with Pravastatin in Ischaemic Disease (LIPID) Study 84
Low density lipoprotein (LDL)
   levels 41, 46, 70–1
   calculating, Friedewald equation 79
   oxidized LDLs (Ox–LDL) 49, 73, 204–5
   physical and chemical characteristics **68**
   role in endothelial dysfunction 202
   structure **67**
   subspecies 74–5
LY333531, oral administration 241

Macroangiopathy 4, 7, 22
   see also Cerebrovascular disease (CVD); Coronary heart disease (CHD); Peripheral vascular disease (PVD)
Macrophages 30
Matrix proteins, AGE-modified 25
Maturity onset diabetes of the young (MODY) 4–5, 139
   pathophysiology 194
Mauriac's syndrome 151, 152
Mesangial cells, glomerulus 51, 52
   hyperplasia 48, 163
      volume fraction increase 250
Mesenteric small arteries
   ACh relaxation 200
   flow-mediated relaxation 201
Metabolic syndrome 113
   and insulin resistance 114–15
   relationships of acute phase markers and cytokines with *124*
Metformin 55
Microalbuminuria 192, 249, 250, 283
   capillary pressure 190, 191
   hypertension, emergence of 22, 253
   insulin resistance 119, 138
   plasma fibrinogen levels 98
   prevention 28, 29, 55
   prothrombotic risk factors elevated in association with *96*
   vWF levels 103
Microangiopathy
   definition microvascular disease 12, 13
   glycaemia, role of 137–54
      atherosclerosis 41
      interventional studies 142–6
      observational studies 140–2
   luxury perfusion, origins of 219–21
   maximal microvascular hyperaemia, limitation in 222–4
   pathogenesis 4, 7, 187–94
      haemodynamic hypothesis 189–91
      microvascular malfunction, indirect evidence 188–9
      pathophysiological framework 194
      pathophysiology of microcirculation in NIDDM 193–4
      reduced microvascular vasodilatory reserve 191
      role of increased microvascular permeability 191–3

Microangiopathy *cont.*
  prevalence 13, 14
  see also Capillary; Nephropathy;
      Neuropathy; Retinopathy
Microcirculation, function 187
Microthrombosis 227
Mitochondrial
  free NADH/NAD$^+$ 169
  reductive stress 173
Monocytes, foam cell formation
      72–3
Multiple insulin injection (MIT)
      therapy 147, **148**, *149*
Multiple Risk Factor Intervention
      Trial (MRFIT) 12, 38, 72, 78
Mulvany–Halpern myograph 199
Munich General Practitioner Project
      22, 29
Myocardial infarction (MI) 10–11,
      22, 95, 104
  albuminuria 98
  factor VII 100
  'insertion/deletion' (I/D)
      polymorphism 253
  plasminogen activator inhibitor
      (PAI–1) levels 49
  time to recurrent 66
  triglycerides 79, 84
Myogenic hypothesis, regulation of
      blood flow in foot 279

N-deacetylase 30, 255
Na$^+$/H$^+$ exchanger 256, 258
NADH/NAD$^+$ *see* Cytosolic free
      NADH/NAD$^+$ ratio;
      Cytosolic reductive stress
NADPH, as cofactor for aldose
      reductase, NO synthase and
      glutathione reductase 171–3
Nail-fold capillary
  blood flow in toe 284, 287
  pressure 190, **191**, 244
National Cholesterol Education
      Program 81, 82
National Health and Nutrition
      Examination Survey
      (NHANES) 10–11
National Hospital Discharge Survey
      66
Neovascularization, retina 188, 233,
      235, 241–2
Nephron number 221
Nephropathy 4, 249–60
  definition 12
  historical perspective 3
  hypertension in diabetes 51–3
  lipid abnormalities 78
  nature of 249–50
  in NIDDM versus IDDM 259–60

pathogenesis 187, 191
  cellular and molecular
      mechanisms 256–9
  derangement of extracellular
      matrix 254–6
  genetic determinants 251
  haemodynamic changes 251–3
  morphological changes 250–1
  selectivity for glomerular size
      and charge 253–4
  TGF-β role 26
plasma fibrinogen levels 98
prevalence 14, 138, 139
progression 214
  interventional studies 143, **144**,
      145–6
  observational studies 141–2
small baby syndrome 120
see also Albuminuria;
      Microalbuminuria
Neuritis, insulin 268
Neurogenic venoarteriolar reflex 286
Neuropathy 221, 267–71
  arteriovenous shunting 188
  definition 12
  experimental nerve ischaemia
      269–70
  human structural and functional
      neurovascular abnormalities
      267–9
  nitric oxide and endothelin, role
      of 271
  pharmacological studies 270–1
  prevalence 14
  vWF levels 103
  see also Foot disease
Niceritrol 270
Nifedipine 57, 270, 288
Nisoldipine 57
Nitric oxide (NO) 197, 220, 225, 280
  chemical inactivation by AGEs
      24–**5**
  decreased production and release
      51
  investigation 198
  mediating vascular dysfunction
      176, 284, 285
  mesangial cell inhibition 52
  role in nephropathy 258–9
  role in neuropathy 271
Nitric oxide synthase, utilization of
      NADPH 172, 173
Nocturnal hypoglycaemia 153
Nodular intercapillary sclerosis 52
Non-enzymatic glycation 165, 174–5,
      238–9, 257
Non-esterified fatty acids (NEFAs)
      127
  metabolism abnormalities 50, 115

single gateway hypothesis 122
Non-insulin-dependent diabetes
      (NIDDM) 4, 5, 42, 51
  ACE inhibitors 56
  blood pressure, loss of circadian
      variation 53
  coagulopathy 41
      atherothrombotic risk *96*, *97*
      factor VII levels 99–100
      fibrinogen levels 97–8
      fibrinolysis 100–1
  coronary heart disease (CHD) 10,
      66
  decreased insulin–induced
      vasodilation 31
  lipid and lipoprotein
      levels, glycaemic control 82
      levels, treatment targets 81
      metabolism 76–8
  macrovascular disease 22
      predictors of death *23*
  maximal microvascular
      hyperaemia, limitation 223
  microangiopathy progression
      changing therapy, retinopathy
          progression **148**, 150
      evidence for tight control 146–50
  nephropathy 4, 53, 259–60
  oral hypoglycaemic agents 55
  pathophysiology of
      microcirculation 193–4
  peripheral vascular disease 8, 9
  venous occlusion
      plethysmographic studies 199
  weight reduction 55
Northwick Park Heart Study 98,
      100, 101
Nurses' Health Study, coronary
      heart disease (CHD) 10, 38

Obesity 45, 46, 49, 125
  and insulin resistance 115
  relationships of acute phase
      markers and cytokines with
      measures of *126*
Oedema
  endoneurial 268
  in foot 278, 279, 283, 287
Oxidative stress 41, 174–5, 203, 204,
      239–40
Oxidized LDLs (Ox-LDL) 49, 73,
      204–5
Oxygen
  consumption, skin 284–5
  supplementation, nerve
      conduction velocity 270

Paris Prospective Study 39, 79
PECAM-1 expression 225

Percutaneous transluminal coronary angioplasty 66
Pericytes
apoptosis 240
diabetic foot 288
p60 component, AGE receptor 239
Peripheral vascular disease (PVD) 7, 29, 37, 38, 39, 66
definitions 8
epidemiology
population-based studies 9
practice-based studies 8
see also Foot disease
Physicians Heart Study 101, 102
Pioglitazone 55
Pittsburgh Epidemiology of Diabetes Complications (EDC) Study 13, 14
Pituitary ablation 152, 242
Plasma
lipid profile 79
viscosity 213, 219
Plasminogen activator inhibitor (PAI–1) 47, 49, 76, 94, 101, 224
genetics of 101–2
PLAT study 100
Platelet factor 4 (PF4) 102
Platelets
abnormalities 48, 73, 102–3, 215, 216
platelet clumping, endoneurial vessels 269
thrombosis formation 95
Plethysmographic studies 188, 198–9, 286
Polyol pathway
hyperglycaemia-associated stimulation 203
retinopathy 238
and pseudohypoxia 256–7
Post-reactive hyperaemia, impaired 280
Postural vasconstriction, impairment 280, 287
Potassium (K) channels, ATP–sensitive, sulphonylurea inhibition 55
Prazocin 270
'Pre-AGE' Amadori glycation products 257
Pre-proliferative retinopathy 233, **234**
'Prediabetic' metabolic state 22
Pregnancy
maternal nutrition 120
protection against abnormality of relaxation to ACh 200

retinopathy progression 152
Prevalence
cerebrovascular disease (CVD) 11, 12
coronary heart disease (CHD) 10, 11, *13*
hypertension 12, *13*
microvascular disease 13, *14*, 138, 139
peripheral vascular disease (PVD) 8, 9, *13*
predicting the future 14–15
Pro-insulin–like molecules 117, 118–19
Probucol 205, 206, 270
PROCAM Study 74, 100
Procoagulant state 48
Proliferative retinopathy 233, **234**
Prorenin 252
Prostacyclin 197
Prostanoids 220, 284
Protein C antigenic levels 49
Protein kinase C activation 27, 28, 50, 51, 220
and cytosolic reductive stress 176–7
increased glomerular 257–8
inhibition 203
Prothrombin fragments F_{1+2} 96
Pseudohypoxia and polyol pathway 256–7
Puberty 152
Pulmonary embolus 95

Radiolabelled
albumin studies 163
microspheres, nerve blood flow studies 270
RAGE *see* AGE–specific cell-surface receptor (AGE–R)
Reactive oxygen species (ROS) 174–5, 176, 220, 239–40
Red cell
aggregation 214, 216
deformability 214, 215, 219
metabolic changes 285
Referral bias 7–8
Renal blood flow changes 162
Renin–angiotensin system 252–3
Retinal blood flow changes 162, 189, 235
causes and effects of 237–8
effect of blood glucose control 236–7
Retinal pigment epithelial cells, lactate/pyruvate ratios 177
Retinopathy 214, 216, 233–42
definition 12
evolution 233–4

historical perspective 3, 4
pathogenesis 187, 234–42
capillary occlusion 216, 240–1
direct effect of hyperglycaemia on retinal vascular cells 238–41
haemodynamic changes 235–8
vascular proliferation 241–2
prevalence 13, 14, 138, 139
progression 214
glycaemic re-entry 150–2
HbA1c levels 147, 150
hypoglycaemia 153
interventional studies 142, 143, **144**, 145, 146–50
observational studies 140–1
vascular endothelial growth factor (VEGF) levels 29, 164, 175–6, 242
vWF levels 103
Rheology *see* Blood flow, changes in
Rotterdam study 97–8

San Luis Valley Colorado study 138
Scavenger receptors 73
Sciatic nerve blood flow, changes 162
Selectins 30
Serotonin 222
Serum albumin 214
Shear stress 215, 238
NO release 198, 200, 220
proximal increase 201
SHEP study 55
Simvastatin 206
Skeletal muscle, glucose disposal 224
Skin, oxygen consumption 284–5
Small baby syndrome 119–21
Small vessel disease, foot problems 282–3
Smoking 98
serum level AGEs 25–6
Sodium-lithium countertransport activity 256, 259
Somatic nerve damage 280
Sorbitol
accumulation 238
pathway metabolism 165–6, 167
cytosolic reductive stress, impact of non-vascular cells on vascular function 177–8
Statins *see* HMG-CoA reductase inhibitors
'Steno' hyperpermeability hypothesis 192
Stockholm Diabetes Intervention Study 143, 145–6
Stroke 11, 12, 22, 37, 38, 39–40, 46

'Strong Heart Study' 11
Sucrose tracer studies 163
Sulphonylureas 55, 82
Superoxide dismutase 204, 206
Sural nerve oxygen tension 268
Sweating, increased 286

Taurine 206
Thiazide diuretics 55–6, 116
    effects on lipid and lipoprotein
        levels *81*
Thiazolidinediones 55
Thrombin-antithrombin complexes
    48
Thrombosis 21, 104, 283
    mechanisms 93–5
Thromboxane B_2 (TXB_2) 102–3
Tissue plasminogen activator (tPA)
    94, 100, 101, 117
    see also Plasminogen activator
        inhibitor (PAI–1)
Tokyo Metropolitan Geriatric
    Hospital series 11
Tolrestat 238
Trandalopril 271
Transcapillary escape rate, albumin
    28
Transforming growth factor β (TGF-
    β) 26, 252, 258
Transperineurial capillary
    abnormalities 268
Triglycerides 74
    predictor of macrovascular
        disease 78–9
Triose phosphates 174
Troglitazone 55

Tumour necrosis factor-α (TNF-α)
    113, 123, 124, 128
    administration of 127
    expression in adipose tissue 125
Type 1 diabetes *see* Insulin-
        dependent diabetes (IDDM)
Type 2 diabetes *see* Non-insulin-
        dependent diabetes (NIDDM)

UK Prospective Diabetes Study
    (UKPDS) 37, 40, 116, 138, 148
University Group Diabetes Program
    (UGDP) 147

Vascular changes
    barrier function 162–3
        pathological significance 163–4
    metabolic imbalances mediating
        164–6
    structural changes 163
    see also Blood flow, changes in
Vascular endothelial growth factor
    (VEGF) 29, 241
    and cytosolic reductive stress
        175–6
    proliferative retinopathy 29, 164,
        175, 242
    upregulation by hypoglycaemia
        153
Vascular smooth muscle cells
    (VSMC)
    IGF-1 synthesis 47
    mesangial cells 51, 52
Vascular tone 197
Verapamil 57
Very low density lipoproteins
    (VLDL) 46, 70, 75

physical and chemical
        characteristics **68**
Veterans Affairs Co–operative
        Studies Program 150
Vitamin C
    concentrations 204
    supplementation 205, 206
Vitamin E
    concentrations 204
    supplementation 205, **206**
Vitreous haemorrhage 153
von Willebrand factor (vWF) 29, 48,
        95, 103–4, 283
    as predictor of neuropathy 269

Weight reduction
    dyslipidaemia 82–3
    hypertension 55
White cells *see* Leucocytes
Whitehall Study 39
Whole blood viscosity 214, 219
Wisconsin Epidemiologic Study 13,
        14
    of Diabetic Retinopathy 40, 141
World health Organization (WHO)
    definition of PVD 8
    Multinational Study 79
Wound healing
    angiogenesis 283–4
    vascular endothelial growth
        factor (VEGF) 29

Z scores, acute phase cluster *123*
Zonula occludens 224–5
Zopolrestat 167